D0887787

OXFORD MEDICAL PUBLICATIONS

Drugs in
Palliative Care

Drugs in Palliative Care

Andrew Dickman MSc MRPharmS

Senior Clinical Pharmacist
Marie Curie Palliative Care Institute
Marie Curie Hospice
Woolton
Liverpool
UK

and

Pharmacy Department
Liverpool Heart and Chest NHS Trust
Liverpool
UK

OXFORD
UNIVERSITY PRESS

OXFORD
UNIVERSITY PRESS

Great Cl... Lun Street Oxford OX2 6DP

Oxford University Press is a department of the University of Oxford.
It furthers the University's objective of excellence in research, scholarship,
and education by publishing worldwide in

Oxford New York

Auckland Cape Town Dar es Salaam Hong Kong Karachi
Kuala Lumpur Madrid Melbourne Mexico City Nairobi
New Delhi Shanghai Taipei Toronto

With offices in

Argentina Austria Brazil Chile Czech Republic France Greece
Guatemala Hungary Italy Japan Poland Portugal Singapore
South Korea Switzerland Thailand Turkey Ukraine Vietnam

Oxford is a registered trade mark of Oxford University Press
in the UK and in certain other countries

Published in the United States
by Oxford University Press Inc., New York

British Library Cataloguing in Publication Data
Data available

Library of Congress Cataloging-in-Publication Data
Data available

Typeset by Glyph International, Bangalore, India
Printed in Italy
on acid-free paper through
L.E.G.O. S.p.A

ISBN 978-0-19-956397-5

10 9 8 7 6 5 4 3 2 1

Foreword

It is widely recognized that palliative care encompasses the physical, psychological, social and spiritual needs of patients, together with support for their carers. Fundamental to this is good symptom control—if patients have uncontrolled symptoms then addressing the other domains of care is often unachievable.

The key elements to symptom control include assessment, diagnosis, and treatment. The treatment falls into pharmacological and non-pharmacological modalities. When pharmacological intervention is deemed appropriate then the knowledge to choose the appropriate drug and the skill to prescribe appropriately is fundamental to good symptom control.

Drugs in Palliative Care aims to support healthcare professionals, including doctors, nurses, and pharmacists involved in the management of palliative care patients, by providing pertinent information in an easily accessible format about many of the medicines likely to be encountered. This information is presented in a logical and comprehensive way, from basic clinical pharmacology through to succinct monographs. There is clear indexing to enable readers to access specific drugs and cross-referencing to other relevant areas.

This book has a place in everyday practice in palliative care, both for the specialist and also the generalist in supporting decision-making and prescribing for palliative care patients. It will enable the healthcare professional to make the most appropriate choice of drug at the right dose for the right symptom. Good palliative care is only as good as the healthcare professionals providing it. This book can play an essential role in supporting healthcare professionals to provide excellent palliative care for patients and their families.

John Ellershaw
Professor of Palliative Medicine
University of Liverpool Director
Marie Curie Palliative Care Institute Liverpool (MCPCIL)

Acknowledgements

I would like to dedicate this book to my wife, Victoria, for without her interminable support, it would not have been possible.

I would also like to thank Margaret Gibbs for her timely contributions to this text.

Contributor

Margaret Gibbs
Specialist Senior Pharmacist
St Christopher's Hospice
London, UK

Contents

Detailed contents

Symbols and abbreviations

📖	cross reference
⤳	dose/dose adjustments
⟐	pharmacology
☺	undesirable side-effects
¥	unlicensed indication
ACE-I	ACE inhbitor
ALP	alkaline phosphatase
ALT	alanine transaminase
ALT DIE	every other day (*alternus die*)
AST	aspartate transaminase
AV	atrioventricular
BD	twice a day (*bis die*)
BNF	*British National Formulary*
BP	blood pressure
BSA	body surface area
BTcP	breakthrough cancer pain
Ca^{2+}	calcium (ion)
CD	controlled drug
CNS	central nervous system
COPD	chronic obstructive pulmonary disease
COX-1	cyclo-oxygenase 1
COX-2	cyclo-oxygenase 2
CrCl	creatinine clearance
CSCI	continuous subcutaneous infusion
CVA	cerebrovascular accident
CYP	cytochrome P450
DVT	deep vein thrombosis
ECOG	Eastern Cooperative Oncology Group
eGFR	estimated glomerular filtration rate
g	gram(s)
G6PD	glucose-6-phosphate dehydrogenase
GEP	gastroenteropancreatic
GFR	glomerular filtration rate
GGT	gamma glutamyl transpeptidase
GI	gastrointestinal
GIST	gastrointestinal stromal tumour

GSL	general sales list (medicine)
GTN	glyceryl trinitrate
H^+	hydrogen (proton)
Hg	mercury
IM	intramuscular
INR	international normalized ratio
IV	intravenous
K^+	potassium (ion)
L	litre(s)
LFT	liver function test
LHRH	luteinizing hormone-releasing hormone
LMWH	low molecular weight heparin
m/r	modified release
MAOI	monoamine oxidase inhibitor
mcg	microgram(s)
mg	milligram(s)
Mg^{2+}	magnesium (ion)
min	minute(s)
mL	millilitre(s)
mm	millimetre(s)
mmol	millimole(s)
µmol	micromole(s)
Na^+	sodium (ion)
NaCl	sodium chloride
NICE	National Institute for Health and Clinical Excellence
NMDA	*N*-methyl-D-aspartate
NRI	noradrenaline reuptake inhibitor
NRT	nicotine replacement therapy
NSAID	non-steroidal anti-inflammatory drug
NSTEMI	non-ST segment elevation myocardial infarction
OD	daily (*omni die*)
OM	in the morning (*omni mane*)
ON	in the evening (*omni nocte*)
OTC	over-the-counter
OTFC	oral transmucosal fentanyl citrate
P	pharmacy only (medicine)
PAH	polycyclic aromatic hydrocarbon
PD	parkinson's disease
PE	pulmonary embolism
PEG	percutaneous endoscopic gastrostomy

P-gp	P-glycoprotein
PM	poor metabolizer
PO	orally (*per os*)
POM	prescription only medicine
PPI	proton pump inhibitor
PR	rectally (*per rectum*)
PRN	when necessary (*pro re nata*)
QDS	four times daily (*quarta die sumendus*)
RLS	restless legs syndrome
s/r	standard release
SC	subcutaneously
SeCr	serum creatinine
SIADH	syndrome of inapproprate antidiuretic hormone hypersecretion
SL	sublingually
SmPC	Summary of Product Characteristics
SPC	Summary of Product Characteristics
SSRI	selective serotonin reuptake inhibitor
stat	immediate(ly)
STEMI	ST segment elevation myocardial infarction
TCA	tricyclic antidepressant
TDS	three times daily (*ter die sumendus*)
TRPV1	transient potential vanilloid 1
U&E	urea and electrolyte
UM	ultra-rapid metabolizer
VTE	venous thromboembolism
WFI	water for injections
WHO	World Health Organization

Clinical pharmacology overview

Introduction

Interpatient variation is a substantial clinical problem when considering drug therapy. Examples of variation include failure to respond to treatment, increased incidence of adverse effects, and increased susceptibility to drug interactions. The concept of 'one dose fits all' is clearly incorrect and is demonstrated by the unacceptable rate of hospital admissions caused by adverse drug reactions (approximately 5% in the UK and 7% in the USA). This variation is hardly surprising, given all the factors that ultimately determine an individual's response to a drug (Fig. 1.1).

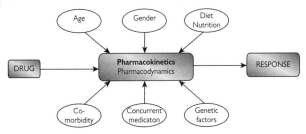

Fig. 1.1 Factors that influence an individual's response to drug therapy.

Pharmacokinetics

The rate and manner that a drug is absorbed, distributed, and eliminated is described by pharmacokinetics, i.e. what the body does to the drug.

Absorption

The bioavailability of a drug describes the proportion of a dose of a drug that enters the systemic circulation, e.g. for IV morphine this would be 100% compared with 15–65% for oral morphine.

For drugs taken orally that are intended for systemic action, a significant proportion of a given dose may not even enter the systemic circulation. This may be due to poor absorption from the GI tract, or metabolism in the gut wall or liver (called first-pass metabolism (Box 1.1)).

Box 1.1 First-pass metabolism

First-pass metabolism is a term used to describe the metabolism that occurs between the gut lumen and the systemic circulation. It can reduce the bioavailability of a drug so much that oral administration is not feasible. Although gastric secretions inactivate certain drugs (e.g. insulin), the main sites of first-pass metabolism are the gut wall and liver.

The cytochrome P450 isoenzyme CYP3A4 (see Box 1.3) is located in the gut wall and liver. It metabolizes many drugs and therefore alterations in CYP3A4 activity can significantly influence bioavailability. It is susceptible to inhibition and induction by a variety of drugs and foods. For example, one glass of grapefruit juice can cause significant inhibition of intestinal CYP3A4, while repeated consumption can interfere with hepatic CYP3A4. The majority of orally administered drugs must pass through the liver before entering the systemic circulation. Some drugs (e.g. lidocaine, fentanyl) are susceptible to extensive first-pass metabolism such that only a small proportion of the oral dose enters the systemic circulation which renders oral administration impossible. (e.g. lidocaine, fentanyl). CYP2C19 is also located in the gut wall and is believed to contribute to first pass metabolism.

First-pass metabolism can be affected by disease, genetic influences, and enzyme inhibition or induction. This helps to explain the wide interpatient variation in drug absorption and hence bioavailability of several drugs (e.g. morphine 15–65%).

Several transporter proteins which influence the absorption of drugs are present in the intestines P-glycoprotein (P-gp) is an efflux transporter molecule that can affect the bioavailability of many drugs (see Box 1.2). Less well categorized influx transporter proteins are also present and their activity may well be influenced by drugs and food.

Box 1.2 The P-glycoprotein (P-gp) drug transporter

P-gp is one of a number of protein transporters that can influence the bioavailability, distribution, and elimination of many drugs relevant to palliative care, e.g. P-gp is believed to be a major determinant of the bioavailability of morphine and tramadol. It is found in the GI tract, kidney, liver, and blood–brain barrier. There is wide patient variation because P-gp is genetically encoded and is subject to polymorphism (📖 Pharmacogenetics, p.11). Drug interactions can occur through induction or inhibition of P-gp, the clinical significance of which is just being realized.

Distribution

Many drugs, such as albumin, bind to plasma proteins. Bound drug is inactive; only unbound drug is available to bind to receptors or cross cell membranes.

Changes in protein binding can alter a drug's distribution, although this is rarely clinically important (exception for phenytoin).

P-glycoprotein is involved in the distribution of several drugs across the blood–brain barrier, e.g. P-gp limits the entry of morphine into the brain.

Elimination

Various processes are involved in drug elimination, although the hepatic and renal processes are the most important.

Drug metabolism

The liver is the main organ of drug metabolism. There are generally two types of reaction (Phase I and Phase II) that have two important effects.
- Make the drug more water soluble—to aid excretion by the kidneys.
- Inactivate the drug—in most cases the metabolite is less active than the parent drug, although in some cases the metabolite can be as active, or more so, than the parent. Prodrugs are inactive until metabolized to the active drug (e.g. codeine is metabolized to morphine).

Phase I metabolism involves oxidation, reduction, or hydrolysis reactions. Oxidation reactions are most common and are catalysed by cytochrome P450 isoenzymes (see Box 1.3) located primarily in the liver. The main exceptions are CYP2C19 and CYP3A4, which are also located in the GI tract (📖 Box 1.1, p.3).

Phase II metabolism involves conjugation reactions, such as glucuronidation or sulphation, which produce more water-soluble compounds, enabling rapid elimination.

Many drugs depend on cytochrome P450 isoenzymes (see end cover) for metabolism and/or elimination. Genetic variations or co-administration of inducers or inhibitors can lead to the development of significant toxicity or lack of effect.

Drug excretion

The main route of excretion of drugs is the kidney. Renal elimination is dependent on many factors including

- Glomerular filtration rate (GFR)
- Active tubular secretion (may involve P-gp)
- Passive tubular secretion

If a drug is metabolized to mainly inactive compounds (e.g. fentanyl), renal function will not greatly affect the elimination. However, if the drug is excreted unchanged (e.g. pregabalin) or an active metabolite is excreted via the kidney (e.g. morphine), changes in renal function will influence the elimination. Dose adjustments may be necessary.

Box 1.3 The cytochrome P450 system

The cytochrome P450 system consists of a large group of over 500 isoenzymes that are involved in the metabolism of endogenous (e.g. steroids, eicosanoids) and exogenous (e.g. drugs) compounds. They are grouped according to amino acid sequence; a family is defined by >40% homology and a subfamily is defined by >55% homology. Five subfamilies (CYP1A, CYP2C, CYP2D, CYP2E, and CYP3A) have a major role in hepatic drug metabolism, with others having a lesser role. The list below briefly describes the isoenzymes involved. See end cover for a list of important substrates, inducers, and inhibitors.

CYP1A subfamily

- CYP1A1—Mainly found in lungs and metabolizes tobacco to potentially carcinogenic substances.
- CYP1A2—Responsible for metabolism of ~15% of drugs; it is induced by tobacco smoke. Also involved in activation of procarcinogens. Polymorphisms exist, but distribution remains undetermined. Important substrates include olanzapine and theophylline.

CYP2A subfamily

- CYP2A6—Metabolizes a small number of drugs including nicotine and the prodrug tegafur. Also metabolizes tobacco to potentially carcinogenic substances. Polymorphisms exist, with 1% of the Caucasian population being poor metabolizers (PMs).

CYP2B subfamily

- CYP2B6—Involved in the metabolism of an increasing number of drugs including ketamine and methadone. Clopidogrel is a potentially potent inhibitor, and rifampicin induces this isoenzyme. Polymorphisms exist, but distribution and consequence remain undetermined.

CYP2C subfamily

- CYP2C8—A major hepatic cytochrome and shares substrates with 2C9. Polymorphisms exist, but their distribution and consequences remain undetermined.

Box 1.3 (cont.)

- CYP2C9—The most important of the CYP2C subfamily. Responsible for the metabolism of many drugs, including warfarin, celecoxib, ibuprofen, diclofenac and phenytoin. Is inhibited by several drugs including fluconazole; rifampicin induces activity of CYP2C9. Polymorphisms exist; 1–3% of Caucasians have reduced activity and are poor metabolizers (PMs).
- CYP2C19—Involved in the metabolism of several drugs, including omeprazole, lansoprazole, diazepam and citalopram. Inhibitors include modafinil, omeprazole and fluoxetine. Carbamazepine can induce this isoenzyme. 3–5% of Caucasians lack the enzyme and are PMs. It has recently been located in the GI tract and is believed to have a role in first-pass metabolism.

CYP2D subfamily
- CYP2D6—No known inducer. Responsible for the metabolism of ~25% of drugs, including codeine, tramadol, and tamoxifen. 5–10% of Caucasians lack this enzyme and are PMs; 1–5% have multiple copies of the gene and are termed ultra-rapid metabolizers (UMs).

CYP2E subfamily
- CYP2E1—Has a minor role in drug metabolism. Main importance is paracetamol metabolism and potential toxicity. Polymorphisms exist, but their distribution and consequences remain undetermined.

CYP3A subfamily
This is the most abundant subfamily in the liver and is responsible for the metabolism of over 50% of drugs, including midazolam and alfentanil. There are four CYP3A genes, although only two are likely to be of importance in human adults. Nonetheless, these isoenzymes are so closely related that they are often referred to collectively as CYP3A. Polymorphisms exist, but their distribution and consequences remain undetermined.
- CYP3A4—Most significant isoenzyme involved in drug metabolism and is frequently implicated in drug interactions. It is located mainly in the liver, but significant amounts are present in the GI tract, where it has an important role in first-pass metabolism. There are several inducers (e.g. carbamazepine, rifampicin) and inhibitors (e.g. clarithromycin, grapefruit juice).
- CYP3A5—Similar substrate spectrum to 3A4, but is possibly less efficient, so is unlikely to have such a dramatic effect on drug metabolism.

Pharmacodynamics

Pharmacodynamics describes the effect of the drug and how it works in terms of its interaction with a receptor or site of action, i.e. what the drug does to the body.

Most drugs act upon proteins.
- Receptor (e.g. morphine and μ-opioid receptor)
- Ion-channel (e.g. lidocaine and Na^+ channel; capsaicin and TRPV1)
- Enzyme (e.g. NSAIDs and cyclo-oxygenase)
- Transporter complex (e.g. SSRIs)

The exceptions include antibiotics, cytotoxic drugs, and immunosuppressants. The term 'receptor' is used loosely to describe the above protein targets.
- Agonists bind to and activate receptors to produce an effect.
- Antagonists also bind to receptors without causing activation. They may prevent the action of, or displace, an agonist.
- Partial agonists activate receptors to a limited extent, but may also interfere with the action of the full agonist. The circumstances in which a partial agonist may act as an antagonist or an agonist depend on both the efficacy (see below) of the drug and the pre-existing state of receptor occupation by an agonist, e.g. buprenorphine will generally act as an antagonist if a patient is using excessive doses of morphine. At lower doses of morphine, buprenorphine will act as an agonist.
- Affinity is a term used to describe the tendency of a drug to bind to its receptors, e.g. naloxone has a higher affinity for opioid receptors than morphine, hence its use in opioid toxicity.
- The intrinsic activity of a drug describes its ability to elicit an effect.
- Efficacy refers to the potential maximum activation of a receptor and therefore the desired response, i.e. a full agonist has high efficacy, a partial agonist has medium efficacy, and an antagonist has zero efficacy.
- Potency refers to the amount of drug necessary to produce an effect, e.g. fentanyl is more potent than morphine since the same analgesic effect occurs at much lower doses (micrograms vs. milligrams).
- Very few drugs are specific for a particular receptor or site of action and most display a degree of relative selectivity. Selectivity refers to the degree by which a drug binds to a receptor relative to other receptors. In general, as doses increase, the relative selectivity reduces such that other pharmacological actions may occur, often manifesting as adverse effects, e.g. meloxicam at doses of 7.5mg/day is selective for COX-2, but at higher doses it loses this selectivity and also binds to COX-1.
- Tolerance is the decrease in therapeutic effect of identical doses of a drug that may occur over a period of time,. Although often expected, this has yet to be conclusively identified for opioid analgesia.
- Tachyphylaxis is the rapid development of tolerance. It can occur with salcatonin (calcitonin), leading to a rebound hypercalcaemia.
- Therapeutic index or margin is the ratio of the dose producing undesired effects to the dose producing therapeutic effects. Drugs with narrow therapeutic margins are often implicated in drug interactions.

- Competitive antagonism describes the situation that occurs when an antagonist competes with the agonist for the binding site of receptors. In such a situation, increasing the concentration of the agonist will favour agonist binding (and vice versa).
- Irreversible competitive antagonism can occur when the antagonist dissociates very slowly, or not at all, from receptors. Increasing the dose of the agonist does not reverse the situation.
- Non-competitive antagonism occurs when the antagonist blocks the effects of the agonist by interaction at some point other than the receptor binding site of the agonist.

Effect of hepatic impairment

Impaired liver function can affect the pharmacokinetics and pharmacodynamics of many drugs. Unlike impaired renal function, there is no simple test that can determine the impact of liver disease on drug handling. A combination of factors need to be considered before such impact can be assessed, including LFTs, diagnosis, and physical symptoms.

In general, the metabolism of drugs is unlikely to be affected unless the patient has severe liver disease. Most problems are seen in patients with jaundice, ascites, and hepatic encephalopathy. Therefore doses of drugs should be reviewed in the following situations.
- Hepatically metabolized drug with narrow therapeutic index
- There is a significant involvement of the cytochrome P450 system (CYP3A4/5 is highly susceptible to liver disease, while CYP2D6 appears relatively refractory)
- INR >1.2
- Bilirubin >100µmol/L
- Albumin <30g/L
- Signs of ascites and/or encephalopathy

Where possible, dosage amendments will be discussed in each monograph.

Effect of renal impairment

The elimination of many drugs and metabolites depends on renal function. Impaired renal function, coupled with rising urea plasma concentrations, induces changes in drug pharmacokinetics and pharmacodynamics. Implications for drug therapy include:
- Increased risk of adverse effects and toxicity through reduced excretion of the drug and/or metabolite(s), e.g. pregabalin, morphine
- Increased sensitivity to drug effects, irrespective of route of elimination e.g. antipsychotics
- Increased risk of further renal impairment, e.g. NSAIDs

Many of these problems can be avoided by simple adjustment of daily dose or frequency of administration. However, in other situations it may be necessary to choose an alternative drug. It is worth noting that patients with endstage renal disease may be at risk of increased drug toxicity due to the reduced activity of CYP3A4/5 and CYP2D6.

Estimating renal function

Unlike liver impairment, the impact of declining renal function is quantifiable. Accurate methods of determining renal function or GFR are unsuitable for routine clinical use. Serum creatinine (creatinine is a product of muscle metabolism) has been used as a simple tool to estimate GFR. However, there are serious limitations to this approach.

- As renal function deteriorates, serum creatinine increases. However, many patients may have reduced GFR but their serum creatinine concentrations fall inside the conventional laboratory normal ranges, e.g. an increase from 50 to 100 μmol/L is still within normal limits, even though renal function has clearly deteriorated.
- Renal function declines with age, but serum creatinine generally remains stable. Thus a 75-year-old may have the same serum creatinine as a 25-year-old, despite having a reduced renal function.

Creatinine clearance (CrCl) serves as a surrogate for GFR. It can be determined from the Cockroft and Gault equation (Box 1.4), which takes weight, age, gender, and serum creatinine (SeCr) into consideration. The majority of dosage-adjustment guidelines in the monographs are based on creatinine clearance. However, there are limitations, with this method as it may report inaccurately for obese and underweight patients.

Box 1.4 Cockcroft and Gault equation for calculating creatinine clearance

$CrCl = ((\,[140-\text{'age'}] \times [\text{'weight (kg)'}] \times F))/(SeCr\,\text{('micromol/l')})$

Where F = 1.23 (male)

1.04 (female)

In the UK, renal function is increasingly being reported in terms of estimated GFR (eGFR), normalized to a body surface area of $1.73m^2$. The formula used to calculate eGFR was derived from the Modification of Diet in Renal Disease (MDRD) study. eGFR assumes that the patient is of average size (assumes an average body surface area of $1.73m^2$), allowing a figure to be determined using only serum creatinine, age, gender, and ethnic origin. It is primarily a tool for determining renal function, of which five categories have been described (see Table 1.1). eGFR is only an estimate of the GFR and has not been validated for use in the following groups or clinical scenarios.

- Children (<18 years old)
- Acute renal failure
- Pregnancy
- Oedematous states
- Muscle-wasting disease states
- Amputees
- Malnourished patients

Table 1.1 Stages of renal failure

Stage	eGFR (mL/min/1.73m^2)
1 Normal GFR*	>90
2 Mild impairment*	60–89
3 Moderate impairment	30–59
4 Severe impairment	15–29
5 Established renal failure	<15

The terms stage 1 and stage 2 chronic kidney disease are only applied when there are structural or functional abnormalities. If there are no such abnormalities, eGFR ≥60mL/min/1.73m^2 is regarded as normal.

While eGFR can be used to determine dosage adjustments in place of creatinine clearance for most drugs in patients of average build, application in palliative care patients may produce erroneous results. For example, eGFR may underestimate the degree of renal impairment in cachectic or oedematous patients, resulting in excessive doses. For palliative care patients, provided that height and weight are known, it would be prudent to calculate the absolute GFR (GFR$_{ABS}$) (Box 1.5) and use this to determine dosage adjustments.

Box 1.5 Calculating absolute GFR (GFRABS) and Body Surface Area (BSA)

$$GFR_{ABS} = eGFR \times \frac{BSA}{1.73}$$

$$BSA = \sqrt{\frac{(height\ (cm) \times weight\ (kg))}{3600}}$$

Pharmacogenetics

If it were not for the great variability among individuals, medicine might as well be a science and not an art.

Sir William Osler, 1892

Just over 50 years ago, two adverse drug reactions were described as being caused by genetic mechanisms. G6PD deficiency and pseudo-cholinesterase deficiency were shown to be manifestations of specific gene mutations. Two years later, in 1959, the term 'pharmacogenetics' was introduced. It was only towards the end of the last century that significant advances were made. As a result of the human genome project, a broader term, 'pharmacogenomics', was introduced (Box 1.6).

Box 1.6 Basic genetic concepts

The human genome consists of 23 pairs of chromosomes (or 22 pairs of *autosomes* and one pair of sex-linked chromosomes) within which are sequences of DNA that are referred to as genes. With the exception of the sex-linked X and Y chromosomes, an individual inherits two copies of each gene, one from each parent. A gene can exist in various forms, or *alleles*. Only 3% of the human genome encodes proteins.

An individual's inherited genetic profile, or genotype, can be described as being:

- Homozygous dominant (i.e. a specific gene consists of two identical dominant alleles)
- Heterozygous (i.e. a specific gene consists of two different alleles, one usually being dominant and the other recessive)
- Homozygous recessive (i.e. a specific gene consists of two identical recessive alleles)

An individual's phenotype describes the observable characteristics that are a result of the genotype and environment. Particular inherited phenotypical traits may be described as being autosomal dominant or recessive.

Pharmacogenetics is the study of how variation in an individual gene affects the response to drugs which can lead to adverse drug reactions, drug toxicity, therapeutic failure, and drug interactions.

Pharmacogenomics is the study of how variation in the human genome can be used in the development of pharmaceuticals.

Polymorphisms refer to commonly occurring genetic variants (i.e. differences in DNA sequences). In most regions of the genome, a polymorphism is of little clinical consequence. However, a polymorphism in a critical coding or non-coding region can lead to altered protein synthesis with clinical implications such as abnormal drug responses.

Genetic variability can affect an individual's response to drug treatment by influencing pharmacokinetic and pharmacodynamic processes, e.g. variations in genes that encode cytochrome P450 isoenzymes, drug receptors, or transport proteins can determine clinical response. Pharmacogenetics can aid in the optimization of drug therapy through the identification of individuals who are likely to respond to treatment, or those who are most likely to be at risk of an adverse drug reaction. Although the exact proportion of adverse drug reactions caused by genetic variability is unclear, emerging evidence suggests an increasing role. Pharmacogenetic testing is currently in early development, but current examples include:

• The need for human epidermal growth factor 2 (HER2) testing before initiating trastuzumab therapy.
• Genetic testing of Han Chinese patients is recommended before commencing carbamazepine therapy because of an association between toxic skin reactions and a specific genotype.

Pharmacogenetic testing has the potential to improve the safety and efficacy of several drugs commonly encountered in palliative care, e.g. analgesics, antidepressants, and antipsychotics.

Genetic influences on pharmacokinetics

Variations in genes that encode transport proteins have been implicated in altered therapeutic response, e.g. P-gp polymorphisms have been associated with altered morphine analgesia. However, the characterization and implications of transporter protein variations are less developed when compared with drug metabolism. There is no doubt that polymorphism of metabolic enzymes has a great effect on interpatient variability.

Several polymorphisms that affect drug metabolism have been identified and there is substantial ethnic variation in distribution. Functional changes as a result of a polymorphism can have profound effects:

• Adverse drug reaction
• Toxicity
• Lack of effect
• Drug interaction

The isoenzymes CYP2C9, CYP2C19, and CYP2D6 are responsible for approximately 40% of cytochrome P450 mediated drug metabolism. They display high levels of polymorphism which have been shown to affect the response of individuals to many drugs (Box 1.7). Pharmaceutical manufacturers have realized the importance of pharmacogenetics; fewer drugs will be developed that are affected by pharmacogenetic factors because potential agents will be discarded at an early stage of development.

Box 1.7 Examples of the effect of P450 polymorphisms on selected drugs

Analgesia
- Codeine—Needs to be metabolized by CYP2D6 to morphine before analgesia is observed. PMs derive no analgesia from codeine. Drugs that inhibit CYP2D6 will mimic the PM phenotype. UMs are at risk of life-threatening adverse drug reactions as codeine is metabolized at a very high rate.
- Methadone—Shows complex pharmacology. Mainly metabolized by CYP3A, but CYP2B6 and CYP2D6 are also involved. PMs of CYP2B6 and CYP2D6 are at risk of developing toxicity if methadone is titrated too quickly.
- NSAIDs—Has been suggested that specific CYP2C8/9 genotypes can cause increased risk of toxicity to NSAIDs.
- Tamoxifen—The active metabolite, endoxifen, is produced by a reaction involving CYP2D6. Patients with a PM phenotype are at risk of therapeutic failure with tamoxifen. Drugs that inhibit CYP2D6 will also mimic the PM phenotype and should be avoided.
- Theophylline—The metabolism of theophylline is highly dependent on CYP1A2 activity, which varies with specific genotypes.
- Tramadol—Is primarily metabolized by CYP2D6 to an active compound M1, which is a more potent opioid agonist. PMs show a poor response to tramadol. As with codeine, drugs that inhibit CYP2D6 can mimic the PM phenotype.

Genetic polymorphisms of cytochrome P450 isoenzymes (Box 1.3) can be divided into four phenotypes.
- Poor metabolizers (PMs) have two non-functional alleles and cannot metabolize substrates
- Intermediate metabolizers (IMs) have one non-functional allele and one low activity allele, so metabolize substrates at a low rate
- Extensive metabolizers (EMs) have one or two copies of a functional allele and metabolize substrates at a normal rate
- Ultrarapid metabolizers (UMs) have three or more copies of a functional allele and metabolize substrates at an accelerated rate

The consequences for a particular phenotype depend upon the activity of the drug. PMs are at increased risk of therapeutic failure (through poor metabolism to an active compound) or adverse effects (because of excessive dose). In contrast, UMs are at increased risk of therapeutic failure with conventional doses because of excessive metabolism; in the case of a prodrug, rapid production of the active compound could lead to toxicity. For example, a patient with UM phenotype for CYP2D6 may rapidly convert codeine to morphine, increasing the risk of developing toxicity, whereas a patient with PM status for CYP2D6 will derive little, if any, analgesic benefit from codeine.

Genetic influences on pharmacodynamics

Genetic polymorphisms of drug receptors, or disease-related pathways, can influence the pharmacodynamic action of drug. These are generally less well categorized than pharmacokinetic consequences. Nonetheless, genetic variations have been shown to be clinically relevant for morphine analgesia and antidepressant therapy. In the latter case, associations between serotonin transport gene polymorphisms and depression have been demonstrated. It has also been shown that genotyping for polymorphisms of certain serotonin or noradrenaline pathways can inform clinical choice of antidepressant, e.g. a patient who fails to respond to citalopram (SSRI) could in fact respond to reboxetine (NRI).

Drug interactions

Be alert to the fact that all drugs taken by patients, including over-the-counter medicines, herbal products, and nutritional supplements, have the potential to cause clinically relevant drug interactions. The patient's diet can also affect drug disposition

The pharmacological actions of a drug can be enhanced or diminished by other drugs, food, herbal products, and nutritional supplements. Clinically relevant and potentially significant drug–drug interactions are included in the monographs.

In a drug-drug interaction, the actions of the object drug are altered by the precipitant in most cases. Occasionally, the actions of both object and precipitant can be affected.

While it is possible to predict the likelihood of a drug interaction, it is often difficult to predict the clinical relevance. Elderly patients or those with impaired renal and/or hepatic function are more at risk. Drug interactions may be overlooked and explained as poor compliance, or even progressive disease. Knowledge of drug interaction processes can aid in the diagnosis of an unexplained or unexpected response to drug therapy.

It is impossible to determine the incidence of drug interactions accurately. Knowledge of many drug–drug interactions comes from isolated case reports and/or small studies in healthy volunteers. However, it is possible to assess a patient's risk indirectly; there are several factors that predispose patients receiving palliative care to a drug interaction (Box 1.8).

Box 1.8 Factors that predispose a patient to drug interactions

- Advancing age
- Multiple medications
- Compromised renal/hepatic function
- More than one prescriber
- Comorbidity

While the majority of risks cannot be reduced, they can be anticipated and managed. For example, a thorough medication history should be taken upon presentation and must include over-the-counter medications, herbal products, and nutritional supplements. In some cases, changes to diet should be enquired about, e.g. the effect of warfarin can be reduced by a diet suddenly rich in leafy green vegetables (a source of vitamin K).

As part of the multidisciplinary team, the pharmacist is an excellent source of information and is often involved in the recording of drug histories.

Two main mechanisms are involved in drug interactions:
- Pharmacokinetic
- Pharmacodynamic

Pharmacokinetic interactions

The precipitant drug alters the absorption, distribution, metabolism, and excretion of the object drug. Pharmacokinetic drug interactions are likely to be encountered in palliative care since many of the drugs used are substrates or inducers/inhibitors of cytochrome P450 isoenzymes (see Metabolism below). These interactions are often difficult to predict.

Absorption

The rate of absorption or amount of object drug absorbed can be altered by the precipitant. Delayed absorption is rarely of clinical relevance unless the effect of the object drug depends upon high peak plasma concentrations (e.g. the effect of paracetamol can be enhanced by combination with metoclopramide). If the amount of drug absorbed is affected, clinically relevant effects can occur.

Absorption interactions involving simple insoluble complex formation can easily be avoided by changing the administration time of the drugs involved, e.g. ciprofloxacin and antacids.

Some interactions involve the induction or inhibition of cytochrome P450 isoenzymes (e.g. CYP3A4), P-gp (Box 1.2) and other transport proteins. The clinical significance of many such interactions remains unclear. CYP3A4, mainly found in the liver, is also present in the gut wall. It is involved in reducing the absorption of many drugs and is subject to both induction and inhibition (see Metabolism below). Grapefruit juice inhibits the action of CYP3A4 in the bowel (and liver with repeated consumption) and can lead to significant increases in bioavailability of several drugs, e.g. ciclosporin, diazepam, sertraline, simvastatin. This interaction is highly variable since the active component of the juice cannot be standardized. This interaction can occur even after consuming just 200mL of grapefruit juice, and inhibition can persist for up to 72 hours. An interaction may occur, whatever the source, e.g. fresh grapefruit and grapefruit juices including fresh, frozen, or diluted from concentrate. Drugs with a narrow therapeutic index are more likely to be affected. Enhanced activity of P-gp will reduce the absorption and bioavailability of a drug. The effect of drugs and food on influx transporters is currently less well categorized but could well contribute to unexplained and unanticipated drug effects.

Distribution

Such interactions are usually of little clinical relevance and often involve alterations in protein binding.

The distribution of some drugs depends on the activity of P-gp, which also appears to act as a component of the blood–brain barrier, e.g. P-gp can limit the entry of hydrophilic opioids into the brain. The clinical significance of the induction or inhibition of P-gp is unclear.

Metabolism

Many drugs are metabolized via the hepatic cytochrome P450 system (Box 1.3) which is subject to both inhibition and induction. CYP3A4 may account for the metabolism of up to 50% of currently used drugs; CYP2D6 may account for up to 25% (see end cover). The effect that smoking can have on drug therapy should not be overlooked (Box 1.9).

Box 1.9 Smoking and potential drug interactions

- Tobacco smoke contains several polycyclic aromatic hydrocarbons (PAHs) that are potent inducers of CYP1A1, CYP1A2, and, to a lesser extent, CYP2E1. PAHs can also induce glucuronide conjugation.
- Induction of CYP1A1 in the lungs causes activation of pro-carcinogens from tobacco smoke and is believed to be a major mechanism in the development of lung cancer.
- Although CYP1A1 is not important for drug metabolism, several drugs are substrates of CYP1A2 (see end cover). Metabolism of these drugs can be induced by tobacco smoke, potentially resulting in increased clearance of the drug and consequent clinically significant reductions in effects. Smokers may require higher doses of these drugs.
- Note that exposure to 'second-hand' smoke can produce similar effects.
- The PAHs cause these pharmacokinetic drug interactions, not the nicotine. Thus nicotine replacement therapy (NRT) will not cause these effects.
- Tobacco smoke and NRT are both implicated in several pharmacodynamic drug interactions. Nicotine can have an alerting effect, thereby countering the action of other drugs.
- The prescriber should consider a dosage reduction of drugs metabolized by CYP1A2 if a patient stops smoking. Similarly, doses of anxiolytics and hypnotics should be reviewed unless NRT is initiated. If a patient starts smoking, doses of drugs metabolized by CYP1A2 may need increasing, whereas doses of anxiolytics and hypnotics may need reviewing.

- Enzyme inhibition is the mechanism most often responsible for life-threatening interactions. It can also result in reduced drug effect where activation of a prodrug is required (e.g. codeine has a reduced analgesic profile when administered with CYP2D6 inhibitors). Inhibition is generally caused by competitive binding for the isoenzyme between object and precipitant. It follows that high doses of the precipitant will cause a greater degree of inhibition. Clinically relevant interactions can be evident within 2 days. The effect of enzyme inhibition generally depends on the half-life of the precipitating drug and the therapeutic index of the object drug. The effect will decrease as blood levels fall. Note that drugs competing for the same isoenzyme can give rise to competitive inhibition. The more drugs that are co-prescribed, the greater the risk of this occurring.

- Induction can occur when the precipitant stimulates the synthesis of more ineffective, increasing metabolic capacity. It can take several days or even weeks to develop and may persist for a similar duration once the precipitant has been withdrawn. Problems with toxicity can occur if doses of the object drug are increased but are not reduced once the precipitant is stopped.
- Many drugs are not always metabolized by one specific pathway and for this reason it is often difficult to precisely predict the outcome of a drug interaction. Nonetheless, although *in vivo* data may not be available for many drugs, *in vitro* evidence of metabolism and specific cytochrome P450 isoenzyme involvement can be used to anticipate and avoid a potentially dangerous drug interaction. The drug monographs (📖 Chapter 3, p.61) note actual and potential drug interactions.

Elimination

In palliative care, it is likely that the most common and potentially more clinically relevant elimination drug interactions will involve renal function. For example, with advancing age, renal function declines but compensatory mechanisms which involve the production of vasodilatory prostaglandins are activated. NSAIDs can significantly impair this compensatory measure, such that there is a marked reduction in renal function and consequential risk of drug interactions.

Pharmacodynamic interactions

The pharmacological actions of the object drug are changed by the presence of the precipitant. Pharmacodynamic interactions can be additive or antagonistic in nature.

Additive

When two or more drugs with similar pharmacodynamic effects are coprescribed, the additive results may result in exaggerated response or toxicity. Additive responses can occur with the main therapeutic action of the drug as well as with the undesirable effects, e.g. SSRI plus tramadol may give rise to the serotonin syndrome (Box 1.10).

Antagonistic

When two drugs with opposing pharmacodynamic effects are coprescribed, there may be a net reduction in response to one or both drugs, e.g. warfarin and vitamin K, NSAIDs and ACE inhibitors, metoclopramide and cyclizine.

Box 1.10 The serotonin syndrome

The serotonin syndrome is a potentially life-threatening condition associated with increased serotonergic activity in the central nervous system (CNS). It can occur as the result of co-administration of drugs that have the net effect of increasing serotonergic neurotransmission. It may also occur after initiation of a single serotonergic drug or by simply increasing the dose of a serotonergic drug.

The syndrome is characterized by a triad of mental, autonomic, and neurological disorders with a sudden onset less than 24 hours after the beginning of treatment. Diagnosis is complex, but includes the addition of a serotonergic agent to an already established treatment (or increase in dosage) and manifestation of at least four major symptoms or three major symptoms plus two minor ones:

- Mental (cognitive and behavioural) symptoms
  - Major symptoms: confusion, elevated mood, coma, or semi-coma
  - Minor symptoms: agitation and nervousness, insomnia
- Autonomic symptoms
  - Major symptoms: fever, hyperhidrosis
  - Minor symptoms: tachycardia, tachypnoea and dyspnoea, diarrhoea, low or high blood pressure
- Neurological symptoms
  - Major symptoms: myoclonus, tremors, chills, rigidity, hyper-reflexia
  - Minor symptoms: impaired coordination, mydriasis, akathisia

Implicated drugs include:

- Citalopram, fluoxetine, paroxetine
- Trazodone, venlafaxine
- Sumatriptan
- Tramadol
- Ondansetron, granisetron

Treatment is largely symptomatic and includes the discontinuation of the serotonergic agents; most patients improve completely within 24 hours upon withdrawal. Benzodiazepines may be used for anxiety and, although effectiveness has not been demonstrated, cyproheptadine or olanzapine (both 5-HT$_{2A}$ antagonists) may be useful.

Prescribing guidance

Unlicensed use of medicines

In the UK, the Medicines and Healthcare Products Regulatory Agency (MHRA) grants a marketing authorization (previously referred to as product licence) to pharmaceutical companies enabling them to market and supply a product for the specific indication(s) mentioned in the summary of product characteristics. It is also possible for pharmaceutical companies to receive a Europe-wide marketing authorization through the European Medicines Evaluation Agency (EMEA).

The Medicines Act 1968 defines the actions of a doctor; this Act ensures that a doctor can legally prescribe unlicensed medicines (those without a marketing authorization) or licensed medicines for 'off-label' purposes (e.g. unlicensed dose, route, or indication). Supplementary prescribers can also prescribe licensed medicines for off-label purposes as well as unlicensed medicines provided that this is part of a patient's clinical management plan. Independent nurse and pharmacist prescribers can prescribe licensed medicines for off-label purposes (must be accepted practice) and have recently been granted authorization to prescribe unlicensed medicines.

Although the use of unlicensed medicines in palliative care is rare, the use of licensed medicines for unlicensed indications, i.e. 'off label', is both common and necessary, and is generally encountered on a daily basis. Off-label use of medicines is highlighted in relevant monographs by the symbol ¥.

The patient should be informed that a drug is to be used beyond its marketing authorization and consent should be documented in the patient's case notes. Although some may feel this is impractical, given the widespread practice in palliative care, certain inpatient units gain consent during the admission process.

Legal categories of medicines

Medicines for human use are classified in the following way. There are three classes of medicine, as defined by the Medicines Act 1968:

- **General Sales List (GSL)**: A medicinal product that can be sold or supplied without the supervision of a pharmacist.
- **Pharmacy Medicine (P)**: A medicinal product that is available for sale from a pharmacy under the supervision of a pharmacist.
- **Prescription-Only Medicine (POM)**: A medicinal product that can be sold or supplied from a pharmacy in accordance with a prescription from an appropriate practitioner.

Controlled drugs (CDs) are further governed by the Misuse of Drugs Regulations 2001, as amended. These drugs are classified into five schedules according to different levels of control.

- **Schedule 1 (CD Lic)**: Production, possession, and supply of drugs in this Schedule are limited in the public interest to purposes of research or other special purposes. Includes drugs such as cannabis, LSD, and ecstasy-type substances which have virtually no therapeutic use.
- **Schedule 2 (CD POM)**: Includes the opioids (e.g. alfentanil, diamorphine, fentanyl, methadone, and morphine) and amphetamines (e.g. methylphenidate). Note that parenteral codeine and dihydrocodeine are classified as Schedule 2 drugs. These drugs are subject to prescription requirements (Box 2.1), safe custody (i.e. CD cupboard), and the need for drug registers.
- **Schedule 3 (CD No Register POM)**: Includes barbiturates, buprenorphine, midazolam, and temazepam. These drugs are subject to prescription requirements (except temazepam), but not safe custody (except temazepam, buprenorphine, flunitrazepam, and diethylpropion), and it is not necessary to keep drug registers (although certain centres may insist upon this as good practice). Note that there is no requirement to store midazolam or phenobarbital in a CD cupboard.
- **Schedule 4 Part 1 (CD Benz POM)**: Includes the benzodiazepines (except midazolam and temazepam), ketamine, and zolpidem. These drugs are not subject to CD prescription or safe storage requirements and a there is no need for a register.
- **Schedule 4 Part 2 (CD Anab POM)**: Includes androgenic and anabolic steroids. These drugs are not subject to CD prescription or safe storage requirements and a there is no need for a register.
- **Schedule 5 (CD Inv POM)**: Includes certain CDs, e.g. codeine, co-phenotrope, pholcodine and morphine, which are exempt from full control when present in medicinal products of low strength.

The quantity of Schedule 2, 3, or 4 CDs to be prescribed at any one time should not exceed 30 days' supply. This represents good practice rather than a legal requirement as there may be circumstances where there is a genuine need to prescribe more than 30 days' supply. Note, however, that prescriptions for Schedule 2, 3, or 4 CDs are only valid for 28 days.

Box 2.1 Prescription requirements for Schedule 2 and 3 controlled drugs

Prescriptions for controlled drugs must be indelible, be signed by the prescriber, be dated, and specify the prescriber's address. The prescription must always state:

- The name and address of the patient
- In the case of a preparation, the form and where appropriate the strength of the preparation
- Either the total quantity (in both words and figures) of the preparation, or the number (in both words and figures) of dosage units to be supplied; in any other case, the total quantity (in both words and figures) of the CD to be supplied
- The dose
- The words 'for dental treatment only' if issued by a dentist

Independent prescribing: palliative care issues

From 1 May 2006 nurse independent prescribing was expanded to enable nurses to prescribe any licensed medicine for any medical condition that a nurse prescriber is competent to treat. This also includes a limited list of controlled drugs (Table 2.1) for restricted indications and routes of administration.

Table 2.1 Controlled drugs which nurse independent prescribers are authorized to prescribe

Drug	Schedule	Indication	Route of administration
Buprenorphine	3	Palliative care	Transdermal
Chlordiazepoxide hydrochloride	4	Treatment of initial or acute withdrawal symptoms caused by the withdrawal of alcohol from persons habituated to it	Oral
Codeine phosphate	5	NA	Oral
Co-phenotrope	5	NA	Oral
Diamorphine hydrochloride	2	Use in palliative care Pain relief in respect of suspected myocardial infarction or for relief of acute or severe pain after trauma, including in either case postoperative pain relief	Oral or parenteral
Dihydrocodeine tartrate	5	NA	Oral
Fentanyl	2	Transdermal use in palliative care	Transdermal
Lorazepam	4	Use in palliative care Tonic–clonic seizures	Oral or parenteral
Midazolam	3	Use in palliative care Tonic–clonic seizures	Parenteral or buccal
Morphine hydrochloride	2	Use in palliative care Pain relief in respect of suspected myocardial infarction or for relief of acute or severe pain after trauma, including in either case postoperative pain relief	Rectal

Table 2.1 (cont.) Controlled drugs which nurse independent prescribers are authorized to prescribe

Drug	Schedule	Indication	Route of administration
Morphine sulphate	2	Use in palliative care, pain relief in respect of suspected myocardial infarction or for relief of acute or severe pain after trauma, including in either case post-operative pain relief	Oral, parenteral or rectal
Oxycodone hydrochloride	2	Use in palliative care	Oral or parenteral administration in palliative care

There are important exclusions that nurse independent prescribers are not authorized to prescribe, which include:

- Alfentanil
- Clobazam
- Clonazepam
- Fentanyl—OTFC, buccal, intranasal, and sublingual products not available
- Hydromorphone
- Ketamine
- Methadone
- Nitrazepam
- Phenobarbital
- Temazepam
- Zolpidem

Pharmacist independent prescribing was also introduced on 1 May 2006. This allows pharmacists to prescribe any licensed medicine for any medical condition that a pharmacist prescriber is competent to treat, with the exception of controlled drugs and unlicensed medicines.

Travelling abroad with medicines

- When planning to travel abroad, patients need to be aware of the laws that govern medicine use in both the UK and their destination(s). It is the patient's responsibility to take the necessary steps to ensure compliance with these laws.
- Note that certain OTC medicines in the UK may be controlled drugs in other countries.
- If any medicines are to be taken abroad (including OTC medicines, e.g. co-codamol 8/500), the patient should contact the Embassy, Consulate, or High Commission of the country or countries to be visited regarding local policies on importing medicines (Box 2.2).
- UK requirements for export/import depend on the medicines in question and the duration of travel abroad.

Box 2.2 Useful contact details

Embassies, Consulates, and High Commissions
- http://www.drugs.homeoffice.gov.uk/publication-search/drug-licences/embassy-list

Application form for personal license
- http://www.drugs.homeoffice.gov.uk/drugs-laws/licensing/personal

Home Office
- Home Office
  Drugs Licensing
  Peel Building
  2 Marsham Street
  LONDON
  SW1P 4DF
- Email: licensing_enquiry.aadu@homeoffice.gsi.gov.uk
- Tel: 0207 035 0467

Less than 3 months
- For all prescription only medicines (POMs), patients are advised to carry a letter from the prescribing doctor that states:
  - patient's name, address and date of birth
  - outbound and inbound dates of travel
  - destination(s)
  - name, form, dose, and total amount of medicine(s) being carried.
- Certain countries may require additional information, such as details of the illness. This information can be obtained from the Embassy, Consulate, or High Commission.

More than 3 months
- Patients carrying any amount of medicines listed in Schedules 2, 3, or 4 (part 1) of the Misuse of Drugs Regulations 2001 will require a personal export/import license. The application form can be downloaded from the Home Office website (see Box 2.2).

- The application must be supported by a covering letter from the prescriber, which should state:
  - patient's name and address
  - quantity of medicine(s) to be carried
  - name, strength, and form of medicine(s) to be carried
  - destination(s)
  - outbound and inbound dates of travel.
- The completed form, together with covering letter, should be sent to the Home Office (see Box 2.2).
- Alternatively, the completed form, together with a scanned copy of the covering letter may be emailed to the Home Office (see Box 2.2).
- The patient must be advised that application for a personal license can take at least 2 weeks.
- Patients taking other POMs abroad are advised to carry a letter from the prescribing doctor that states:
  - patient's name, address and date of birth
  - outbound and inbound dates of travel
  - destination(s)
  - name, form, dose, and total amount of medicine(s) being carried.
- Certain countries may require additional information, such as details of the illness. This information can be obtained from the Embassy, Consulate, or High Commission.
- When travelling by air, POMs should be carried:
  - in original packaging
  - in hand luggage*
  - with a valid personal license (if applicable)
  - with a covering letter from the prescriber, unless a personal license is held.

*Because of liquid restrictions, airport and airline regulations must be checked prior to departure. As of June 2008, medicines essential for the journey may be permitted in quantities greater than 100mL. The patient must have secured the prior agreement of the airline and airport, in addition to having the documentation described above.

Management of pain

- The pain experience is a multifaceted process which can be due to a multitude of factors
- The International Association for the Study of Pain defines pain as: 'an unpleasant sensory and emotional experience associated with actual or potential tissue damage, or described in terms of such damage'
- There are many different ways to classify pain; common terms are shown in Table 2.2.

Table 2.2 Common types of pain

Type of pain	Definition
Acute pain	Typically of short duration, arbitrarily taken to be <3 months. It serves as a warning for injury, or potential for further harm. It subsides as healing occurs. Responds well to analgesia.
Chronic pain	Chronic pain serves no purpose and generally does not relate to injury (except cancer pain) persisting beyond the usual healing period. Response to analgesia can be unpredictable.
Total pain	The total pain that the patient experiences is influenced by emotional, psychological, and spiritual factors, in addition to the physical pain caused by the disease.
Nociceptive pain	Caused by noxious stimuli in the periphery. Inflammatory mediators, such as prostaglandins, sensitize nociceptors. Types of nociceptive pain include somatic pain (e.g. skin, bone) and visceral pain (e.g. bowel). Generally responds well to analgesia.
Somatic pain	Often described as aching or throbbing, somatic pain is generally localized and constant. Usually responds well to classic analgesics, although occasionally adjuvant analgesics are required, e.g. bone pain (bisphosphonates).
Visceral pain	May be described as a constant sharp pain (e.g. bowel colic). It is often diffuse and poorly localized, and may be referred to other non-visceral areas. Usually responds well to classic analgesics, although occasionally adjuvant analgesics are required, e.g. bowel colic (hyoscine butylbromide). Nausea may accompany visceral pain.
Neuropathic pain	Caused by damage to, or changes in, the central or peripheral nervous system. Typically responds poorly to common analgesics; adjuvant analgesics generally required. Described by a variety of terms depending upon the nerve affected, e.g. hot/cold, sharp, shooting, stabbing, itch.
Breakthrough cancer pain	A transient exacerbation of pain that occurs either spontaneously or in relation to a specific predictable or unpredictable trigger, experienced by patients who have relatively stable and adequately controlled background pain.

Cancer pain is traditionally managed using the WHO analgesic ladder (Fig. 2.1).

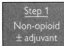
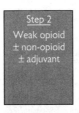

Step 3
Strong opioid
± non-opioid
± adjuvant

Step 2
Weak opioid
± non-opioid
± adjuvant

Step 1
Non-opioid
± adjuvant

e.g. NSAID, paracetamol

- Prescribe paracetamol regularly
- Refer to 🕮 p. 31 (selection of an NSAID) for advice on choosing a NSAID

e.g. Codeine, dihydrocodeine, tramadol

- Do not prescribe paracetamol if combination products are used (e.g. co-codamol)
- Codeine is metabolised to morphine
- Check for drug interactions with codeine and tramadol– effect can be greatly reduced
- Anti-emetic and laxative(s) may need prescribing

e.g. Morphine, fentanyl, oxycodone

- Anti-emetic and laxative(s) should be prescribed

Fig. 2.1 Based on the WHO analgesic ladder.

Management of pain: selection of an NSAID

Summary

- All NSAIDs have significant cardiovascular and GI toxicity.
- Consider whether alternative treatment would be appropriate
- Prescribe the lowest effective dose of NSAID for the shortest time necessary. Review response to treatment after 14 days. Discontinue if no improvement.
- COX-2 inhibitors are contraindicated for use in patients with established ischaemic heart disease and/or cerebrovascular disease and also in patients with peripheral arterial disease. Although NSAIDs are presently licensed for use in these conditions, they should be used with extreme caution.
- Renal function should be assessed prior to and within 7 days of starting an NSAID/COX-2 inhibitor or increasing the dose.
- All patients receiving long-term treatment with an NSAID/COX-2 inhibitor should receive gastroprotective therapy, i.e. PPI, misoprostol. Use PPIs with caution in patients receiving clopidogrel.

Table 2.3 suggests an NSAID selection strategy, which is discussed below:

Is an NSAID/COX-2 necessary?

- Try alternatives first, as follows:
  - Topical NSAID.
  - Tramadol 50 mg modified release BD + paracetamol 1g QDS.
  - Increase tramadol to 100mg BD if no improvement within 2 days. Continue to increase tramadol to maximum 200 mg BD.

  OR
  - Tramacet® 1–2 tablets QDS.
  - Review after 5 days and consider changing to an equivalent dose of modified-release tramadol and regular paracetamol.

Patients at risk of, or with established cardiovascular disease

- The risk of a cardiovascular event associated with COX-2 inhibitors is relatively low; the number of additional events per year has been shown to be 3 per 1000 patients, but the mortality is unknown. Compare this with 1 in 500 perforations, ulcers, or gastroduodenal bleeds that occur with NSAIDs after just 2 months' treatment. In addition, 1 in 1200 patients may die from gastroduodenal complications of NSAIDs after receiving 2 months' treatment. The choice of treatment will depend upon the prescriber's assessment of the individual's risk factors. Nonetheless, COX-2 inhibitors (e.g. celecoxib) are contraindicated for use in patients with established disease and the cardiovascular safety of conventional NSAIDs remains controversial (e.g. diclofenac has been shown to be similar to etoricoxib in terms of cardiovascular toxicity).

- If alternative treatment is unsuccessful, consider the following options:
  - Naproxen + misoprostol or PPI (NB. Caution with PPI if patient on clopidogrel)

OR

  - Ibuprofen + misoprostol or PPI (NB: caution with PPI if patient on clopidogrel)

OR

  - Nabumetone + misoprostol or PPI (NB: caution with PPI if patient on clopidogrel)

Patients at risk of GI toxicity with no cardiovascular risks

- If alternative treatment is unsuccessful, consider the following options:
  - COX-2 inhibitor + misoprostol or PPI (NB: caution with PPI if patient on clopidogrel)

OR

  - Nabumetone + misoprostol or PPI (NB: caution with PPI if patient on clopidogrel)

Patients not at risk of GI toxicity and no cardiovascular risks

- If alternative treatment is unsuccessful, consider the following options:
  - Ibuprofen + misoprostol or PPI (NB: caution with PPI if patient on clopidogrel)

OR

  - Nabumetone + misoprostol or PPI (NB: caution with PPI if patient on clopidogrel)

Table 2.3 Selection of NSAID according to cardiovascular history and gastrointestinal risk factors

Step	CV history ☒ GI risk ☒	CV history ☒ GI risk ☑	CV history ☑ GI ris k ☒	CV history ☑ GI risk ☑
1	Alternative analgesia e.g. topical NSAID, paracetamol, tramadol	Alternative analgesia e.g. topical NSAID, paracetamol, tramadol	Alternative analgesia e.g. topical NSAID, paracetamol, tramadol	Alternative analgesia e.g. topical NSAID, paracetamol, tramadol
2	Ibuprofen + PPI or nabumetone + PPI	COX-2 inhibitor + PPI	Ibuprofen + PPI or naproxen + PPI	Ibuprofen + PPI or naproxen + PPI
3	Non-selective NSAID (e.g. naproxen) + PPI	Ibuprofen + PPI or nabumetone +PPI	Nabumetone + PPI	Nabumetone + PPI
4	COX-2 inhibitor + PPI	Non-selective NSAID (e.g. naproxen) + PPI		

Management of pain: opioid substitution

- Morphine is the strong opioid of choice in palliative care. It may become necessary to switch to another route of administration, or indeed another opioid, because of problems such as:
  - intolerable undesirable effects (e.g. nausea, constipation, hallucinations, myoclonus)
  - dysphagia
  - renal impairment
  - patient request (e.g. reduction of tablet load)
  - malabsorption.
- Before considering opioid substitution, consider simple measures such as:
  - dose reduction
  - rehydration
  - adjuvant medications to improve undesirable effects, e.g. haloperidol for hallucinations, methylnaltrexone for constipation
  - check for drug interactions (e.g. erythromycin and fentanyl).
- Equivalent doses of opioids are shown in Table 2.4. These are an approximate guide since equianalgesic doses are difficult to ascertain due to wide interpatient variations and non-interchangeability of products. The prescriber is ultimately responsible for his/her own actions.
- When converting from one opioid (or route) to another, the suggested equianalgesic dose gradually becomes less precise as the dose increases, especially if there has been recent rapid dose escalation. Therefore, when converting at relatively high doses, initial dose conversions should be conservative. It may be appropriate to reduce the equianalgesic dose by 25–50% since it is preferable to underdose the patient and use rescue medication for any shortfalls.
- In addition, there are several factors that must be considered before simply adopting the equianalgesic dose, e.g.:
  - concurrent morbidity
  - drug interaction (e.g. converting from morphine to an equianalgesic dose of fentanyl in a patient taking carbamazepine may result in worsening pain; converting a patient from morphine to an equianalgesic dose of oxycodone in a patient taking erythromycin may actually result in opioid toxicity due to increased production of the more potent active metabolite)
  - hepatic impairment
  - renal impairment.
- Once the dose of opioid has been decided, the choice of formulation and associated chronological profile need to be considered. For example, consider a patient receiving an oral modified-release morphine preparation twice daily who is being converted to a transdermal fentanyl patch. The patch will be applied at the same time as the last oral dose of morphine.
- Ensure appropriate rescue medication is prescribed to ensure titration of background analgesia.

Table 2.4 Equianalgesic ratios

Opioid	Conversion ratio* (opioid:oral morphine)	Notes
Alfentanil (SC)	1:30	
Buprenorphine (TD)	75:1 to 115:1	Refer to monograph
Codeine (PO)	10:1	
Diamorphine (SC)	1:3	
Dihydrocodeine (PO)	10:1	
Fentanyl (TD)	1:100	Manufacturer recommends 1:150
Hydromorphone (PO)	1:7.5	
Methadone (PO)	Refer to monograph	
Morphine (SC)	1:2	
Oxycodone (PO)	1:1.5	Manufacturer recommends 1:2
Oxycodone (SC)	1:2	PO oxycodone: SC oxycodone is 1.5:1; manufacture states 2:1

*Examples: Morphine 60mg PO in 24 hours = Alfentanil 2mg via CSCI over 24 hours
Morphine 60mg PO in 24 hours = Oxycodone 40mg PO in 24 hours
Codeine 240mg PO in 24 hours = Morphine 24mg PO in 24 hours
Hydromorphone 16mg PO in 24 hours = Morphine 120mg PO in 24 hours

Management of pain: breakthrough cancer pain (BTcP)

Summary

- BTcP episodes can be:
  - unpredictable, e.g. caused by involuntary actions such as coughing (non-volitional incident pain)
  - predictable, e.g. precipitated by a specific activity like walking (volitional incident pain) or dressing change (procedural pain)
  - idiopathic, with no known precipitant (spontaneous pain).
- BTcP episodes typically reach peak intensity in as little as 3min and last an average of 30min, with a median of 2–4 episodes per day.
- Opioids are considered the drugs of choice for most episodes of BTcP.
- There is no correlation between background analgesic dose and the rescue dose for BTcP.
- The use of a short-acting opioid with quick onset and short duration of action is the most appropriate treatment for the majority of BTcP episodes.

Introduction

Pain is a common symptom of cancer with a prevalence of up to 90% in patients with advanced disease. In most cases, background pain (also referred to as baseline or persistent pain) can be treated successfully with the use of long-acting opioid formulations and adjuvant drugs such as gabapentin, pregabalin, or amitriptyline.

In addition to background pain, cancer patients can experience pain of fast onset and short duration that can occur in a predictable or spontaneous manner, which is referred to as breakthrough pain. There is no universally accepted definition of breakthrough pain and this lack of consensus undoubtedly results in inadequate assessment and subsequent suboptimal treatment which impacts on the patient's quality of life.

Breakthrough pain is widely used erroneously to describe any pain episode that occurs in the presence of background pain, i.e. pain that 'breaks through' background analgesia. Traditional treatment has been guided by the WHO analgesic ladder where fixed doses of oral standard-release opioids, based on background requirements, are administered to treat any exacerbation of pain. Adjustments to the background dose are considered, depending on the number of doses of standard-release opioid given in the preceding 24 hours, without any regard to the nature of the exacerbation.

Definition

The term breakthrough cancer pain (BTcP) has been introduced to describe a transient exacerbation of pain, which occurs either spontaneously or in relation to a specific predictable or unpredictable trigger, experienced by patients who have relatively stable and adequately controlled background pain. There are essentially two subtypes of BTcP.

- Incident pain is the most common and is precipitated by movement or activity; it is further divided into volitional pain (i.e. predictable pain caused by voluntary event, e.g. walking), non-volitional pain (i.e. unpredictable pain caused by involuntary actions, e.g. coughing, sneezing), and procedural pain (i.e. pain caused by a particular therapeutic intervention, e.g. wound dressing).
- spontaneous pain, also referred to as idiopathic pain, generally lasts longer than incident pain and is of unknown cause.

Characteristics

Clinical features can vary between patients in that some patients may only experience one type of pain, while others may experience several distinct pains. Furthermore, the clinical features can vary within a patient during the course of the disease.

BTcP is usually of moderate to severe intensity and the pathophysiology is often, but not always, the same as the background pain; it can be neuropathic, nociceptive, or a combination of both. The prevalence of BTcP varies widely and is difficult to determine given the lack of accepted definition. Nonetheless, it is suggested that BTcP:
- is experienced by 65% of patients with background pain, particularly in advanced disease
- typically reaches a maximum intensity after 3–5min
- has an average duration of 15–30min, with a median of 24 episodes per day.

Poorly controlled BTcP pain has a profound impact on quality of life and there are a number of consequences:
- impairment of daily activities,e.g. walking, working
- anxiety and depression
- interference with sleep
- reduced social interaction
- higher pain severity
- dissatisfaction with overall pain management
- greater healthcare costs.

Management

The patient must be assessed in order to differentiate between exacerbations of uncontrolled background pain and BTcP because subsequent treatment modalities are completely different. It is important that BTcP is considered separately from background pain and its treatment must be individualizd. The treatment of BTcP primarily involves pharmacotherapy, although consideration should be given to non-pharmacological interventions such as massage, application of heat or cold,and distraction or relaxation techniques.

Successful management of BTcP includes the following:
- assessment of the characteristics of both pain (e.g. temporal profile, aetiology) and patient (e.g. disease, preferences)
- treatment of the underlying cause (e.g. radiotherapy, chemotherapy, surgery)
- avoidance of precipitating factors

- adjustment of background analgesia (e.g. addition of adjuvant analgesics)
- reassessment.

Opioids are considered the drugs of choice for the treatment of BTcP. Note that opioids are unlikely to control all types of BTcP, and alternative strategies may need to be adopted. There is no correlation between background analgesic dose and the rescue dose of opioid needed to control BTcP successfully. This must be determined by individual titration.

Oral standard-release opioid formulations are unlikely to be of benefit for BTcP. The pharmacokinetic profiles do not complement the temporal characteristics of most episodes of BTcP (onset of action 20–30min, peak analgesia 60–90min). There is also the prolonged duration of action to consider (e.g. 4 hours with morphine) which can potentially manifest with undesirable effects such as drowsiness. Nonetheless, such an approach would be suitable for BTcP of slower onset and duration of an hour or more.

The use of a short-acting opioid with quick onset and short duration of action is the most appropriate treatment for most cases of BTcP. There are presently four products licensed for the treatment of BTcP (📖 Fentanyl, p.181). In addition, an unlicensed alfentanil product is available (📖 Alfentanil, p.65).

Non-opioid analgesics (e.g. paracetamol, NSAIDs, ketamine) and non-pharmacological techniques (e.g. massage, heat/cold, and relaxation) have been used to treat BTcP, although there is presently very little evidence to support their use. A variety of interventional techniques for the treatment of BTcP can be considered (e.g. neural blockade, neuroablation).

Management of pain: neuropathic pain

- The WHO analgesic ladder should be followed.
- Contrary to the common belief of poor efficacy in neuropathic pain, opioids have been found useful in several neuropathic conditions.
- Strong opioids should be titrated against response. If the patient experiences intolerable undesirable effects or poor efficacy during titration with an opioid:
  - try an alternative opioid (📖 Opioid substitution, p.33)
  - consider using a psychostimulant (e.g. modafinil, methylphenidate) if there is excessive fatigue
  - the pain may be opioid-insensitive.
- A suggested approach to the selection of an adjuvant for neuropathic pain is shown in Fig. 2.2.

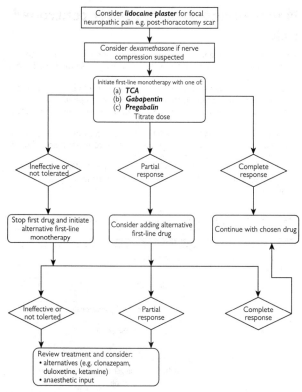

Fig. 2.2 Suggested approach for the use of adjuvant analgesics for neuropathic pain.

Management of pain: poorly controlled pain

- Occasions may be encountered whereby traditional approaches to pain relief do not work, or the patient simply derives little benefit from pharmacotherapy.
- Cancer pain is often multimodal (i.e. components of neuropathic and nociceptive pain). Simply increasing the dose of an opioid will not necessarily control a patient's pain; high doses of opioids can actually cause worsening pain.
- The use of adjuvant analgesia will be necessary in cases of difficult pain. When introducing an adjuvant, the dose of concomitant opioid should be reviewed as a dose reduction may be necessary.
- Table 2.5 lists some of the commonly encountered difficult pains and suggested treatments. Refer to the individual drug monographs for further information.

Table 2.5 Suggested treatment for a selection of difficult pain

Pain	Suggested treatment
Headache associated with brain tumour	Dexamethasone
Malignant bone pain	Radiotherapy NSAIDs Bisphosphonate (e.g. pamidronate, zoledronic acid) Gabapentin/pregabalin
Mucositis	Antifungal. e.g. fluconazole if oral candidiasis suspected Gelclair® (an oral gel classed as a dressing) Topical (dia)morphine
Painful wounds	Topical (dia)morphine
Smooth muscle spasm e.g. bowel colic e.g. rectal pain	Hyoscine butylbromide Hyoscine hydrobromide GTN, nifedipine
Skeletal muscle spasm	Baclofen Diazepam

Management of nausea and vomiting

- Many patients with advanced cancer (up to 60%) can experience nausea and vomiting. There are many causes, some of which are reversible (see Box 2.3).

Box 2.3 Common causes of nausea and vomiting in advanced cancer

Anxiety	Gastritis
Autonomic neuropathy	Gastroparesis
Biochemical (e.g. $\uparrow Ca^{2+}$)	Infection
Bowel obstruction	Pain
Constipation	Raised intracranial pressure
Cough	Renal failure
Drugs	Vestibular disturbance

- The choice of anti-emetic depends on the cause, although many patients may have multiple irreversible causes. Suggested choices are shown in Table 2.6.

Table 2.6 Suggested drug choices for nausea and vomiting

Cause	First-line drug	Second-line drug*	Notes
Unknown	Cyclizine ± haloperidol or Levomepromazine	–	–
Gastric stasis	Domperidone or Metoclopramide	–	Antimuscarinic drugs and 5-HT$_3$ antagonists may reduce the prokinetic effect
Gastric irritation (e.g. drugs, tumour infiltration)	Domperidone or Metoclopramide	Levomepromazine or Ondansetron	Consider PPI or ranitidine if NSAID induced
Total bowel obstruction	Haloperidol ± hyoscine butylbromide or Hyoscine hydrobromide or Glycopyrronium	Add cyclizine or Levomepromazine or Add ondansetron	In difficult cases, consider dexa-methasone 8–12mg daily (SC) and review after 5 days Octreotide ± glycopyrronium may be beneficial if vomiting large volumes Consider NG tube or venting gastrostomy

Table 2.6 (cont.) Suggested drug choices for nausea and vomiting

Cause	First-line drug	Second-line drug*	Notes
Partial bowel obstruction (without colic)	Domperidone *or* Metoclopramide	Add dexamethasone	Consider faecal softener (e.g. docusate sodium)
Chemoreceptor trigger zone (e.g. drugs, hypercalcaemia)	Haloperidol *or* Metoclopramide	Add cyclizine *or* Levomepromazine	The prokinetic effect of metoclopramide may be inhibited by cyclizine
Raised intra-cranial pressure	Dexamethasone + cyclizine	Levomepromazine + dexamethasone	Do not administer dexamethasone and levomepromazine together via the same CSCI

*Substitute the first-line drug with the second-line agent unless the table states otherwise.

Management of constipation

- Constipation should be defined by the patient, not the practitioner.
- Patients with ECOG1 performance status 3 or 4 are at a high risk of developing constipation (i.e. patients confined to bed or chair for more than 50% of waking hours or totally confined to bed or chair).
- Patients receiving opioids are at a high risk of developing constipation. Note that the risk is independent of dose.
- Common causes of constipation are shown in Box 2.4. Where possible, address reversible causes.
- The suggested treatment of constipation is shown in Fig. 2.3.

Box 2.4 Common causes of constipation in advanced cancer

Anal fissure	Environmental
Bowel obstruction	Haemorrhoids
Brain tumour	Hypercalcaemia
Confusion	Immobility
Dehydration	Poor food intake
Depression	Spinal cord compression
Drugs	Weakness
(e.g. anti-cholinergics, 5-HT$_3$ antagonists)	

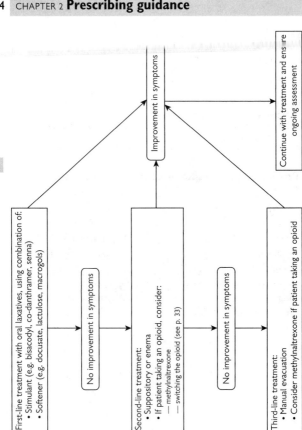

First-line treatment with oral laxatives, using combination of:
• Stimulant (e.g. bisacodyl, co-danthramer, senna)
• Softener (e.g. docusate, lactulose, macrogols)

No improvement in symptoms

Second-line treatment:
• Suppository or enema
• If patient taking an opioid, consider:
  — methylnaltrexone
  — switching the opioid (see p. 33)

No improvement in symptoms

Third-line treatment:
• Manual evacuation
• Consider methylnaltrexone if patient taking an opioid

Improvement in symptoms

Continue with treatment and ensure ongoing assessment

Fig. 2.3 Suggested management of constipation.

Discontinuing and/or switching antidepressants

Summary
- All antidepressants can cause discontinuation symptoms if stopped abruptly or if doses are missed.
- If antidepressants are taken regularly for 8 weeks or more they should generally be discontinued by tapering the dose over at least 4 weeks.
- Longer-term maintenance therapy may need to be discontinued over a 6 month period.
- Fluoxetine has a long plasma half-life; doses ≤20mg OD may be stopped abruptly without dose tapering, although gradual withdrawal may be necessary at higher doses.
- Care is required when switching between antidepressants.
- When switching between SSRIs, TCAs, and related antidepressants, the ideal method would be to incrementally reduce the dose of the first antidepressant and discontinue it before starting the second. This is not always possible in the palliative care setting and cross-tapering or immediate switching may need to be considered.
- The potential for medication errors with complicated switching regimens should be considered.

Discontinuation

If a patient has been taking antidepressants for 8 weeks or more, because of the risk of withdrawal symptoms the antidepressant should not be stopped abruptly unless:
- the drug has caused a serious adverse effect, e.g. a cardiac arrhythmia in association with a TCA
- the patient is entering the terminal phase.

Onset of withdrawal symptoms can occur within a few days, although missing a single dose can precipitate symptoms in susceptible individuals. Problems are more likely with high doses or long courses. Withdrawal symptoms can usually be avoided by tapering the dose of the antidepressant rather than abruptly stopping it. Symptoms should not usually last longer than 1–2 weeks. The antidepressant can be restarted if the symptoms are severe or prolonged, after which withdrawal symptoms usually resolve within 24 hours. More gradual tapering can then be commenced.

Withdrawal symptoms experienced depend on the type of antidepressant and can vary in form and intensity. For SSRIs the most common symptoms include flu-like illness, dizziness exacerbated by movement, insomnia, excessive (vivid) dreaming, and irritability. For TCAs, withdrawal symptoms include rebound cholinergic effects such as headache, restlessness, diarrhoea, and nausea/vomiting. Refer to individual monographs for further detail.

In general, when discontinuing an antidepressant, the following should be applied:
- if taken for <8 weeks, taper dose over 1–2 weeks
- if taken for ≥8 weeks, taper dose over 4 weeks.

One exception is fluoxetine. At a dose of 20mg daily this can be stopped abruptly because of the long plasma half-life of the active metabolite, but at higher doses gradual withdrawal may be required.

Switching antidepressants

Switching antidepressants can increase the risk of undesirable effects due to the potential for interaction between drugs (e.g. serotonin syndrome); there is also the likelihood of withdrawal symptoms developing due to discontinuation of the first antidepressant.

In the palliative care setting there may be limited time to achieve an improvement in the mood of the patient and hence in their quality of life. A more rapid switch under close medical supervision may be indicated.

Before switching antidepressants, several factors must be considered:
- What is the need and urgency for the switch?
- What is the patient's condition?
- What is the current dose of the antidepressant to be withdrawn?
- What is the duration of treatment of the antidepressant to be withdrawn? If ≤8weeks, it may be possible to shorten the withdrawal period or stop the drug abruptly.
- Is there a risk of serotonin syndrome? (◻ Box 1.10, p.19)
- Could the switch result in medication error?

There are several approaches to switching antidepressants that can be considered. Whichever method is used, the patient should be closely monitored.

Method 1—Withdrawal and switch
- Involves gradual withdrawal of the first antidepressant over several weeks, followed by initiation (at low doses) of the new antidepressant, with or without a washout period.
- If the first antidepressant has been taken for:
  - ≥8weeks, dose taper over 4 weeks
  - <8weeks, dose taper over 1–2 weeks.
- Potential risks of administering two antidepressants together include pharmacokinetic interaction (e.g. increased clomipramine levels with paroxetine due to CYP2D6 inhibition) and pharmacodynamic interactions, such as the serotonin syndrome. This method is suggested for switches where there is considerable risk of serious drug interaction.
- Switching from fluoxetine requires careful consideration. Refer to Table 2.7 for advice and further examples.

Method 2—Cross-taper
- The dose of the first antidepressant is gradually reduced while the dose of the second is introduced at a low initial level and gradually increased. The speed of the cross-taper may need to be adjusted according to how well the patient tolerates the process.

- Some drugs should never be co-administered because of the risk of serious drug interactions (see above) and in these cases cross-tapering should be avoided.
- Cross-taper is generally not suitable for fluoxetine because of its long half life (see below).
- See Table 2.7 for specific examples.

Method 3—Immediate switch

- The current antidepressant is stopped abruptly and the new anti-depressant is introduced at a low dose, with or without a washout period.
- Useful if switching between two very similar antidepressants, e.g. two SSRIs. The first drug should be discontinued and the new drug intro-duced at a low dose.
- This is the usual method to adopt when swapping from fluoxetine.
- This process may put a patient at a greater risk of developing with-drawal symptoms.
- See Table 2.7 for specific examples.

Table 2.7 A guide to switching and stopping antidepressants

From \ To	SSRI	TCA*	Venlafaxine	Duloxetine	Mirtazapine
SSRI (except fluoxetine)	*Method 1* Withdraw first SSRI. Initiate new SSRI at low dose the following day or *Method 3* Immediate switch	*Method 1* Withdraw SSRI. Initiate TCA at low dose the following day. If the SSRI being stopped is paroxetine or fluvoxamine, ideally have washout period of 2–3 days *Method 2* Cross-taper cautiously	*Method 2* Cross-taper cautiously or *Method 3* Immediate switch	*Method 1* Withdraw SSRI. Initiate duloxetine 60mg on alternate days the following day and increase dose slowly or *Method 3* Immediate switch	*Method 2* Cross-taper cautiously
Fluoxetine 20mg daily	*Method 3* Immediate switch Stop fluoxetine abruptly. In tiate second SSRI at half the normal starting dose 4–7 days later	*Method 3* Immediate switch Stop fluoxetine abruptly. Initiate TCA at low dose 4–7 days later and increase dose very slowly	*Method 3* Immediate switch. Stop fluoxetine abruptly. Initiate venlafaxine 37.5mg daily 4–7 days later	*Method 3* Immediate switch Stop fluoxetine abruptly. Initiate duloxetine 60mg on alternate days 4–7 days later	*Method 3* Immediate switch. Stop fluoxetine abruptly. Initiate mirtazapine 4–7 days later
TCA*	*Method 2* Gradually reduce the dose of TCA to 25–50mg daily and then start SSRI at usual dose. Withdraw TCA over next 5–7 days*	*Method 2* Cross-taper cautiously	*Method 2* Cross-taper* cautiously, starting with venlafaxine 37.5mg daily	*Method 2* Cross-taper using a starting dose of duloxetine 60mg on alternate days and increase dose slowly	*Method 2* Cross-taper cautiously

	SSRI	TCA	Venlafaxine	Duloxetine	Mirtazapine
Venlafaxine	*Method 2* Cross-taper and initiate SSRI at half normal dose or *Method 3* Immediate switch	*Method 2* Cross-taper* using a low starting dose of TCA, e.g. amitriptyline 25mg daily		*Method 1* Withdraw venlafaxine. Initiate duloxetine 60mg on alternate days the following day and increase dose slowly	*Method 2* Cross-taper cautiously
Duloxetine	*Method 1* Withdraw duloxetine. Initiate SSRI the following day	*Method 2* Cross-taper using a low starting dose of TCA	*Method 1* Withdraw duloxetine. Initiate venlafaxine the following day		*Method 1* Withdraw duloxetine. Initiate mirtazapine the following day
Mirtazapine	*Method 2* Cross-taper cautiously	*Method 1* Withdraw mirtazapine. Initiate TCA the following day	*Method 2* Cross-taper cautiously	*Method 1* Withdraw mirtazapine. Initiate duloxetine 60mg on alternate days the following day and increase dose slowly	

Adapted from UK Medicines Information (UKMI). Switching between tricyclic, SSRI and related antidepressants, from National Electronic Library for Medicines 2009 Available from: http://www.nelm.nhs.uk. (Accessed 22nd November 2009.)

Continuous subcutaneous infusions

Important considerations

- At least four devices are available; ensure familiarity with the selected device.
- The MS16A, MS26 and MP Daily all deliver a length of fluid (mm) in a given time period; the T34 delivers a volume (mL) in a given time period.
- In general, use a 20mL Luer-Lok® syringe as the minimum size. There are occasions when a 10mL syringe may be adequate, but always check local guidelines.
- Mixtures can be diluted with either NaCl 0.9% or WFI. Refer to local policies.
- The CSCI can be started at the time the next oral modified-release opioid dose is due.
- Transdermal opioid patches should remain *in situ* and additional analgesia should be added to a CSCI.

Syringe drivers/pumps

- Continuous subcutaneous infusions (CSCIs) are an effective method of drug administration and are particularly useful in palliative care, whether for end-of-life care or continued symptom relief earlier in the disease.
- There are presently at least four devices that are used to deliver CSCIs in the UK:
  - Smiths Medical MS26
  - Smiths Medical MS16A
  - Micrel MP Daily
  - McKinley T34.

Smiths Medical MS16A and MS26

- Until recently, these were the only two devices available. Many centres have adopted the use of one device only to avoid confusion.
- The MS26 is GREEN and the MS16A is BLUE and there are important differences.
- The flow rate is determined in the same way on both devices, i.e. millimetres of syringe travel over time:
  - MS16A delivers at a rate of mm/hour
  - MS26 delivers at a rate of mm/24 hours.
- Unlike most infusion devices, it is the length of liquid within the syringe, not the volume, which determines the rate of delivery with these syringe drivers. The rate is set by simply turning two screws on the front of the device. For example:
  - Syringe length 48mm and daily infusion
    MS16A, rate of infusion = 48mm/24 hours = 2mm/hour
    MS26, rate of infusion = 48mm/1 day = 48mm/day

- Since the rate of infusion is determined by length, it allows greater flexibility in the choice of brand and size of syringe.
- The maximum length than can be infused per infusion is 60mm and syringes of varying sizes can be attached, with 35mL being the largest (which permits up to 25mL to be infused, depending on the brand).
- The MS26 has a 'boost' button which should not be used as the amount delivered is pointless. However, from a safety point of view, although there is an alarm after 10 seconds of continual use, the whole contents of the syringe could be delivered in a matter of minutes.
- Both devices are powered by a 9V PP3 battery, which delivers approximately 50 infusions.

Micrel MP Daily
- The MP Daily is very similar to the MS26, in that it delivers the length of liquid over a 24 hour period.
- The rate has to be calculated as for the MS26 and input manually.
- The maximum length that can be infused is 60mm and syringes of varying sizes can be attached with 30mL being the largest (which permits up to 22mL to be infused, depending on the brand).
- It is more sophisticated than the MS26, in that infusion rates are set electronically, allowing them to be fixed, limited, or zoned. Once the infusion has started, the rate cannot be changed.
- This device has a range of alarms with and it is powered by six AAA batteries, which deliver approximately 50 infusions.

McKinley T34
- The T34 differs from the above devices in that the delivery rate is based on volume, rather than length.
- It is more sophisticated and complicated than the other syringe drivers, but it is inherently safer.
- A 50mL syringe will fit comfortably on the device, allowing a volume of up to 38mL to be infused, depending upon the brand.
- The T34 detects the syringe size and automatically determines the rate of infusion; the user has to input the brand of syringe.
- The T34 offers a range of advantages over the other devices:
  - a record of infusion activity is maintained
  - the device has a range of alarms
  - less likely to need complicated 12-hourly infusions given the volume that can be infused
- It is powered by a 9V PP3 battery, but this will only last for 3–4 infusions, making it the most expensive device to maintain.

Practical points
- WFI can be used to dilute all mixtures, although this may precipitate infusion site reactions. Anecdotally, NaCl 0.9% may reduce the incidence of infusion site reactions, and it can be used to dilute most mixtures except those containing:
  - cyclizine (use WFI)
  - diamorphine >40mg/mL (use WFI).

- To reduce the incidence of infusion site reactions, the following are suggested:
  - dilute the solution with NaCl 0.9% using a minimum 20 mL Luer-Lok® syringe
  - in the case of cyclizine, consider using a 10mL syringe as this may be more appropriate since dilution with WFI may produce a hypotonic solution (which itself can cause site reactions)
  - rotate the site at least every 72 hours
  - use non-metal cannulae
  - review the drug combination
  - consider the addition of 1mg dexamethasone, after checking compatibility.
- If a patient is being transferred from an oral modified-release opioid formulation, for practical purposes the CSCI can be started at the time the next oral dose is due, although a rescue dose may be necessary. Some centres choose to start the CSCI 4 hours beforehand to maintain adequate analgesia.
- If a CSCI is necessary for a patient using transdermal buprenorphine or fentanyl patches, it is considered best practice to leave these *in situ*; any further analgesic requirements can be added to the CSCI.

Use of drugs in end-of-life care

- Symptoms commonly experienced by patients in the dying phase are:
  - pain
  - nausea and vomiting
  - restlessness
  - respiratory tract secretions
  - dyspnoea.
- Anticipatory prescribing of drugs is essential for the control of symptoms at the end of life.
- All medication should be reviewed and non-essential drugs should be discontinued.
- In the case of type 1 diabetic patients, the patient should be maintained on insulin, but at a reduced dose in order to limit the risk of symptomatic ketoacidosis (e.g. reduced by 30–50%). For type 2 patients, oral hypoglycaemics and/or insulin should be discontinued.
- Unless corticosteroids are used for symptom management (e.g. pain, headache, seizures), it is usually appropriate for them to be withdrawn
- An alternative method of drug administration will invariably be required in order to maintain adequate symptom control. The sub-cutaneous route is usually employed and most symptoms experienced at the end of life can be adequately controlled with a small number of drugs. Administration via a CSCI is a safe, practical, and effective solution.

Managing pain

- Morphine is generally considered the first-line opioid for subcutaneous administration at the end of life, unless the patient is already established on an alternative opioid. Initial doses depend upon current opioid requirements. A suitable dose of morphine for an opioid-naive patient would be rescue doses of 2.5–5 mg SC 2–4 hourly PRN. A CSCI should be initiated if ≥2 rescue doses are required in a 24-hour period.
- Occasionally, diamorphine may be used as the opioid of first choice for subcutaneous administration if opioid requirements are excessive.
- Patients established on a regular dose of oral opioid should be converted to an appropriate dose for CSCI as shown below.

Oral morphine to subcutaneous morphine (2:1)

- Divide the total daily dose of oral morphine by 2 to give the equivalent daily dose of subcutaneous morphine. For example, morphine m/r 90 mg PO BD is equivalent to:
  - 180 mg oral morphine daily
  - 90 mg subcutaneous morphine daily.

Oral morphine to subcutaneous diamorphine (3:1)
- Divide the total daily dose of oral morphine by 3 to give the equivalent daily dose of subcutaneous diamorphine. For example, morphine m/r 90mg PO BD is equivalent to:
    180mg oral morphine daily
    60mg subcutaneous diamorphine daily.

Oral oxycodone to subcutaneous oxycodone (1.5:1)
- Divide the total daily dose of oral oxycodone by 1.5 to give the equivalent daily dose of subcutaneous oxycodone (NB: manufacturer states divide by 2). For example, oxycodone m/r 45mg PO BD is equivalent to:
    90mg oral oxycodone daily
    60mg subcutaneous oxycodone daily.

Oral hydromorphone to subcutaneous hydromorphone (2:1)
- Note that parenteral formulations of hydromorphone are currently unlicensed in the UK.
- Divide the total daily dose of oral hydromorphone by 2 to give the equivalent daily dose of subcutaneous hydromorphone. For example, hydromorphone m/r 24mg PO BD is equivalent to
    48mg oral hydromorphone daily
    24mg subcutaneous hydromorphone daily.
- If a patient has been using oral methadone and a CSCI is required, halve the oral dose, although some patients may require a fairly rapid dose escalation as the ratio approaches 1:1.
- If it is necessary to change to an alternative opioid, initial dose conversions should be conservative because equianalgesic doses are difficult to determine in practice because of wide interpatient variation. The lowest equianalgesic dose should be chosen if a range is stated. Refer to 📖 Management of pain: opioid substitution, p.33 for conversion between opioids.
- The use of opioids at the end of life is summarized in Fig. 2.4.
- Morphine and diamorphine should be used cautiously in patients with renal impairment because of accumulation of active metabolites. In patients displaying signs of opioid toxicity, such as myoclonus, agitation, restlessness, and worsening pain, conversion to alfentanil for use in a CSCI may be appropriate.
- If a patient is receiving analgesic treatment with a transdermal patch (i.e. buprenorphine or fentanyl), this should remain *in situ* with further analgesic requirements being administered using rescue doses of SC morphine (or alternative) and subsequent CSCI. Suitable rescue doses for transdermal buprenorphine and fentanyl patches are shown in Tables 2.8 and 2.9, respectively.

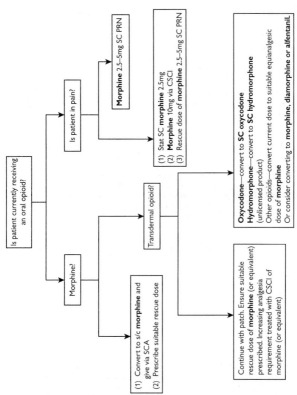

Fig. 2.4 Management of pain with opioids at the end of life.

- BTcP should be managed as described on 📖 Breakthrough cancer pain, p.35. The products currently available can be used successfully during end-of-life care.
- Unresolved pain can present problems during end-of-life care. The vast majority of adjuvant analgesics cannot be administered subcutaneously. Some of the adjuvants, such as tricyclic antidepressants, will have a relatively long half-life, so their actions may persist for several days after discontinuation. Drugs such as clonazepam, ketamine, and ketorolac can be administered via CSCI and may be considered for the treatment of unresolved pain.

Table 2.8 Determination of subcutaneous rescue doses of diamorphine, morphine, and oxycodone for patients using a transdermal buprenorphine patch

Buprenorphine patch strength (mcg/hr)	Morphine or oxycodone subcutaneous rescue dose*(mg)	Diamorphine subcutaneous rescue dose (mg)
35	5–10	2.5–5
52.5	10	5–10
70	10–15	5–10
105	15–25	10–15
140	20–30	15–20

*Based on a conversion of 1:1 between subcutaneous morphine and oxycodone (📖 Opioid substitution, p.33)

Table 2.9 Determination of subcutaneous rescue doses of diamorphine, morphine and oxycodone for patients using a transdermal fentanyl patch.

Fentanyl patch strength (mcg/hr)	Morphine or oxycodone subcutaneous rescue dose* (mg)	Diamorphine subcutaneous rescue dose (mg)
12	2.5	2.5
25	5	2.5–5
50	10	5–10
75	15	10
100	20	15

*Based on a conversion of 1:1 between subcutaneous morphine and oxycodone (📖 Opioid substitution, p.33)

Managing nausea and vomiting

- The choice of anti-emetic will depend upon the cause of nausea and vomiting.
- If there is no identifiable cause, levomepromazine 6.25–12.5mg SC OD or via CSCI over 24 hours may be the most appropriate treatment for nausea and vomiting during end-of-life care.
- Alternatively, cyclizine 100–150mg and haloperidol 3–5mg via CSCI over 24 hours can also be used.
- Note that cyclizine can exacerbate congestive heart failure and should be avoided in such patients.
- Haloperidol alone may be preferred for patients with chronic renal impairment.
- If large volumes are being vomited, the use of anti-secretory drugs such as octreotide 500mcg ± glycopyrronium 1.2mg (or hyoscine butylbromide 120mg) via CSCI over 24 hours can be considered.
- The 5-HT3 antagonists (e.g. granisetron, ondansetron) are suitable second-line choices if the cause of nausea and vomiting is due to renal failure or damage to GI enterochromaffin cells, i.e. recent radiotherapy/chemotherapy, bowel obstruction or gastric cancers.
- Dexamethasone can be used in resistant cases and often produces an indirect anti-emetic effect, particularly in bowel obstruction.
- Ranitidine via CSCI has been used to treat dyspepsia.

Managing restlessness

- Agitation and delirium contribute to the condition known as 'terminal restlessness'. Treatment is defined by the symptoms displayed.
- Reversible causes should be corrected where possible or appropriate:
  - alcohol/nicotine withdrawal
  - biochemical abnormalities (e.g. hypercalcaemia, hypoglycaemia)
  - brain tumour/metastases
  - constipation
  - drugs (e.g. as renal/liver function deteriorate)
  - emotional distress (e.g. fear, anxiety)
  - infection
  - pain
  - urinary retention.
- Non-pharmacological measures may be useful and include a quiet room and the avoidance of isolation or loneliness.
- Benzodiazepines are considered first-line choice for management of agitation. Note that they can exacerbate symptoms associated with delirium. If the patient shows signs of delirium (e.g. paranoia, hallucinations, altered cognition), an antipsychotic may be more appropriate first-line treatment.

Managing agitation

- Begin with midazolam 2.5–5mg SC PRN.
- If two or more PRN doses are administered in a 24 hour period consider adding to or commencing a CSCI. A suitable dose would be 10mg via CSCI over 24 hours. Continue to administer appropriate PRN doses and review requirements daily.

- Alternatively, clonazepam 0.5mg SC PRN may be used. If two or more PRN doses are administered in a 24 hour period consider adding to or commencing a CSCI. A suitable starting dose would be 1mg via CSCI over 12 hours.
- The dose can be increased as necessary, up to an arbitrary dose of 30mg midazolam via CSCI over 24 hours or 1.5–2mg clonazepam via CSCI over 12 hours. Further dose increases should only occur after thorough assessment.
- If partial response to the benzodiazepine, consider adding levomepromazine 25mg to the CSCI (check for compatibility). Increase the dose as necessary in 25–50mg increments up to a maximum of 200mg over 24 hours. It is a useful adjunct to a benzodiazepine for uncontrolled agitation.
- If there is no response to the benzodiazepine, change to levomepromazine 25mg via CSCI over 24 hours. In patients with cerebral tumours, midazolam should be continued since levomepromazine may lower the seizure threshold.
- In refractory cases, phenobarbital may be used for the management of agitation at the end of life.

Managing delirium
- Begin haloperidol 0.5–2.5mg SC PRN.
- Consider adding to or commencing a CSCI if two or more PRN doses are administered in a 24 hour period. A suitable starting dose would be 2.5mg via CSCI over 24 hours. Increase the dose as necessary up to a maximum of 10mg over 24 hours.
- If there is no, or partial, response, levomepromazine as detailed above may be used in place of haloperidol.
- In rare instances, olanzapine has been administered via a CSCI.
- In refractory cases, phenobarbital may be used.

Managing respiratory tract secretions
- The management of respiratory tract secretions in the dying patient is primarily aimed at minimizing the distress of relatives or carers, rather than the patient.
- Non-pharmacological measures are an important part of the management of respiratory tract secretions and may include repositioning the patient and suction.
- The main treatment of terminal secretions involves the use of anticholinergic drugs:
  - hyoscine butylbromide 20mg SC PRN and 60–180mg via CSCI over 24 hours
  - glycopyrronium 0.2mg SC PRN and 0.6–1.2mg via CSCI over 24 hours
  - hyoscine hydrobromide 0.4mg SC PRN and 1.2–2.4mg via CSCI over 24 hours
- There is no evidence to support the superiority of any one drug.
- A PRN dose should be administered as soon as symptoms develop. Anticholinergic drugs do not relieve symptoms from secretions that are already present. Regular administration or a CSCI should be started as soon as possible.

Managing dyspnoea

- The aim of treatment is to reduce the level of anxiety and alter the perception of breathlessness, ensuring that the patient remains comfortable.
- Non-pharmacological measures, such as a fan passing cool air over the face or a calming hand, are important and should not be overlooked.
- Terminal secretions may contribute to the development of terminal dyspnoea and should be treated as described above.
- Pharmacological treatment can involve:
  - midazolam 2.5–5 mg SC PRN. If two or more PRN doses are administered in a 24 hour period consider adding to or commencing a CSCI.
  - morphine 1.25–2.5 mg SC PRN (for opioid-naive patients). If two or more PRN doses are administered in a 24 hour period consider adding to or commencing a CSCI (suitable starting dose 5–10 mg via CSCI over 24 hours). For patients established on opioids, use PRN doses initially based on one-sixth of the background dose and amend as necessary.
  - Other options include levomepromazine, promethazine, and furosemide. The evidence for these is weaker.

Chapter 3

Drug monographs A–Z

Monographs

The monographs are divided into sections as described below. The layout has been designed to provide the healthcare professional with quick access to useful, practical, and relevant information. If more in-depth pharmacological information is required, other reference sources should be consulted.

Products available

- Information about the brand(s) and generic formulations (where applicable), including legal category, available strengths, and the quantity of tablets, capsules, etc. per original pack (where available).
- The legal classification of medicines is shown on 📖 Legal classification of medicines, p.23.
- Some brands are included in the drug monographs. These do not constitute recommendations and other brands may be available. It is not practical to include brand names for all countries and we regret any inconvenience to overseas reader.

Indications

- Lists the indications for which the drug is used in palliative care. This can include both licensed and unlicensed uses; the latter are clearly marked with the symbol ⱽ. Readers should refer to 📖 Unlicensed use of medicines, p.22 for information on the use of licensed drugs for unlicensed purposes

Contraindications and precautions

- A selection of contraindications and precautions are presented in this section. The reader should refer to a product's Summary of Product Characteristics (SPC) for a complete list. Note that it assumed that hypersensitivity to the drug is a contraindication and is not included in each monograph.

☺ Undesirable effects

- Describes a selection of undesirable effects that have been reported.
- The monographs classify undesirable effects as per the SPC:
  - very common (≥10%)
  - common (≥1%, <10%)
  - uncommon (≥0.1%, <1%)
  - rare (≥0.01%, <0.1%)
  - very rare (<0.01%)
  - unknown.
- Certain SPCs have not been updated and do not use this system. In such cases, the frequency of undesirable effects as described in the SPC has been included.
- The reader is referred to the SPC for a complete list.

Drug interactions

- Provides a list of potential and actual pharmacokinetic and pharmacodynamic drug interactions. The reader should read 📖 Chapter 1 in order to appreciate this section fully. Information relating to cytochrome involvement is provided as this can be used to anticipate or identify drug interactions. The table on the inside back cover provides a quick reference guide to cytochrome substrates, inducers, and inhibitors. Be aware that some drugs are metabolized by many cytochrome pathways, and while one drug interaction may seem unimportant, if additional drugs are co-prescribed that block other metabolic pathways, this interaction may assume greater significance.

Dose

- Information for each indication described in the second section is provided. Unlicensed indications are shown by the symbol ✴.

Dose adjustments

- A quick guide to dosage adjustments that may be required in the elderly or those with hepatic/renal impairment. For complete information, the reader is referred to the SPC.

Additional information

- Further relevant information about the practical use of the drug is found here.
- Although brief CSCI stability information is also provided here, this does not indicate stability for all ranges of concentrations. For more in depth information, the reader is referred to Dickman A et al., *The Syringe Driver* (2nd edn), Oxford University Press, 2005.

Pharmacology

- A synopsis of the pharmacology is included in the monograph.

Alfentanil

Rapifen® (CD POM)
Injection: 500mcg/mL (10 × 2mL; 10 × 10mL)

Rapifen Intensive Care® (CD POM)
Injection: 5mg/mL (10 × 1mL)

Generic (CD POM)
Injection: 500mcg/mL (10 × 2mL; 10 × 10mL)

Unlicensed special (CD POM)
Nasal spray: 5mg/5mL (5mL; each actuation delivers 0.14mg in 0.14mL; attachment supplied for sublingual or buccal administration).

See additional information below for supply issues.

Alfentanil is a Schedule 2 controlled drug (see 📖 Legal categories of medicines, p.23 for further information. Independent prescribers are **NOT** authorized to prescribe alfentanil (📖 Independent prescribing: palliative care issues, p.25).

Indications
- ¥ Alternative analgesic for subcutaneous administration, especially in renal failure.
- ¥ Management of BTcP. Refer to 📖 Breakthrough cancer pain, p.35 for guidance relating to BTcP.
- Refer to 📖 Use of drugs in end-of-life care, p.53 for end-of-life care issues.

Contraindications and precautions
- Use caution if the patient received an MAOI within the previous 2 weeks.
- May cause hypotension; use caution If the patient is ambulatory.
- Empirical dose adjustment may be necessary in hepatic impairment (see 📖 Dose adjustments).
- Metabolized by CYP3A4 and is susceptible to drug interactions (see below).
- Alfentanil may modify reactions and patients should be advised not to drive (or operate machinery) if affected.

☺ Undesirable effects
Strong opioids tend to cause similar undesirable effects, albeit to varying degrees(see also 📖 Morphine, p.340).

Very common
- Constipation
- Nausea
- Vomiting

Common
- Bradycardia
- Drowsiness
- Postural hypotension

Uncommon
- Headache
- Pruritus

Rare
- Respiratory depression

Unknown
- Irritation/local reaction (nasal spray)

Drug interactions

Pharmacokinetic
- Alfentanil is metabolized by CYP3A4.
- *Erythromycin*—increased risk of alfentanil toxicity; dose reduction may be necessary
- *Fluconazole*—may inhibit the metabolism of alfentanil (although more likely to occur when fluconazole doses >200mg daily)
- The clinical significance of co-administration with other CYP3A4 inhibitors or inducers (📖 end cover) is unknown. The prescriber should be aware of the potential for interactions and that dosage adjustments may be necessary.

Pharmacodynamic
- *Antihypertensives*—increased risk of hypotension.
- *CNS depressants*—risk of excessive sedation.
- *Haloperidol*—may be an additive hypotensive effect.
- *Ketamine*—there is a potential opioid-sparing effect with ketamine; the prescriber should be aware of the need to reduce the opioid dose.
- *Levomepromazine*—may be an additive hypotensive effect.

💊 Dose

¥ Analgesia
- For opioid-naïve patients, typical starting dose is 250–500mcg SC PRN, or 1mg via CSCI over 24 hours.
- Refer to 📖 Opioid substitution, p.33 for information regarding opioid dose equivalences.
- Given the short duration of action of alfentanil (<15min), it is unusual to titrate persistent background pain with PRN doses of this opioid. Typically, an equivalent dose of an alternative opioid (e.g. oxycodone) is used, based on one-sixth of the 24 hour alfentanil requirements. Note that it may be necessary to make empirical dose adjustments of the alternative opioid in renal impairment. For example:
  - 3mg alfentanil via CSCI =
    5–10mg oxycodone SC PRN (normal renal function)
    2.5–5mg oxycodone SC PRN (impaired renal function).

¥ BTcP

- There is no correlation between the dose of opioid used for persistent background pain and the dose needed to treat BTcP.
- The patient must be using opioids for persistent background pain.
- No validated treatment schedule exists. A suggested starting dose is 250–500mcg SC or 140–280mcg using the nasal spray (equivalent to 1–2 sprays) and increase as necessary.
- In the case of the nasal spray, the prescriber should consider any coexisting oral or nasal condition.

Dose adjustments

Elderly

- No specific guidance is available. Dose requirements should be individually titrated.

Hepatic/renal impairment

- No specific guidance available.
- In hepatic impairment, the half-life and free fraction of alfentanil increase. An empirical dose reduction may be necessary as the effect can be more prolonged and pronounced. This is of particular importance if changing from another opioid using conventional equianalgesic values.
- Alfentanil is the drug of choice in renal disease. Although the clearance is unaltered, the free fraction of alfentanil is raised in renal impairment. Dose requirements should be individually titrated.

Additional information

- Alfentanil spray is available from the manufacturing unit at Torbay Hospital. Delivery can take up to 5 working days (Tel 01803 664707; Fax 01803 664354)
- Via CSCI, alfentanil is reportedly compatible with clonazepam, dexamethasone, glycopyrronium, haloperidol, hyoscine butylbromide, hyoscine hydrobromide, levomepromazine, metoclopramide, midazolam, octreotide, and ondansetron. There is a possible concentration-dependent compatibility issue with cyclizine.

⊕ Pharmacology

Alfentanil is a synthetic opioid, chemically related to fentanyl, and is more lipophilic than morphine. It is a suitable alternative to morphine for use in a CSCI, particularly in patients with renal failure. Alfentanil is approximately 10 times as potent as diamorphine (given subcutaneously). It is extensively metabolized in the liver by the CYP3A4 isoenzyme to inactive compounds. Drugs that inhibit or induce CYP3A4 (📖 end cover) could alter responses to alfentanil. Note that although patients requiring a CSCI of alfentanil are unlikely to be using most of these drugs, their effect on alfentanil metabolism may persist for several days even after cessation.

Allopurinol

Zyloric® (POM)
Tablet: 100mg (100); 300mg (28)

Generic (POM)
Tablet: 100mg (28); 300mg (28)

Indications
- Prophylaxis of:
  - gout
  - hyperuricaemia associated with cancer chemotherapy
  - renal stones.

Contraindications and precautions
Allopurinol should be withdrawn immediately if a skin rash or other evidence of sensitivity occurs as this could result in more serious hypersensitivity reactions (e.g Stevens-Johnson syndrome).

- Allopurinol treatment should not be started until an acute attack of gout has completely resolved.
- Acute attacks of gout may be precipitated during allopurinol use. It is advisable to give prophylaxis treatment during early treatment (e.g. until 1 month after hyperuricaemia corrected) with an NSAID or colchicine. Allopurinol need not be discontinued.
- Patients should be adequately hydrated to prevent xanthine deposition in the urinary tract (of particular importance during chemotherapy).
- Use with caution in patients with hepatic and renal impairment (see 📖 Dose adjustments).

☹ Undesirable effects
Common
- Rash (withdraw treatment; can re-introduce gradually if mild but withdraw permanently if recurs).

Uncommon
- Altered LFTs
- Hypersensitivity reactions
- Nausea/vomiting (can be avoided by taking after meals).

Rare
- Stevens-Johnson syndrome
- Toxic epidermal necrolysis
- Hepatitis

Drug interactions
Pharmacokinetic
- Metabolized by xanthine oxidase (the cytochrome P450 system is not involved).
- *Aspirin/salicylates*—may reduce the effectiveness of allopurinol.
- *Azathioprine/6-mercaptopurine*—azathioprine is a prodrug of 6-mercaptopurine; allopurinol inhibits the metabolism of 6-mercaptopurine. Doses of both azathioprine and 6-mercaptopurine should be reduced by 75%.

- *Ciclosporin*—plasma concentration of ciclosporin may increase.
- *Theophylline*—plasma levels of theophylline may increase.

Pharmacodynamic
- None reported.

Dose
- Initial dose 100mg PO OD
- Usual maintenance dose:
  - 100–200mg PO daily (mild conditions)
  - 300–600mg PO daily (moderate conditions)
  - 700–900mg PO daily (severe conditions)
- Doses over 300mg are given in two or more divided doses (to reduce GI intolerance).

Dose adjustments
Elderly
- The lowest effective dose should be used.

Hepatic/renal impairment
- In hepatic impairment, the manufacturer advises that reduced doses should be used. Periodic LFTs should be performed.
- In mild to moderate renal impairment, a maximum dose of 100mg PO OD is recommended and should only increase if response is inadequate. In severe renal impairment, doses should not exceed 100mg PO OD, or the dosing interval should be increased.

Additional information
- Tablets can be dispersed in water immediately prior to administration if necessary.

Pharmacology
Allopurinol (and its main metabolite oxipurinol) inhibits the enzyme xanthine oxidase, blocking the conversion of hypoxanthine and xanthine to uric acid. It is rapidly absorbed from the upper GI tract and the majority of a dose is eliminated through metabolism; less than 10% is excreted unchanged.

Amitriptyline

Generic (POM)
- **Tablet**: 10mg (28); 25mg (28); 50mg (28)
- **Oral solution**: 25mg/5mL (150mL); 50mg/5mL (150mL)

Indications
- Depression
- Nocturnal enuresis
- ⅍ Neuropathic pain
- ⅍ Bladder spasm

Contraindications and precautions
- Amitriptyline is contraindicated for use in the following:
  - arrhythmias
  - mania
  - porphyria
  - recent myocardial infarction
  - severe liver disease.
- Do not use with an irreversible MAOI, or within 14 days of stopping one, or at least 24 hours after discontinuation of a reversible MAOI (e.g. moclobemide, linezolid). Note that in exceptional circumstances linezolid may be given with paroxetine, but the patient must be closely monitored for symptoms of serotonin syndrome (🕮 Box 1.10, p.19)
- Amitriptyline should be used with caution in patients with:
  - cardiovascular disorders
  - epilepsy
  - hepatic impairment
  - hyperthyroid patients or those receiving thyroid medication (enhances response to antidepressant)
  - narrow-angle glaucoma
  - prostatic hypertrophy
  - urinary retention.
- Elderly patients are more susceptible to undesirable effects (see 🕮 Dose adjustments, p.72).
- Depression is associated with an increased risk of suicidal thoughts, self-harm, and suicide which persists until remission. Note that that the risk of suicide may increase during initial treatment.
- Hyponatraemia should be considered in all patients who develop drowsiness, confusion, or convulsions while taking an antidepressant. Hyponatraemia has been associated with all types of antidepressants, although it is reportedly more common with SSRIs.
- Avoid abrupt withdrawal as symptoms such as nausea, headache, and malaise can occur. Although generally mild, they can be severe in some patients. Withdrawal symptoms usually occur within the first few days of discontinuing treatment and they usually resolve within 2 weeks, although they can persist in some patients for up to 3 months or longer. See 🕮 Discontinuing and/or switching antidepressants, p.45 for information about switching or stopping antidepressants.

If withdrawal symptoms emerge during discontinuation, raise the dose to stop symptoms and then restart withdrawal much more gradually.
- Amitriptyline may modify reactions and patients should be advised not to drive (or operate machinery) if affected.

☺ Undesirable effects

The frequency is not defined, but reported undesirable effects include:

- Abnormal LFTs
- Arrhythmias
- Blurred vision
- Confusion
- Constipation
- Convulsions
- Delirium (particularly in elderly)
- Difficulty with micturition
- Dizziness
- Dry mouth
- Galactorrhoea
- Gynaecomastia
- Hallucinations
- Headache
- Hypomania or mania
- Hyponatraemia
- Increased appetite and weight gain
- Movement disorders
- Nausea
- Postural hypotension
- Sedation
- Sexual dysfunction
- Stomatitis
- Sweating
- Tachycardia
- Taste disturbances
- Tinnitus
- Tremor

Drug interactions

Pharmacokinetic

- Amitriptyline is metabolized by CYP1A2, CYP2C9, CYP2C19, CYP2D6 (major), and CYP3A4. Given the range of metabolic pathways, other factors may be necessary before single-drug interactions become significant (e.g. co-administration of other interacting drugs).
- *Fluconazole*—may increase the plasma concentrations of amitriptyline.
- *Methylphenidate*—may inhibit the metabolism of amitriptyline as a degree of competitive inhibition may develop.
- The clinical significance of co-administration with inhibitors of CYP2D6 (📖 end cover) is unknown. The prescriber should be aware of the potential for interactions and that dosage adjustments may be necessary.
- The clinical significance of co-administration with inducers or inhibitors of CYP1A2, CYP2C9, CYP2C19 and CYP3A4 (📖 end cover) is unknown. The prescriber should be aware of the potential for interactions and that dosage adjustments may be necessary.

Pharmacodynamic

- Amitriptyline may cause prolongation of the QT interval. There is a potential risk that co-administration with other drugs that also prolong the QT interval (e.g. *amiodarone*, *erythromycin*, *haloperidol*, *quinine*) may result in ventricular arrhythmias.
- *Anticholinergics*—increased risk of undesirable effects.
- *Anti-epileptics*—amitriptyline antagonizes the effect.
- *Antihypertensives*—possible increased risk of hypotension.
- β$_2$-*agonists*—combination may predispose patients to cardiac arrhythmias.

- *CNS depressants*—additive sedative effect.
- *Domperidone*—may inhibit prokinetic effect.
- *MAOIs*, including *linezolid*, should be avoided (see *Contraindications and precautions*).
- *Metoclopramide*—may inhibit prokinetic effect.
- *Nefopam*—increased risk of anticholinergic undesirable effects.
- *Serotonergic drugs*—caution is advisable if amitriptyline is co-administered with serotonergic drugs (e.g. *methadone*, *mirtazapine*, *SSRIs*, *tramadol*, *trazodone*) due to the risk of serotonin syndrome (📖 Box 1.10, p.19).
- *SSRIs*—increased risk of seizures and serotonin syndrome.
- *Tramadol*—increased risk of seizures and serotonin syndrome.

Dose

- All indications:
  - 10–25mg PO ON, increasing as necessary to a maximum of 150mg PO daily in divided doses.

Dose adjustments

Elderly

- Elderly patients are particularly susceptible to undesirable anticholinergic effects, with an increased risk for cognitive decline and dementia. No specific dose reductions are recommended by manufacturers. However, it is suggested that elderly patients are initiated on the lower end of the usual range, i.e. 10mg ON, and the dose increased as necessary and as tolerated.

Hepatic/renal impairment

- There are no specific instructions for dose reduction in hepatic impairment. It is contraindicated for use in severe liver disease and should be used with caution in patients with hepatic impairment. If the drug has to be used, the patient should be closely monitored and the lowest effective dose should be prescribed.
- There are no specific instructions for dose adjustment in renal impairment. The lowest effective dose should be prescribed.

Additional information

- May have immediate benefits in treating insomnia or anxiety; antidepressant action may be delayed 2–4 weeks.

Pharmacology

Amitriptyline is a tertiary amine tricyclic antidepressant with strong anticholinergic activity. It undergoes first-pass metabolism to the primary active metabolite nortriptyline. Both amitriptyline and its active metabolite block the reuptake of noradrenaline and serotonin. The interference with the reuptake of noradrenaline and serotonin is believed to explain the mechanism of the antidepressant and analgesic activity of amitriptyline.

Amoxicillin

Amoxil® (POM)
Capsule: 250mg (21); 500mg (21)
Sachet (*sugar-free*): 3g (2)
Injection: 500mg (5; 10); 1g (5; 10)

Generic (POM)
Capsule: 250mg (21); 500mg (21)
Sachet (*sugar-free*): 3g (2)
Oral suspension (*as powder for reconstitution*): 125mg/5mL (100mL); 250mg/5mL (100mL).
Note: Sugar-free formulations are available
Injection (*as powder for reconstitution*): 250mg (10); 500mg (10); 1g (10)

Indications
- Refer to local guidelines.
- Broad-spectrum antibiotic indicated for the treatment of commonly occurring bacterial infections.
- *Helicobacter pylori* eradication.

Contraindications and precautions
- Contraindicated for use in patients with penicillin hypersensitivity.
- Use with caution in renal impairment (risk of crystalluria). Maintain adequate hydration with high doses.

☺ Undesirable effects
Common
- Diarrhoea
- Nausea
- Skin rash

Uncommon
- Pruritus
- Urticaria
- Vomiting

Very rare
- Antibiotic-associated colitis
- Crystalluria
- Hepatitis
- Interstitial nephritis

Drug interactions
Pharmacokinetic
- Oral contraceptives—reduced efficacy.
- *Warfarin*—possible increase in INR.

Pharmacodynamic
- *Allopurinol*—possible increase in skin reactions.

⚕ Dose

Standard doses are described here. Refer to local guidelines for specific advice.

- 250mg PO TDS, increasing to 500mg PO TDS in severe infections. Higher doses (1g PO TDS) have been used.
- 500mg IV injection or infusion TDS, increasing to 1g IV injection or infusion QDS in severe infections. Higher doses (2g IV injection or infusion 4 hourly have been used for serious infections).

⚕ Dose adjustments

Elderly

- No dose adjustment necessary.

Hepatic/renal impairment

- No specific guidance is available for use in hepatic impairment. Use the lowest effective dose.
- Patients in severe renal impairment may need dose adjustments, although no specific guidance is available. Standard adult doses should be tolerated; only the high doses for severe infections may need reducing.

Additional information

- Once reconstituted, the **oral solution** must be discarded after 14 days
- To reconstitute the **injection**, add 5mL WFI to 250mg vial (final volume 5.2mL), 10mL WFI to 500mg vial (final volume 10.4mL), or 20mL WFI to 1g vial (final volume 20.8mL)
- Administer IV **injection** over 3–4 minutes; administer IV **infusion** in 50–100mL NaCl 0.9% (or glucose 5%) over 30–60 minutes

⊙ Pharmacology

Amoxicillin is a broad-spectrum antibiotic active against a wide range of Gram-positive bacteria, with a limited range of Gram-negative cover. It is well absorbed following oral administration, particularly in comparison with other β-lactam antibiotics. Amoxicillin is bactericidal in that it interferes with the synthesis of the bacterial cell wall. As a result, the cell wall is weakened and the bacterium swells and then ruptures.

Anastrozole

Arimidex® (POM)
Tablet: 1mg (28)

Indications
- Treatment of advanced breast cancer in postmenopausal women

Contraindications and precautions
- Anastrozole is contraindicated for use in:
  - premenopausal women
  - pregnant or lactating women
  - patients with severe renal impairment (creatinine clearance <20mL/min)
  - patients with moderate or severe hepatic disease
- Avoid concurrent administration of tamoxifen (see 📖 *Drug interactions* p.75)
- Asthenia and drowsiness have been reported with the use of anastrozole. Caution should be observed when driving or operating machinery while such symptoms persist.

☺ Undesirable effects
Very common
- Asthenia
- Headache
- Hot flushes
- Joint pain
- Nausea
- Rash

Common
- Alopecia
- Anorexia
- Carpal tunnel syndrome
- Diarrhoea
- Drowsiness
- Hypercholesterolaemia
- Vaginal bleeding

Uncommon
- Altered LFTs (GGT and bilirubin)
- Hepatitis
- Urticaria

Rare
- Erythema multiforme

Drug interactions
Pharmacokinetic
- Unlikely to be involved in pharmacokinetic interactions

Pharmacodynamic
- *Oestrogens*—may antagonize the effect of anastrozole
- *Tamoxifen*—may reduce the beneficial effect of anastrozole

Dose
- 1mg PO OD

Dose adjustments
Elderly
- No dosage adjustments necessary.

Hepatic/renal impairment
- No dose change is recommended in patients with mild hepatic disease, but anastrozole is contraindicated for use in patients with moderate or severe hepatic disease.
- No dose change is recommended in patients with mild or moderate renal impairment, but anastrozole is contraindicated for use in patients with severe renal impairment (creatinine clearance <20mL/min).

Pharmacology
Anastrozole is a potent and selective non-steroidal aromatase inhibitor which does not possess any progestogenic, androgenic, or oestrogenic activity. It is believed to work by significantly lowering serum oestradiol concentrations through inhibition of aromatase (converts adrenal androstenedione to oestrone, which is a precursor of oestradiol). Many breast cancers have oestrogen receptors and growth of these tumours can be stimulated by oestrogens.

Baclofen

Lioresal® (POM)
Tablet: 10mg (84)
Liquid (*sugar-free*): 5mg/5mL (300mL)

Generic (POM)
Tablet: 10mg (84)
Liquid*: 5mg/5mL (300mL)

*Check each generic product for sugar content

Indications
- Relief of spasticity of voluntary muscle
- ⃰ Hiccup

Contraindications and precautions
- Avoid in patients with active peptic ulceration.
- Baclofen should be used cautiously in the following conditions since it may lead to exacerbations:
  - confusional states
  - depressive or manic disorders
  - epilepsy
  - Parkinson's disease
  - schizophrenia.
- Baclofen should also be used cautiously in the following conditions:
  - cerebrovascular accident
  - diabetes mellitus (baclofen may cause rise in blood glucose)
  - hepatic impairment (baclofen may elevate LFTs)
  - hypertension (see 📖 *Drug interactions*, p.78)
  - renal impairment (see 📖 *Dose adjustments*, p.78)
  - respiratory impairment (see 📖 *Undesirable effects*, p.78)

- Do not withdraw baclofen abruptly as symptoms such as anxiety, confusions, convulsions, dyskinesia, hallucinations, mania, paranoia, psychosis, and tachycardia can occur. In addition, rebound temporary aggravation of spasticity can also occur. Treatment should always be discontinued over a period of about 1–2 weeks by gradual dosage reduction, unless a serious adverse event has occurred. If such symptoms occur, the dose should be increased and a longer withdrawal should be planned.

- Baclofen may modify reactions and patients should be advised not to drive (or operate machinery) if affected.

☺ Undesirable effects
Very common
- Nausea
- Sedation
- Somnolence

Common

- Ataxia
- Confusion
- Constipation
- Depression
- Diarrhoea
- Dizziness
- Dry mouth
- Dysuria
- Euphoria
- Fatigue
- Hallucinations
- Headache

- Hypotension
- Insomnia
- Light-headedness
- Muscular weakness
- Myalgia
- Nightmares
- Nystagmus
- Polyuria
- Respiratory depression
- Sweating
- Tremor
- Visual disturbances

Rare

- Abnormal LFTs
- Abdominal pain
- Paraesthesia
- Urinary retention

Drug interactions

Pharmacokinetic

- *ACE Inhibitors*—may reduce renal excretion of baclofen.
- *NSAIDs*—may reduce renal excretion of baclofen.

Pharmacodynamic

- *Antihypertensives*—additive hypotensive effect.
- *CNS depressants*—increased risk of undesirable effects such as sedation and respiratory depression.

Dose

- For both indications:
  - Initial dose 5mg PO TDS, increasing by 5mg PO TDS every 3 days until satisfactory control is achieved, or a dose of 20mg PO TDS is reached. The dose can be increased further under supervision to a maximum daily dose of 100mg.
  - Patients may require a slower titrating schedule if undesirable effects become problematic.

Dose adjustments

Elderly

- No specific dose reductions are necessary, but lower initial doses may be necessary (e.g. 2.5–5mg PO BD). Further titration should be cautious. Also refer to renal impairment below.

Hepatic/renal impairment

- For liver impairment, no specific guidance is available. Dose requirements should be individually titrated.
- Baclofen is substantially excreted by the kidney and dose reductions will be necessary in those with impaired renal function. The manufacturer recommends that an initial low dose (e.g. 5mg PO OD) should

be used and the patient should be observed for signs of toxicity if the dose is increased further. Only use in endstage renal failure if perceived benefit outweighs the risk.

Additional information
- If the patient develops hypotonia which is considered problematic during the day, increasing the evening dose and reducing the daytime dose(s) may overcome this issue.

✲ Pharmacology
Baclofen is a gamma-aminobutyric acid derivative that is a specific agonist at GABA-B receptors. The precise mechanism of action is not fully understood and there is no conclusive evidence that actions on GABA systems lead to the clinical effects. Nonetheless, it inhibits reflexes at the spinal level and actions at supraspinal sites may also occur. The clinical effect in hiccups may be due to a direct effect on the diaphragm. Baclofen is rapidly and extensively absorbed and is excreted primarily by the kidney in unchanged form (approximately 85% of the dose is excreted unchanged).

Betahistine

Serc® (POM)
Tablet: 8mg (120); 16mg (*scored*; 84)

Generic (POM)
Tablet: 8mg (84; 120); 16mg (84)

Indications
- Ménière's syndrome
- Tinnitus
- Vertigo

Contraindications and precautions
- Contraindicated for use in patients with phaeochromocytoma.
- Use with caution in patients with patients with a history of
  - asthma
  - peptic ulcer.

☹ Undesirable effects
The frequency is not defined, but reported undesirable effects include:
- Headache
- Dyspepsia
- Nausea
- Peptic ulcer disease

Drug interactions
Pharmacokinetic
- None known.

Pharmacodynamic
- H_1 antihistamines—theoretical risk of reduction in effect of betahistine

Dose
- Initial dose 16mg PO TDS. Dose can be increased as necessary to 24–48mg PO daily in divided doses.

Dose adjustments
Elderly
- No specific guidance available.

Hepatic/renal impairment
- No specific guidance available. However, betahistine is excreted unchanged so the prescriber should be aware that dose reductions may be necessary.

Additional information
- Tablets can be crushed and dispersed in water immediately prior to administration if necessary.

✦ Pharmacology
Betahistine is a specific histamine agonist and it appears to act on the precapillary sphincter in the stria vascularis of the inner ear, reducing the pressure in the endolymphatic space.

Bicalutamide

Casodex® (POM)
Tablet: 50mg (28); 150mg (28)

Indications
- Treatment of advanced prostate cancer in combination with LHRH analogue therapy or surgical castration (50mg).
- Locally advanced prostate cancer at high risk of disease progression, either alone or as adjuvant treatment to prostatectomy or radiotherapy (150mg).
- Locally advanced non-metastatic prostate cancer when surgical castration or other medical intervention is inappropriate (150mg).

Contraindications and precautions
- Contraindicated for use in women and children.
- Should only be initiated by or under the supervision of a specialist.
- Use with caution in patients with liver disease (see 📖 *Dose adjustments*, p.83)
- Bicalutamide inhibits CYP3A4; the manufacturer advises caution when co-administered with drugs metabolized predominantly by CYP3A4.

☺ Undesirable effects

Very common
- Breast tenderness
- Gynaecomastia

Common
- Alopecia
- Altered LFTs (manufacturer recommends checking LFTs periodically)
- Anaemia
- Asthenia
- Cholestasis
- Decreased libido
- Dry skin
- Hot flushes
- Impotence
- Jaundice
- Nausea
- Pruritus
- Weight gain

Uncommon
- Depression
- Dyspepsia
- Haematuria
- Hypersensitivity reactions

Drug interactions

Pharmacokinetic
- Bicalutamide is an inhibitor of CYP3A4.
- The clinical significance of co-administration with substrates of CYP3A4 (📖 end cover) is unknown. Caution is advised if bicalutamide is co-administered with drugs that are predominantly metabolized by CYP3A4 (e.g. *midazolam*). The prescriber should be aware of the potential for interactions and that dosage adjustments may be necessary, particularly of drugs with a narrow therapeutic index.

- *Warfarin*—may be displaced from protein binding sites; check INR if bicalutamide started in patient already on warfarin.

Pharmacodynamic
- No clinically important interactions

Dose
- Treatment of advanced prostate cancer in combination with LHRH analogue therapy or surgical castration:
  - 50mg PO OD
  - treatment should be started at least 3 days before commencing treatment with an LHRH analogue, or at the same time as surgical castration.
- Locally advanced prostate cancer:
  - 150mg PO OD
  - should be taken for at least 2 years, or until the disease progresses.

Dose adjustments
Elderly
- Dosage adjustments are unnecessary.

Hepatic/renal impairment
- Bicalutamide is extensively metabolized in the liver. However, dosage adjustments are not required for patients with mild hepatic impairment. Increased accumulation may occur in patients with moderate to severe hepatic impairment, although no specific guidance is available. Patients should be closely monitored for signs of deteriorating liver function.
- Dosage adjustments are not required for patients with renal impairment.

Additional information
- Although tablets may be crushed and dispersed in water prior to administration, this is not recommended because of the risk of exposure.

Pharmacology
Bicalutamide is a non-steroidal anti-androgen which blocks the action of androgens of adrenal and testicular origin that stimulate the growth of normal and malignant prostatic tissue. It is well absorbed following oral administration, is highly protein bound, and is extensively metabolized. The metabolites are eliminated via the kidneys and bile.

Bisacodyl

Generic (P)
Tablet: 5mg (500; 1000)
Suppository: 10mg (12)

Indications
- Treatment of constipation

Contraindications and precautions
- Abdominal pain of unknown origin
- Acute inflammatory bowel diseases
- Anal fissure (suppository)
- Ileus
- Intestinal obstruction
- Severe dehydration
- Ulcerative proctitis (suppository)

☺ Undesirable effects
Common
- Abdominal cramps and discomfort
- Diarrhoea
- Nausea

Uncommon
- Vomiting

Unknown
- Colitis

Drug interactions
Pharmacokinetic
- *Antacids*—may remove the enteric coat and increase the risk of dyspepsia

Pharmacodynamic
- *Anticholinergics*—antagonize the laxative effect.
- *Cyclizine*—antagonizes the laxative effect.
- *Opioids*—antagonize the laxative effect.
- *5-HT$_3$ antagonists*—antagonize the laxative effect.
- *Tricyclic antidepressants*—antagonize the laxative effect.

♣ Dose
- Initial dose 5–10mg PO ON. Can be increased as necessary to a maximum of 20mg PO ON.
- ¥ Higher doses may be necessary.
- Alternatively, 10mg PR OM.
- ¥ Additional doses may be needed.

⌃ Dose adjustments

Elderly

• No specific dose adjustments recommended by the manufacturer.

Hepatic/renal impairment

• No specific dose adjustments recommended by the manufacturer.

Additional information

• Suppositories are usually effective in about 30 minutes; tablets take effect after 6–12 hours
• Tablets must not be crushed because of risk of dyspepsia.

⌖ Pharmacology

Bisacodyl is a locally acting laxative which undergoes bacterial cleavage in the colon to produce stimulation of the both the large intestine and rectum, causing peristalsis and a feeling of rectal fullness.

Bisoprolol

Cardicor® (POM)
Tablet: 1.25mg (28); 2.5mg (scored, 28); 3.75mg (scored, 28); 5mg (scored, 28); 7.5mg (scored, 28); 10mg (scored, 28)

Emcor® (POM)
Tablet: 5mg (scored, 28); 10mg (scored, 28).

Generic (POM)
Tablet: 1.25mg (28); 2.5mg (28); 5mg (28); 10mg (28)

Indications
- Adjunctive treatment of stable chronic moderate to severe heart failure (Cardicor®)
- Angina
- Hypertension

Note: Cardicor® is only licensed for use in the treatment of heart failure.

Contraindications and precautions
- Bisoprolol is contraindicated for use in patients with:
  - acute heart failure
  - AV block of second or third degree (without a pacemaker)
  - bradycardia with less than 60 beats/min before the start of therapy
  - hypotension (systolic blood pressure less than 100mmHg)
  - late stages of peripheral arterial occlusive disease
  - metabolic acidosis
  - Raynaud's syndrome
  - severe bronchial asthma or severe chronic obstructive pulmonary disease
  - sick sinus syndrome
  - sinoatrial block
  - untreated phaeochromocytoma
- Bisoprolol must be used with caution in:
  - asthma
  - AV block of first degree
  - diabetes mellitus (may mask signs of hypoglycaemia)
  - obstructive airways diseases
  - peripheral arterial occlusive disease
  - Prinzmetal's angina
  - psoriasis (bisoprolol may exacerbate).
- Treatment with bisoprolol should not be stopped abruptly unless clearly indicated, especially in patients with ischaemic heart disease.
- There is a risk that sensitivity to allergens is increased with bisoprolol.

☺ Undesirable effects
Common
- Cold/numb extremities
- Constipation
- Diarrhoea

- Dizziness
- Exhaustion
- Headache
- Nausea
- Tiredness
- Vomiting

Uncommon
- Bradycardia
- Bronchospasm
- Cramps
- Depression
- Muscular weakness
- Sleep disturbances
- Postural hypotension
- Worsening of heart failure

Drug interactions

Pharmacokinetic
- Bisoprolol is metabolized by CYP3A4.
- The clinical significance of co-administration with CYP3A4 inhibitors, or inducers (📖 end cover) is unknown. The prescriber should be aware of the potential for interactions and that dosage adjustments may be necessary.
- The effect of grapefruit juice on the bioavailability of bisoprolol is unknown, but excessive amounts should be avoided.

Pharmacodynamic
- *Antihyperstensives*—increased risk of hypotension.
- *Digoxin*—increased risk of bradycardia.
- *Diltiazem*—increased risk of hypotension and AV block.
- *Haloperidol*—potential increased risk of hypotension.
- *Insulin/oral antidiabetic drugs*—symptoms of hypoglycaemia may be masked.
- *Levomepromazine*—potential increased risk of postural hypotension.
- *NSAIDs*—may reduce hypotensive effect of bisoprolol.
- *Verapamil*—increased risk of hypotension and AV block.

💊 Dose

- Adjunct in stable moderate to severe heart failure:
  - initial dose 1.25mg PO OM for 7 days; if necessary increase the dose to 2.5mg PO OM for 7 days then 3.75mg PO OD for 7 days, then 5mg PO OD for 4 weeks, then 7.5mg PO OM for 4 weeks, then 10mg PO OM; maximum dose 10mg PO daily.
- Angina and hypertension:
  - initial dose 10mg PO OM, increased as necessary to maximum 20mg PO daily.

┋ Dose adjustments

Elderly

- No dose adjustment necessary, although 5mg daily may be a more suitable starting dose for hypertension/angina.

Hepatic/renal impairment

- In patients with liver impairment or severe renal impairment (CrCl <20mL/min) the dose should not exceed 10mg daily.

Additional information

- Tablets may be crushed and dispersed in water immediately prior to administration.

⟐ Pharmacology

Bisoprolol is a competitive highly selective β_1-adrenergic receptor antagonist and is generally not expected to influence the airway resistance. This selectivity extends beyond the therapeutic range. It is well absorbed orally with a bioavailability of 90%; excretion is divided evenly between metabolism (mainly by CYP3A4) and renal elimination of unchanged drug. The metabolites are inactive and are also excreted renally.

Buprenorphine

Temgesic® (CD No Register POM)
Sublingual tablet: 200mcg, 400mcg.

BuTrans® (CD No Register POM)
Patch: 5mcg/hour for 7 days (2); 10mcg/hour for 7 days (2); 20mcg/hour for 7 days (2).

Transtec® (CD No Register POM)
Patch: 35mcg/hour for 96 hours (4); 52.5mcg/hour for 96 hours (4); 70mcg/hour for 96 hours (4).

Generic (CD No Register POM)
Injection: 300mcg/mL (10 × 1mL).

Buprenorphine is a Schedule 3 controlled drug (see 📖 Legal categories for medicines, p.23 for further information). Independent prescribers are **NOT** authorized to prescribe parenteral or sublingual buprenorphine (📖 Independent prescribing: palliative care issues, p.25).

Indications
- Alternative analgesic for acute pain (tablets and injection)—rarely used in palliative care.
- Management of severe pain unresponsive to non-opioid analgesics (*BuTrans®* patches).
- Management of moderate to severe cancer pain and severe pain unresponsive to non-opioid analgesics (*Transtec®* patches).
- End-of-life care issues (📖 Use of drugs in end-of-life care, p.53).

Contraindications and precautions
- Buprenorphine has both opioid agonist and antagonist properties, so in theory could precipitate withdrawal symptoms including pain in patients using other opioids.
- Its actions are only partially reversed by naloxone.
- Dose adjustments may be necessary in hepatic impairment
- Not recommended for use if the patient has received an MAOI within the previous 2 weeks.
- Should not be used in opioid-naive patients, or for the treatment of acute or intermittent pain.
- Not recommended for use if the patient has received an MAOI within the previous 2 weeks.
- Use with caution in patients with:
  - severe respiratory disease
  - concurrent CYP3A4 inhibitors (see 📖 *Drug interactions*, p.90)
  - hepatic impairment (empirical dose adjustment may be necessary—see 📖 *Dose adjustments*
  - pyrexia (transdermal route only—increased buprenorphine delivery rate)

- Patients should be advised to avoid exposing the patch application site to direct heat sources such as hot-water bottles, electric blankets, heat lamps, saunas, or baths because of the risk of increased fentanyl absorption.
- Patients who experience serious adverse events should have the patches removed immediately and should be monitored for up to 24 hours after patch removal.
- Buprenorphine may modify reactions and patients should be advised not to drive (or operate machinery) if affected.

☺ Undesirable effects

- Strong opioids tend to cause similar undesirable effects, albeit to varying degrees (see also ▣ Morphine, p.340).

Very common
- Constipation
- Dizziness
- Drowsiness
- Dry mouth
- Headache
- Nausea
- Vomiting

Common
- Anorexia
- Confusion
- Depression
- Dyspnoea
- Erythema
- Insomnia
- Nausea
- Nervousness
- Pruritus

Uncommon
- Postural hypotension
- Sleep disorder
- Tachycardia

Rare
- Hallucinations
- Respiratory depression
- Visual disturbances

Drug interactions

Pharmacokinetic
- Buprenorphine is metabolized by CYP3A4.
- *Ketoconazole* significantly increases the plasma concentration of buprenorphine so its dose should be halved if starting treatment with ketoconazole.

- The clinical significance of co-administration with other CYP3A4 inhibitors or inducers (📖 end cover) is unknown. The prescriber should be aware of the potential for interactions and that dosage adjustments may be necessary.

Pharmacodynamic

- *Antihypertensives*—increased risk of hypotension.
- *CNS depressants*—risk of excessive sedation.
- *Haloperidol*—may be an additive hypotensive effect.
- *Ketamine*—there is a potential opioid-sparing effect with ketamine; the prescriber should be aware of the need to reduce the opioid dose.
- *Levomepromazine*–there may be an additive hypotensive effect.

⁙ Dose

- For moderate to severe acute pain:
  - 200–400mcg SL every 6–8 hours (but rarely used in palliative care)
  - Alternatively 300–600mcg IM or slow IV injection (but rarely used in palliative care).
- For severe pain unresponsive to non-opioids, i.e suitable for opioid-naive patient:
  - using *BuTrans*® patches, initial dose 5mcg/hour patch for 7 days.
  - the analgesic effect should not be evaluated for at least 72 hours after application in order to allow for gradual increase in plasma-buprenorphine concentration.
  - the dose can be adjusted, if necessary, at 3-day intervals using a patch of the next strength or two patches of the same strength (applied at the same time to avoid confusion).
  - a maximum of two patches can be used at any one time.
- For moderate to severe cancer pain and severe pain unresponsive to non-opioids:
  - using *Transtec*® patches, initial dose of buprenorphine is based upon previous opioid requirements. For opioid-naive patients, the manu-facturer recommends 35mcg/hour for 96 hours.
  - the analgesic effect should not be evaluated for at least 24 hours after application in order to allow for gradual increase in plasma-buprenorphine concentration.
  - the dose can be adjusted, if necessary, at intervals of no longer than 96 hours using a patch of the next strength or two patches of the same strength (applied at same time to avoid confusion).
  - a maximum of two patches can be used at any one time.
- For guidance relating to BTcP refer to 📖 Breakthrough cancer pain, p.25.

⁙ Dose adjustments

Elderly

- No dosage adjustments are necessary, although dose requirements should be individually titrated.

Hepatic/renal impairment
- Buprenorphine is metabolized in the liver so although no specific instructions are available, dose reduction should be considered in patients with hepatic impairment, especially if switching from another opioid using conventional equianalgesic values. Alternative treatment should be considered for patients with severe hepatic impairment.
- No dosage adjustments are necessary for patients with renal impairment, although dose requirements should be individually titrated.

Additional information
- If buprenorphine is taken orally, first-pass metabolism reduces it to a weakly active metabolite.
- Patches should be applied to clean dry non-irritated skin and sites rotated regularly to reduce the chance of skin reactions. The same site should be avoided for at least 6 days (*Transtec®*) or at least 3 weeks (*BuTrans®*).
- After removal of a buprenorphine patch, significant plasma concentration persists and a substitute background opioid should not be started until 24 hours after patch removal.
- It is appropriate to use alternative pure opioid agonists as rescue doses for BTcP or for dose titration.

✜ Pharmacology
Buprenorphine is a partial agonist at the μ-opioid receptor, in addition to being an antagonist at the δ- and κ-opioid receptors. It displays high affinity and low intrinsic activity at the μ-opioid receptor and can displace other opioid agonists (e.g. morphine, oxycodone). Although buprenorphine, when administered transdermally or sublingually, is at least 75 times as potent as oral morphine, it is unable to elicit a full opioid agonist effect at the μ-opioid receptor. The agonist effects of buprenorphine reach a maximum and do not increase in a linear fashion with increasing doses; this is known as a ceiling effect.

If overdose requiring intervention occurs, naloxone may be effective, but other supportive measures such as doxapram have been used. Peaks in plasma concentration are often associated with nausea and vomiting, limiting the usefulness of the buccal product, but the smooth plasma concentration curves provided by transdermal administration offer a useful route of administration to patients needing lower-dose opioids and who have problems with swallowing or concordance.

Carbamazepine

Different preparations may vary in bioavailability. Therefore it is recommended that patients should remain on the same product once treatment has been stabilized. Inclusion of the brand name on the prescription is suggested.

Standard release
Tegretol® *(POM)*
Tablet (*scored*): 100mg (84); 200mg (84); 400mg (56)
Chewtab: 100mg (56); 200mg (56)
Liquid (*sugar-free*): 100mg/5mL (300mL)
Suppository: 125mg (5); 250mg (5)

Generic (POM)
Tablet: 100mg (28); 200mg (28); 400mg (28)
Includes branded generics

Modified release
Tegretol Retard® *(POM)*
Tablet (*scored*): 200mg (56); 400mg (56)

Carbagen SR® *(POM)*
Tablet (*scored*): 200mg (56); 400mg (56)

Indications
- Generalized tonic–clonic and partial seizures
- Trigeminal neuralgia
- ¥ Neuropathic pain

Contraindications and precautions
- Carbamazepine is contraindicated for use in patients with:
  - Acute porphyria
  - AV block
  - History of bone marrow depression
- Agranulocytosis and aplastic anaemia have been associated with carbamazepine. Ensure patients and/or their carers can recognize signs of blood, liver, or skin disorders, and advise them to seek immediate medical attention if symptoms such as fever, sore throat, rash, mouth ulcers, bruising, or bleeding develop.
- Use with caution in the following circumstances:
  - Angle-closure glaucoma
  - Cardiac disease
  - Elderly (see 📖 *Dose adjustments*, p.96)
  - Han Chinese and Thai population (patient should be screened for HLA-B*1502 before initiating treatment due to association with risk of developing Stevens-Johnson syndrome)
  - Hepatic impairment
  - Renal impairment
- Manufacturer recommends LFTs should be performed before initiating treatment and periodically thereafter, particularly in patients with a

history of liver disease and elderly patients. Carbamazepine should be withdrawn immediately in cases of aggravated liver dysfunction or acute liver disease.

- It can cause altered LFTs, such as elevations of GGT and ALP. In the absence of other signs or symptoms, carbamazepine does not need to be withdrawn.
- Carbamazepine has weak anticholinergic activity. It may precipitate confusion or agitation in the elderly.
- It may modify reactions and patients should be advised not to drive (or operate machinery) if affected.

☻ Undesirable effects

Very common
- Altered LFTs (raised GGT/ALP)
- Ataxia
- Dizziness
- Drowsiness
- Fatigue
- Leucopenia
- Nausea and vomiting
- Urticaria

Common
- Dry mouth
- Eosinophilia
- Headache
- Hyponatraemia (SIADH)
- Oedema
- Thrombocytopenia
- Visual disturbances (e.g. diplopia)
- Weight increase

Uncommon
- Dystonia
- Exfoliative dermatitis
- Nystagmus
- Tremor

Rare
- Gynaecomastia
- Systemic lupus erythematosus

Drug interactions

Pharmacokinetic
- Carbamazepine is metabolized by CYP3A4, and is a strong inducer of CYP1A2, CYP2B6, CYP2C8/9, CYP2C19, and CYP3A4
- Carbamazepine may lower the plasma concentration, diminish, or even abolish the activity of many drugs through enzyme induction. Several interactions are listed below (📖 end cover for a list of drugs that may potentially be affected).
- *Clonazepam*—effect of clonazepam may be reduced.
- *Codeine*—risk of opioid toxicity.

- *Corticosteroids*—effect of corticosteroids reduced; higher doses necessary (possibly double or more).
- *Erythromycin*—risk of carbamazepine toxicity (avoid combination or monitor closely).
- *Fentanyl*—risk of reduced analgesic benefit.
- *Fluconazole*—possible risk of carbamazepine toxicity and/or loss of activity of fluconazole.
- *Haloperidol*—effect of haloperidol reduced.
- *Levothyroxine*—increased metabolism may precipitate hypothyroidism.
- *Mirtazapine*—effect of mirtazapine may be reduced.
- *Modafinil*—effect of modafinil may be reduced.
- *Oxycodone*—possible risk of reduced analgesic benefit.
- *Paracetamol*—may increase the risk of hepatoxicity of paracetamol.
- *Tramadol*—reduced analgesic effect.
- The clinical significance of co-administration with other substrates of CYP1A2, CYP2B6, CYP2C8/9, and CYP3A4 (⬚ end cover) is unknown. Caution is advised if carbamazepine is co-administered with drugs that are predominantly metabolized by these isoenzymes. The prescriber should be aware of the potential for interactions and that dosage adjustments may be necessary, particularly for drugs with a narrow therapeutic index.
- The clinical significance of co-administration with CYP3A4 inducers or inhibitors (⬚ end cover) is unknown. The prescriber should be aware of the potential for interactions and that dosage adjustments may be necessary.
- Avoid excessive amounts of grapefruit juice as it may increase the bioavailability of carbamazepine through inhibition of intestinal CYP3A4.

Pharmacodynamic
- *Antipsychotics*—seizure threshold lowered.
- *Antidepressants*—seizure threshold lowered.
- *CNS depressants*—risk of excessive sedation.
- *MAOIs*—avoid concurrent use.
- *Tramadol*—seizure threshold lowered.

⚡ Dose

Carbamazepine induces its own metabolism after several days. Always start with a low dose and increase gradually in increments of 100–200mg every 2 weeks.
- All indications:
  - initial dose 100–200mg PO OD or BD (using standard- or modified-release formulation)
  - increase dose gradually (see above) until response is obtained (usually 400–600mg PO BD)
  - alternatively, 125–250mg PR BD OD or BD. Recommended maximum duration of treatment via rectal route is 7 days; recommended maximum dose is 250mg PR QDS.

Dose adjustments

Elderly

- No specific guidance available. Use with caution because of the potential risk of drug interactions. Carbamazepine has anticholinergic activity and the elderly have been shown to be at an increased risk for cognitive decline and dementia with such drugs.

Hepatic/renal impairment

- No specific guidance available. Manufacturer advises caution in hepatic impairment; lower doses may be necessary.
- Normal doses can be used in renal impairment.

Additional information

- Standard-release oral formulations can be taken TDS/QDS if necessary to reduce risk of undesirable effects. Alternatively, the modified-release formulation can be used.
- Carbamazepine standard-release tablets can be dispersed in water prior to use if necessary.
- Therapeutic plasma concentration range: 4–12mcg/mL, or 17–50micromol/L. Plasma samples are taken immediately prior to next dose (at steady state).

Pharmacology

Carbamazepine is structurally related to tricyclic antidepressants. The mechanism of action is believed to be mediated by blockade of use-dependent sodium channels. It has a range of other pharmacological properties, including anticholinergic, antidiuretic, muscle relaxant, and antidepressant actions. Carbamazepine is well absorbed a fter oral administration (>85%) and is extensively metabolized by CYP3A4; it is a potent inducer of CYP1A2, CYP2B6, CYP2C8/9, CYP2C19, and CYP3A4. Many drugs are affected (See ☐ *Drug interactions*, p.94–5).

Carbocisteine

Mucodyne® (POM)
Capsule: 375mg (120)
Oral liquid: 125mg/5mL (300mL); 250mg/5mL (300mL)

Indications
• Reduction of sputum viscosity (e.g. for use in COPD).

Contraindications and precautions
• Contraindicated for use in active peptic ulceration.

☺ Undesirable effects
The frequency is not defined, but reported undesirable effects include:
• GI bleeding (rare)
• Skin rashes (rare)

Drug interactions
Pharmacokinetic
• None known

Pharmacodynamic
• None known

♣ Dose
• Initial dose 750mg PO TDS, reducing to 750mg PO BD when a satisfactory reduction in cough and sputum production is evident.

♣ Dose adjustments
Elderly
• No dose adjustments are necessary

Hepatic/renal impairment
• No specific guidance available.

⟿ Pharmacology
Carbocisteine affects the nature and amount of mucus glycoprotein which is secreted by the respiratory tract, reducing the viscosity and allowing easier expectoration.

Celecoxib

Celebrex® (POM)
Capsule: 100mg (60); 200mg (30)

Indications
- Symptomatic relief of osteoarthritis, rheumatoid arthritis, and anky-losing spondylitis.
- * Pain associated with cancer.

Contraindications and precautions
- Celecoxib is contraindicated for use in patients with:
  - active peptic ulceration or GI bleeding
  - congestive heart failure (NYHA II–IV)
  - established ischaemic heart disease, peripheral arterial disease, and/or cerebrovascular disease
  - hypersensitivity reactions to ibuprofen, aspirin, or other NSAIDs
  - hypersensitivity to sulphonamides
  - inflammatory bowel disease
  - severe hepatic dysfunction (serum albumin <25g/L or Child–Pugh score ≥10)
  - severe renal impairment (estimated creatinine clearance <30mL/min)
- Use the minimum effective dose for the shortest duration necessary in order to reduce the risk of cardiac and GI events.
- Elderly patients are more at risk of developing undesirable effects.
- Treatment should be reviewed after **2 weeks**. In the absence of benefit, other options should be considered.
- Use with caution in the following circumstances:
  - concurrent use of diuretics, corticosteroids, and NSAIDs (see 📖 *Drug interactions*, p.100)
  - congestive heart failure and/or left ventricular dysfunction
  - diabetes mellitus
  - established ischaemic heart disease, peripheral arterial disease, and/or cerebrovascular disease need careful consideration because of the increased risk of thrombotic events
  - hepatic impairment
  - hyperlipidaemia
  - hypertension (particularly uncontrolled)
  - recovery from surgery
  - renal impairment
  - smoking
- Patients known to be CYP2C9 poor metabolizers should be treated with caution. Similarly, drugs that inhibit CYP2C9 should be used with caution (see 📖 *Drug interactions*, p.100).
- Discontinue treatment at the first appearance of skin rash, mucosal lesions, or any other sign of hypersensitivity.
- Celecoxib may prevent the development of signs and symptoms of inflammation/infection (e.g. fever).

- Consider co-prescription of misoprostol or a PPI if:
  - long-term NSAID therapy
  - concurrent use of drugs that increase the risk of GI toxicity (see 📖 *Drug interactions*, p.100)
- Refer to (📖 *Selection of an NSAID*, p.31) for further information, including selection.

☺ Undesirable effects

Very common
- Hypertension (at doses of 400mg daily)

Common
- Abdominal pain
- Cough
- Diarrhoea
- Dizziness
- Insomnia
- Myocardial infarction
- Peripheral oedema
- Pharyngitis
- Rash
- Sinusitis
- Upper respiratory tract infection
- Urinary tract infection

Uncommon
- Anaemia
- Anxiety
- Blurred vision
- CVA
- Depression
- Drowsiness
- Gastritis
- Heart failure
- Hyperkalaemia
- Leg cramps
- Stomatitis

Rare
- Confusion
- Duodenal ulceration
- Gastric ulceration
- Leucopenia
- Melaena
- Oesophagitis
- Oesophageal ulceration
- Thrombocytopenia

Unknown
- Acute renal failure
- Bronchospasm
- Conjunctivitis

- Headache
- Hepatic failure
- Hyponatraemia
- Stevens–Johnson syndrome
- Toxic epidermal necrolysis

Drug interactions

Pharmacokinetic

- Celecoxib is metabolized by CYP2C9; it is an inhibitor of CYP2C19 and CYP2D6.
- *Carbamazepine*—can reduce the effectiveness of celecoxib.
- *Clopidogrel*—antiplatelet action may be reduced (avoid combination).
- *Fluconazole*—use half-recommended doses of celecoxib as plasma levels increased.
- *Rifampicin*—can reduce the effectiveness of celecoxib.
- The clinical significance of co-administration with other CYP2C9 inducers or inhibitors (📖 end cover) is unknown. The prescriber should be aware of the potential for interactions and that dosage adjustments may be necessary.
- The clinical significance of co-administration of CYP2C19 or CYP2D6 substrates (📖 end cover) is unknown. Caution is advised if celecoxib is co-administered with drugs that are predominantly metabolized by CYP2C19 or CYP2D6. The prescriber should be aware of the potential for interactions and that dosage adjustments may be necessary, particularly for drugs with a narrow therapeutic index.
- The clinical significance of co-administration with prodrugs metabolized by CYP2D6 (e.g. codeine, tramadol) is unknown. The prescriber should be aware of the potential for interactions and that a change in therapy may be indicated.

Pharmacodynamic

- *Anticoagulants*—increased risk of bleeding.
- *Antihypertensives*—reduced hypotensive effect.
- *Antiplatelet drugs*—increased risk of bleeding.
- *Corticosteroids*—increased risk of GI toxicity.
- *Ciclosporin*—increased risk of nephrotoxicity.
- *Diuretics*—reduced diuretic effect.
- *Rosiglitazone*—increased risk of oedema.
- *SSRIs*—increased risk of GI bleeding.

💊 Dose

Osteoarthritis, rheumatoid arthritis, and ankylosing spondylitis

- Initial dose 100mg PO BD or 200mg PO OD. Increase if necessary to 200mg PO BD. If no benefit after **two weeks** discontinue treatment and review.

¥ Cancer pain

- Initial dose 100mg PO BD or 200mg PO OD. Increase if necessary to 200mg PO BD. If no benefit after **two weeks** discontinue treatment and review.

⚗ Dose adjustments

Elderly
- Usual adult doses recommended. Note that the elderly are particularly susceptible to undesirable effects. Use the lowest effective dose for the shortest duration possible.

Hepatic/renal impairment
- Initial dose 100mg PO OM in patients with established moderate hepatic impairment with a serum albumin of 25–35g/L.
- Use of celecoxib in severe renal impairment is contraindicated. No specific guidance is available for use in mild to moderate renal impairment. Use the lowest effective dose for the shortest duration possible. Close monitoring of renal function is recommended.

Additional information
- Contents of the capsule can be dispersed in water or fruit juice if necessary prior to administration.
- Despite contraindication, several studies have shown that celecoxib can be used safely in patients with aspirin/NSAID sensitivity. However, there is a risk of cross-sensitivity. If celecoxib is used, it should be monitored closely.

⟿ Pharmacology
Like traditional NSAIDs, the mechanism of action of celecoxib is believed to be due to inhibition of prostaglandin synthesis. However, unlike most NSAIDs, celecoxib is a selective non-competitive inhibitor of COX-2. Celecoxib is mainly eliminated by metabolism, with less than 1% of the dose being excreted unchanged in urine. Celecoxib metabolism is primarily mediated via CYP2C9 to form three inactive metabolites.

Ciprofloxacin

Ciproxin® (POM)
Tablet (scored): 250mg (10; 20); 500mg (10; 20); 750mg (10)
Suspension (for reconstitution with provided diluent): 250mg/5mL (100mL)
Injection: 100mg/50mL; 200mg/100mL; 400mg/200mL

Generic (POM)
Tablet: 250mg (10; 20); 500mg (10; 20); 750mg (10)
Injection: 100mg/50mL; 200mg/100mL; 400mg/200mL

Indications
- Refer to local guidelines.
- Broad-spectrum antibiotic indicated for the treatment of infections caused by susceptible organisms (mainly Gram-negative, see below)

Contraindications and precautions
- Ciprofloxacin should not be used to treat infections caused by Gram-positive organisms (e.g. *Streptococcus pneumonia*) because of poor activity.
- Concurrent use of duloxetine and tizanidine is contraindicated.
- Use with caution in the following:
  - concurrent use of CYP1A2 substrates, or drugs that prolong the QT interval (see 📖 *Drug interactions*, p.103)
  - epilepsy
  - glucose-6-phosphate dehydrogenase deficiency
  - renal impairment (risk of crystalluria)
- Ciprofloxacin may modify reactions and patients should be advised not to drive (or operate machinery) if affected.

☺ Undesirable effects
Common
- Diarrhoea
- Nausea

Uncommon
- Abdominal pains
- Abnormal LFTs (raised bilirubin, AST)
- Anorexia
- Asthenia
- Dizziness
- Dyspepsia
- Flatulence
- Headache
- Musculoskeletal pain
- Renal impairment
- Sleep disorders
- Taste disorders
- Vomiting

Rare
- Anaemia
- Antibiotic-associated colitis
- Confusion
- Crystalluria
- Depression
- Hallucinations
- Hyperglycaemia
- Seizures
- Thrombocytopenia
- Tremor

Drug interactions

Pharmacokinetic
- Ciprofloxacin is an inhibitor of CYP1A2.
- Concurrent use of *duloxetine* and *tizanidine* is contraindicated (due to CYP1A2 inhibition).
- *Diazepam*—possible increase in effect.
- *Ropinirole*—significant increase in effect requiring dose adjustment.
- *Sucralfate*—marked reduction in oral absorption of ciprofloxacin; avoid by 2 hours.
- *Theophylline*—plasma concentrations of theophylline can be markedly increased.
- *Warfarin*—possible increase in INR.
- The clinical significance of co-administration with substrates of CYP1A2 (📖 end cover) is unknown. Caution is advised if ciprofloxacin is co-administered with drugs that are predominantly metabolized by CYP1A2. The prescriber should be aware of the potential for interactions and that dosage adjustments may be necessary, particularly for drugs with a narrow therapeutic index.

Pharmacodynamic
- Ciprofloxacin can cause dose-related prolongation of the QT interval. There is a potential risk that co-administration with other drugs that also prolong the QT interval (e.g. *amiodarone*, *erythromycin*, *haloperidol*, *quinine*) may result in ventricular arrhythmias.
- *CNS depressants*—additive sedative effect

Dose
- Dose depends on infection. Refer to local guidelines.
- Typical doses:
  - urinary tract infections, 250–500mg PO BD
  - respiratory tract infections, 250–750mg PO BD
  - by IV infusion, 200–400mg BD

⚕ Dose adjustments

Elderly

- Dose adjustments are not required.

Hepatic/renal impairment

- Dose adjustments are not required in hepatic impairment.
- Dose adjustments are necessary for patients with renal impairment (Table 3.1).

Table 3.1 Dose adjustments for ciprofloxacin

Creatinine clearance (mL/min/1.73m^2)	Serum creatinine (µmol/L)	Oral dose (mg)
>60	<124	Usual dosage
30–60	124–168	250–500mg/12hr
<30	>169	250–500mg/24hr
Patients on haemodialysis	>169	250–500mg/24hr (after dialysis)
Patients on peritoneal dialysis	>169	250–500mg/24hr

Additional information

- The tablets can be dispersed in water immediately prior to administration if necessary.
- The suspension is unsuitable for administration through a feeding tube (may block).
- Once reconstituted, the oral suspension should be used within 14 days.
- A 200mg IV infusion should be administered over 30–60 minutes, 400mg over 60 minutes.
- Each 100mL of IV infusion contains 15.4mmol of sodium.

⚕ Pharmacology

Ciprofloxacin is a broad-spectrum antibiotic active against a wide range of Gram-negative organisms, with a limited range of Gram-positive cover. It is bactericidal and works by inhibiting bacterial DNA gyrase, an enzyme involved with DNA synthesis. Ciprofloxacin is well absorbed following oral administration and has good penetration into tissues and cells.

Citalopram

Cipramil® (POM)
Tablet: 10mg (28); 20mg (28); 40mg (28)
Oral drops (*sugar-free*): 40mg/mL (15mL) (see *Dose*)

Generic (POM)
Tablet: 10mg (28); 20mg (28); 40mg (28)

Indications
• Depression
• Panic

Contraindications and precautions
• Do not use with an irreversible MAOI, or within 14 days of stopping one, or at least 24 hours after discontinuation of a reversible MAOI (e.g. moclobemide, linezolid). At least 7 days should elapse after discontinuing citalopram treatment before starting an MAOI or reversible MAOI. Note that in exceptional circumstances linezolid may be given with citalopram, but the patient must be closely monitored for symptoms of serotonin syndrome (📖 Box 1.10, p.19).
• Depression is associated with an increased risk of suicidal thoughts, self-harm, and suicide which persists until remission. Note that that the risk of suicide may increase during initial treatment.
• Hyponatraemia should be considered in all patients who develop drowsiness, confusion, or convulsions while taking an antidepressant. Hyponatraemia has been associated with all types of antidepressants, although it is reportedly more common with SSRIs.
• May precipitate psychomotor restlessness, which usually appears during early treatment.
• Use with caution in:
  • diabetes (alters glycaemic control)
  • elderly (greater risk of hyponatraemia)
  • epilepsy (lowers seizure threshold)
  • hepatic impairment (see below).
• Avoid abrupt withdrawal, as symptoms such as agitation, anxiety, dizziness, nausea, sleep disturbance (e.g. insomnia, intense dreams), and tremor can occur. Although generally mild, they can be severe in some patients. Withdrawal symptoms usually occur within the first few days of discontinuing treatment and generally resolve within 2 weeks, although they can persist for up to 3 months or longer in some patients (📖 Discontinuing and/or switching antidepressants, p.45 for information about switching or stopping antidepressants).
• Citalopram may increase the risk of haemorrhage (see 📖 *Drug interactions*, p.106–7).
• Citalopram may modify reactions and patients should be advised not to drive (or operate machinery) if affected.

☺ Undesirable effects

Frequent

- Agitation
- Constipation
- Diarrhoea
- Dizziness
- Drowsiness
- Dry mouth
- Headache
- Insomnia
- Nausea
- Nervousness
- Sweating
- Tremor

Less frequent

- Anorexia and weight loss
- Anxiety
- Confusion
- Postural hypotension
- Pruritus
- Rash
- Rhinitis
- Sexual dysfunction
- Sleep disorder
- Suicide
- Visual disturbances

Rare

- Convulsions
- Cough
- Euphoria
- Myalgia
- Psychomotor restlessness
- Tinnitus

Drug interactions

Pharmacokinetic

- Citalopram is a weak inhibitor of CYP2C19 and CYP2D6; it is metabolized by CYP2C19 and CYP3A4. Unexpected effects may be explained by the fact that up to 5% of the Caucasian population are CYP2C19 poor metabolizers.
- The clinical significance of co-administration with inducers or inhibitors of CYP2C19 (Ⅲ end cover) is unknown. The prescriber should be aware of the potential for interactions and that dosage adjustments may be necessary.
- The clinical significance of co-administration with other CYP3A4 inducers or inhibitors (Ⅲ end cover) is unknown. The prescriber should be aware of the potential for interactions and that dosage adjustments may be necessary.
- Avoid excessive amounts of grapefruit juice as it may increase the bioavailability of citalopram through inhibition of intestinal CYP3A4.

Pharmacodynamic
- *Anticoagulants*—potential increased risk of bleeding.
- *Carbamazepine*—increased risk of hyponatraemia.
- *Cyproheptadine*—may inhibit the effects of serotonin reuptake inhibitors.
- *Diuretics*—increased risk of hyponatraemia.
- *MAOIs*—risk of serotonin syndrome (see *Contraindications and precautions*).
- *NSAIDs*—increased risk of GI bleeding.
- *Serotonergic drugs* (e.g. duloxetine, methadone, mirtazapine, tramadol, TCAs, and trazodone)—risk of serotonin syndrome (💷 Box 1.10, p.19).
- *Tramadol*—increased risk of seizures and serotonin syndrome.

Dose
Note: 8mg of Cipramil® oral drops (four drops) can be considered equivalent in therapeutic effect to a 10mg citalopram tablet. The drops should be mixed with water, orange juice, or apple juice before taking.

Depression
- Initial dose:
  - tablets—20mg PO OD. The dose should be reviewed after 2–3 weeks and increased if necessary in 20mg increments to a maximum of 60mg PO OD.
  - oral drops—16mg PO OD (8 drops). The dose should be reviewed after 2–3 weeks and increased if necessary in 16mg increments to a maximum of 48mg PO OD (24 drops).

Pain
- Initial dose
  - tablets—10mg PO OD. The dose can be increased in 10mg increments to the recommended dose of 20–30mg PO OD. Further dose increases in careful increments up to 60mg PO OD may be necessary.
  - oral drops—8mg PO OD (4 drops). The dose can be increased in 8mg increments to the recommended dose of 16–24mg PO OD (8–12 drops). Further dose increases in careful increments up to 48mg PO OD (24 drops) may be necessary.

Dose adjustments
Elderly
- Initial doses unchanged, but the maximum dose should not exceed 40mg PO OD.

Hepatic/renal impairment
- In hepatic impairment, doses should be maintained at the lower end of the range.
- In mild or moderate renal impairment, no dosage adjustment is necessary. Information is unavailable for severe renal impairment (creatinine clearance <20mL/min).

Additional information

Response in depression may be evident within the first week of treatment; generally, an effect is seen in at least the second week of treatment.

- Symptoms of anxiety or panic may worsen on initial therapy. This can be minimized by using lower starting doses.
- If withdrawal symptoms emerge during discontinuation, increase the dose to prevent symptoms and then start withdrawal more slowly.

♦ Pharmacology

Citalopram is a highly selective inhibitor of neuronal serotonin reuptake, with only very minimal effects on noradrenaline and dopamine neuronal reuptake. It has a weak affinity for muscarinic receptors, but little affinity for α_1, α_2, D_2, 5-HT$_1$, 5-HT$_2$, and H$_1$ receptors. Citalopram is metabolized primarily by CYP2C19 and CYP3A4 to active metabolites, but they are unlikely to contribute to the overall antidepressant effect. Citalopram is excreted mainly via the liver, with less than 20% via the kidneys.

Clonazepam

Rivotril® (CD Benz POM)
Tablet (*scored*): 500mcg (100); 2mg (100)
Injection: 1mg/mL with 1mL WFI (10) (see 📖 *Additional information*, p.111)

Unlicensed Special (CD Benz POM)
Liquid: 500mcg/5mL; 2mg/5mL

Note: Independent prescribers are **NOT** authorized to prescribe clonazepam (📖 Independent prescribing: palliative care issues, p.25)

See *Additional information* below for supply issues.

Indications
- Epilepsy
- Myoclonus
- ⃰ Neuropathic pain
- ⃰ Restless legs syndrome
- ⃰ Terminal restlessness
- For end-of-life care issues see 📖 Use of drugs in end-of-life care, p.53.

Contraindications and precautions
- Contraindicated for use in patients with myasthenia gravis or severe hepatic impairment.
- Suicidal ideation and behaviour have been reported with anti-epileptics.
- Clonazepam should be used with caution in patients with chronic respiratory disease, renal impairment, or moderate hepatic impairment.
- Dose reductions may be necessary in the elderly (see 📖 *Dose adjustments*).
- Avoid abrupt withdrawal, even if short duration treatment. In epileptic patients, status epilepticus may be precipitated. In addition, prolonged use of benzodiazepines may result in the development of dependence with subsequent withdrawal symptoms on cessation of use, e.g. agitation, anxiety, confusion, headaches, restlessness, sleep disturbances, sweating, and tremor. The risk of dependence increases with dose and duration of treatment. Gradual withdrawal is advised.
- Clonazepam may modify reactions and patients should be advised not to drive (or operate machinery) if affected.

☹ Undesirable effects
- The frequency is not defined, but commonly reported undesirable effects include:
  - ataxia
  - coordination disturbances
  - dizziness
  - drowsiness
  - fatigue
  - light-headedness
  - muscle weakness.

- Other reported undesirable effects include:
  - anterograde amnesia
  - headache
  - sexual dysfunction.

Drug interactions

Pharmacokinetic

- Clonazepam is metabolized by CYP3A4.
- The clinical significance of co-administration with inducers or inhibitors of CYP3A4 (🕮 end cover) is unknown. The prescriber should be aware of the potential for interactions and that dosage adjustments may be necessary.
- Avoid excessive amounts of grapefruit juice as it may increase the bioavailability of clonazepam through inhibition of intestinal CYP3A4.

Pharmacodynamic

- *Alcohol*—may precipitate seizures.
- *Antidepressants*—reduced seizure threshold.
- *Antipsychotics*—reduced seizure threshold.
- *CNS depressants*—additive sedative effect.

♣ Dose

Epilepsy/myoclonus

- initial dose 1mg PO ON, increased as necessary up to 8mg PO in 2–4 divided doses.
- ¥ Alternatively, 0.5–4mg via CSCI **every 12 hours** (see 🕮 *Additional information*).

¥ Neuropathic pain

- Initial dose 0.5mg PO ON, increased as necessary up to 8mg PO daily in 2–4 divided doses.
- Alternatively, 0.5–4mg via CSCI **every 12 hours** (see 🕮 *Additional information*, p.111).

¥ Restless legs syndrome

- Initial dose 0.5mg PO ON, increased as necessary to 2mg PO ON.

¥ Terminal restlessness

- 1–4mg via CSCI **every 12 hours** (see 🕮 *Additional information*, p.111).

♣ Dose adjustments

Elderly

- No specific dose reductions stated, but initial doses should not exceed 1mg PO daily.

Hepatic/renal impairment

- No specific guidance available. The dosage of clonazepam must be carefully adjusted to individual requirements.

Additional information

- Clonazepam oral suspension is available from Rosemont Pharmaceuticals Ltd as an unlicensed special (Tel: 0113 244 1999).
- Clonazepam tablets disperse in water after a short period of time.
- The 1mg/mL injection of clonazepam must be diluted with the supplied WFI prior to parenteral administration. However, if clonazepam is to be administered via CSCI, this is not necessary.
- Clonazepam may adsorb to PVC. The clinical significance remains unknown but the manufacturer recommends the use of non-PVC equipment for infusions. The manufacturer also states that the stability of diluted clonazepam is maintained for up to 12 hours. Until further information becomes available, it is recommended that CSCIs containing clonazepam should only run for a maximum of 12 hours.
- Clonazepam via CSCI is reportedly compatible with alfentanil, cyclizine, dexamethasone, diamorphine, glycopyrronium, haloperidol, hyoscine butylbromide, hyoscine hydrobromide, levomepromazine, metoclopramide, morphine sulphate, midazolam, octreotide, and oxycodone.

☼ Pharmacology

The exact mechanism of action is unknown, but it is believed to act via enhancement of GABA-ergic transmission in the CNS. It is extensively metabolized by CYP3A4 to inactive metabolites.

Co-danthramer

Co-danthramer (Generic–POM)
Capsule: 25/200, dantron 25mg + poloxamer '188' 200mg (60).
Suspension: 25/200 in 5mL, dantron 25mg, poloxamer '188' 200mg/5mL (300mL; 1000mL).

Co-danthramer strong (Generic–POM)
Capsule: 37.5/500, dantron 37.5mg + poloxamer '188' 500mg (60)
Suspension: 75/1000 in 5mL, dantron 75mg, poloxamer '188' 1g/5mL (300mL).

Note: Co-danthramer suspension, 5mL = 1 × co-danthramer capsule; strong co-danthramer suspension 5mL = 2 × strong co-danthramer capsules.

Indications
• Treatment of constipation in terminally ill patients.

Contraindications and precautions
• Contraindicated in intestinal obstruction.
• Avoid in patients with abdominal pain of unknown origin.
• Use with caution in incontinent patients (both urinary and faecally) because of the risk of superficial sloughing of the skin.

☺ Undesirable effects
• Co-danthramer may cause a temporary and harmless pink or red colouring of the urine and perianal skin.
• Prolonged contact with the skin can lead to superficial sloughing of the skin (co-danthramer 'burn'). This should be prevented by application of a barrier cream in susceptible patients.

Drug interactions

Pharmacokinetic
• No known pharmacokinetic interactions.

Pharmacodynamic
• *Anticholinergics*—antagonizes the laxative effect.
• *Cyclizine*—antagonizes the laxative effect.
• *Opioids*—antagonizes the laxative effect.
• *5-HT$_3$ antagonists*—antagonizes the laxative effect.
• *Tricyclic antidepressants*—antagonizes the laxative effect.

∴ Dose

Table 3.2 Co-danthramer dosage

	Co-danthramer capsules	Co-danthramer suspension	Co-danthramer strong capsules	Co-danthramer strong suspension
Initial dose	1–2 PO ON	5–10mL PO ON	1–2 PO ON	5mL PO ON
Dose adjustment *(following doses are higher than licensed)*	¥ Increase as necessary to max 2 PO BD. Consider changing to co-danthramer strong if no response	¥ Increase as necessary to max 10mL PO BD. Consider changing to co-danthramer strong if no response	¥ Increase as necessary to max 3 PO BD. Review treatment if no response.	¥ Increase as necessary to max 10mL PO BD. Review treatment if no response.

∴ Dose adjustments

Elderly
● No specific dose adjustments recommended by the manufacturer.

Hepatic/renal impairment
● No specific dose adjustments recommended by the manufacturer.

Additional information

● Warn patients that urine may be coloured red/orange.

⊕ Pharmacology

Co-danthramer consists of dantron poloxamer 188. Dantron is an anthraquinone derivative chemically related to the active principle of cascara and senna. It is believed to stimulate muscles of the large intestine through action on the myenteric plexus. Griping should not occur as the small intestine is not affected. Poloxamer 188 is a surfactant that improves the penetration of water into faecal material and also has a lubricant effect.

Codeine

Generic (CD Inv POM)
Tablet: 15mg (28); 30mg (28); 60mg (28)
Syrup: 25mg/5mL (100mL)
Linctus: 15mg/5mL (100mL)
Note: Sugar-free linctus is available
Injection: 60mg/mL (10) (*CD POM*)

Combination products
Certain products containing <15mg codeine and paracetamol are available OTC.

Co-codamol 8/500 (CD Inv P)
Tablet: codeine phosphate 8mg, paracetamol 500mg (30).
Capsule: codeine phosphate 8mg, paracetamol 500mg (10; 20).
Effervescent or dispersible tablet: codeine phosphate 8mg, paracetamol 500mg (100).

Co-codamol 15/500 (CD Inv POM)
Caplet: codeine phosphate 15mg, paracetamol 500mg (100) (Codipar®).

Co-codamol 30/500 (CD Inv POM)
Tablet: codeine phosphate 30mg, paracetamol 500mg (100) (Kapake®).
Caplet: codeine phosphate 30mg, paracetamol 500mg (100) (Solpadol®).
Capsule: codeine phosphate 30mg, paracetamol 500mg (100) (Kapake®, Solpadol®, Tylex®).
Effervescent or dispersible tablet: codeine phosphate 30mg, paracetamol 500mg (32; 100) (Kapake®, Solpadol®, Tylex®).

Co-codaprin 8/400 (CD Inv POM)
Dispersible tablet: codeine phosphate 8mg, aspirin 400mg (100).

Note: Independent prescribers are **NOT** authorized to prescribe parenteral codeine (📖 Independent prescribing: palliative care issues, p.25).

Indications
- Management of mild to moderate pain
- Treatment of diarrhoea
- Cough (linctus)

Contraindications and precautions
- Use codeine with caution in the following instances:
  - acute alcoholism
  - arrhythmias
  - asthma (can release histamine)
  - bowel obstruction
  - concurrent use with CYP2D6 inhibitors (see 📖 Drug interactions, p.116)
  - diseases of the biliary tract (e.g. gallstones)
  - elderly

- head injury
- hepatic impairment
- obstructive airways disease
- pancreatitis
- paralytic ileus
- raised intracranial pressure
- renal impairment
- prostatic hypertrophy
- respiratory depression.

- Effervescent formulations contain up to 16.9mmol Na^+/L (check individual product). Avoid in renal impairment and use with caution in patients with hypertension or congestive heart failure.
- Codeine may modify reactions and patients should be advised not to drive (or operate machinery) if affected.

- Ultra-rapid metabolizers convert codeine into its active metabolite, morphine more rapidly and completely than other people, which can result in higher than expected plasma morphine concentrations. Even at usual doses, ultra-rapid metabolizers may experience symptoms of overdose, such as extreme sleepiness, confusion, or shallow breathing.
- Poor metabolizers or those taking concurrent CYP2D6 inhibitors (see 📖 *Drug interactions*, p.116) may derive little or no analgesic benefit from codeine. Titration of an alternative opioid is recommended, rather than substitution to an equianalgesic dose.

☺ Undesirable effects

- The frequency is not defined, but commonly reported undesirable effects include:
  - constipation
  - drowsiness
  - headache
  - nausea and/or vomiting
  - pruritus
  - rash
- Less commonly reported undesirable effects include:

  - abdominal pain
  - biliary spasm
  - confusion
  - decreased libido
  - dizziness
  - dry mouth
  - flushing
  - hallucinations

  - hypotension
  - paraesthesia
  - paralytic ileus
  - respiratory depression
  - sweating
  - ureteric spasm
  - urinary retention
  - visual disturbance

Drug interactions

Pharmacokinetic

- Codeine is a prodrug and is metabolized by CYP2D6 to morphine. A minor pathway involves CYP3A4.
- Co-administration with CYP2D6 inhibitors may alter the analgesic effect of codeine.
- The efficacy of codeine may be altered by other CYP2D6 inhibitors, such as duloxetine, fluoxetine, haloperidol, levomepromazine and paroxetine. The clinical implications of co-administration with these drugs are unknown; the prescriber should be aware of the potential for altered response.
- It is possible that co-administration of CYP3A4 inducers (📖 end cover) may increase analgesic response and/or risk of undesirable effects due to the increase in formation of an active metabolite.

Pharmacodynamic

- *Antihypertensives*—increased risk of hypotension.
- *CNS depressants*—risk of excessive sedation.
- *Haloperidol*—may be an additive hypotensive effect.
- *Ketamine*—there is a potential opioid-sparing effect with ketamine and the dose of codeine may need reducing.
- *Levomepromazine*—may be an additive hypotensive effect.

⚕ Dose

Pain

- 30–60mg PO or IM every 4 hours when necessary for pain to a maximum of 240mg daily
- ＊ Alternatively, codeine can be given either 30–60mg SC every 4 hours when necessary, or via CSCI over 24 hours
- Combination products—co-codamol 8/500, 15/500 and 30/500: 1–2 tablets PO every 4 hours (maximum 8 daily because of paracetamol).

Diarrhoea

- 30mg PO TDS–QDS. Higher doses have been used (e.g. 30–60mg every 4 hours).

Cough

- 5–10mL (of linctus) PO TDS-QDS.

⚕ Dose adjustments

Elderly

- No specific guidance is available, although lower starting doses may be preferable. Dose requirements should be individually titrated.

Hepatic/renal impairment

- No specific guidance is available, although in patients with hepatic impairment, the plasma concentration is expected to be increased. In view of its hepatic metabolism, caution is advised when giving dihydrocodeine to patients with hepatic impairment. Lower starting doses may be preferable and dose requirements should be individually titrated.

- No specific guidance is available for patients with renal impairment. However, in view of the fact that metabolites are renally excreted, lower starting doses may be preferable and dose requirements should be individually titrated.

Additional information

- Poor CYP2D6 metabolizers (up to 10% of the Caucasian population) cannot produce the active metabolite of codeine—morphine. Drug interactions can affect the metabolism of codeine via inhibition of CYP2D6. The clinical consequences of genotype and drug interaction are unknown Genetic variations lead to the possibility of a modified undesirable effect profile and varied analgesic response with tramadol.
- Codeine is included in a number OTC preparations for coughs, colds, and pain, so drug histories must include remedies that patients may have self-selected.

❧ Pharmacology

Codeine is a naturally occurring weak opioid agonist derived from opium. By mouth, it has similar potency to dihydrocodeine; parenterally it is considered to be half as potent as dihydrocodeine. Normally regarded as being about one-tenth as potent as morphine, it is demethylated to morphine in the liver by CYP2D6. A percentage of the Caucasian population (5–10%) are poor metabolizers of CYP2D6, so codeine will be less effective or even ineffective in this group. Co-administration of CYP2D6 inhibitors produces similar effects. A minor pathway involving CYP3A4 usually produces an active metabolite in very small amounts. However, this pathway becomes important in poor metabolizers and with CYP2D6 inhibition or CYP3A4 induction. The metabolites are renally excreted.

Cyclizine

Valoid®
Tablet (*scored*) (*P*): 50mg (100)
Injection (*POM*): 50mg/mL (5)

Unlicensed (POM)
Suppositories: 12.5mg; 25mg; 50mg; 100mg
Available on a named-patient basis as manufactured special

Indications
- Prevention and treatment of nausea and vomiting
- For end-of-life care issues see 📖 Use of drugs in end-of-life care, p.53.

Contraindications and precautions
- Avoid in patients with porphyria
- Cyclizine should be used with caution in patients with:
  - glaucoma
  - severe congestive heart failure
  - prostatic hypertrophy.
- The anticholinergic effect can be additive with other drugs and may precipitate delirium or cognitive impairment in susceptible patients, especially the elderly.
- Cyclizine may modify reactions and patients should be advised not to drive (or operate machinery) if affected.

☻ Undesirable effects
The frequency is not defined, but reported undesirable effects include:
- Blurred vision
- Confusion
- Constipation
- Delirium
- Drowsiness
- Dry mouth
- Extrapyramidal motor disturbances (rare)
- Hallucinations (especially with higher doses)
- Headache
- Hypersensitivity reactions (rare)
- Nervousness
- Restlessness
- Tachycardia
- Urinary retention

Drug interactions
Pharmacokinetic
- No recognized pharmacokinetic interactions.

Pharmacodynamic
- *Anticholinergics*—increased risk of undesirable effects.
- *CNS depressants*—increased risk of CNS undesirable effects.
- *Domperidone*—may inhibit prokinetic effect.

- *Metoclopramide*—may inhibit prokinetic effect.
- *Nefopam*—increased risk of anticholinergic undesirable effects.
- *TCAs*—increased risk of anticholinergic undesirable effects.

⚕ Dose
- Initial dose 50–100mg PO or SC¥ BD–TDS PRN. Alternatively, 100–150mg via CSCI over 24 hours.
- Maximum daily dose 200mg¥ PO or SC.

⚕ Dose adjustments
Elderly
- The manufacturer indicates that the normal adult dosage is appropriate. Note that the elderly may be more susceptible to the central and anticholinergic effects of cyclizine (which may be additive with concomitant drugs); there may be an increased risk for cognitive decline and dementia.

Hepatic/renal impairment
- No specific guidance available. Dose requirements should be individually titrated.
- In hepatic impairment, empirical dose adjustments may be necessary since cyclizine is undergoes hepatic clearance.
- The manufacturer states that dose reductions may be necessary in renal impairment.

Additional information
- The anti-emetic effect should occur within 2 hours of oral administration and lasts approximately 4 hours. Parenteral administration would be expected to produce a much quicker response.
- Cyclizine should be avoided in severe congestive heart failure because it can cause a reduction in cardiac output associated with increases in heart rate, mean arterial pressure and pulmonary wedge pressure.
- Cyclizine injection must be diluted with WFI. It is incompatible with NaCl 0.9% and in solutions with pH ≥6.8.
- Cyclizine and diamorphine mixtures are chemically and physically stable in WFI up to concentrations of 20mg/mL over 24 hours. If the diamorphine concentration exceeds 2mg/mL, crystallization may occur unless the concentration of cyclizine is ≤10mg/mL. Similarly, if the concentration of cyclizine exceeds 20mg/mL, crystallization may occur unless the concentration of diamorphine is ≤15mg/mL.
- There are concentration-dependent compatibility issues with alfentanil, dexamethasone, glycopyrronium, hyoscine butylbromide, metoclopramide, and oxycodone, although the specific details are unknown.
- Cyclizine via CSCI is compatible with clonazepam, diamorphine (see above), dihydrocodeine, haloperidol, hyoscine hydrobromide, levomepromazine, midazolam, morphine, octreotide, and ondansetron.

⊙ Pharmacology

Cyclizine is a histamine H_1 receptor antagonist and has a low incidence of drowsiness. It also possesses anticholinergic activity. The exact mechanism by which cyclizine can prevent or suppress nausea and vomiting from various causes is unknown, but it may have an inhibitory action within part of the midbrain referred to as the vomiting centre. Cyclizine also increases lower oesophageal sphincter tone and reduces the sensitivity of the labyrinthine apparatus. It is metabolized in the liver to a relatively inactive metabolite.

Cyproheptadine

Periactin® (POM)
Tablet (scored): 4mg (30)

Indications
- Symptomatic relief of allergy (e.g. hayfever, allergy)
- Vascular headache and migraine
- * Symptomatic relief of serotonin syndrome
- * Appetite stimulant (other treatments preferred)
- * Management of diarrhoea associated with carcinoid syndrome (octreotide generally preferred)

Contraindications and precautions
- Contraindicated for use in patients with:
  - glaucoma
  - pyloroduodenal obstruction
  - stenosing peptic ulcer
  - symptomatic prostatic hypertrophy
  - predisposition to urinary retention or bladder neck obstruction.
- Use cautiously in patients with:
  - bronchial asthma
  - increased intraocular pressure
  - hyperthyroidism
  - cardiovascular disease
  - hypertension.
- Avoid concurrent use with MAOIs (see 📖 *Drug interactions*, p.121)
- Cyproheptadine may modify reactions and patients should be advised not to drive (or operate machinery) if affected.

☻ Undesirable effects
The frequency is not defined, but commonly reported undesirable effects include:
- Abdominal pain
- Appetite stimulation
- Diarrhoea
- Dizziness
- Drowsiness (should improve within 1 week of treatment)
- Dry mouth
- Thickening of bronchial secretions
- Fatigue
- Headache
- Nausea
- Nervousness
- Weight gain

Drug interactions
Pharmacokinetic
- Mechanism of hepatic metabolism unspecified.
- No known pharmacokinetic interactions.

Pharmacodynamic
- *SSRIs*—antidepressant effect may be reduced by cyproheptadine
- *CNS depressants*—risk of excessive sedation
- *MAOIs*—may cause hallucinations

Dose

Symptomatic relief of allergy
- Initial dose 4mg PO TDS. Dose can be increased to a maximum of 32mg PO daily.

Vascular headache and migraine
- Initial dose 4mg PO, repeated if necessary after 30 minutes. Patients who respond usually obtain relief with 8mg, and this dose should not be exceeded within a 4–6 hour period.
- Usual maintenance dose is 4mg PO every 4–6 hours.

¥ Symptomatic relief of serotonin syndrome
- Initial dose 4–8mg PO. Can be repeated in 2 hours. If no response is seen after 16mg, it should be discontinued. If there is a response then it may be continued in divided doses up to 32mg/day (e.g. up to 8mg four times daily).

Dose adjustments

Elderly
- Elderly patients are more likely to experience undesirable effects such as dizziness, sedation, and hypotension. The UK manufacturer contraindicates the use of cyproheptadine in elderly patients. However, for the treatment of serotonin syndrome, the lowest effective dose should be used.

Hepatic/renal impairment
- No specific guidance available. Dose requirements should be individually titrated.

Additional information

Tablets can be crushed and dispersed in water prior to administration if necessary.

Pharmacology

Cyproheptadine is a piperidine antihistamine with weak anticholinergic properties. In addition, it also antagonizes serotonin receptors. This latter effect makes cyproheptadine particularly useful in the symptomatic treatment of serotonin syndrome. The drug is extensively metabolized, with the metabolites being excreted renally. The exact mechanism of metabolism is unknown, but may involve the cytochrome P450 system.

Cyproterone

Cyp..ostat® (POM)
Tablet (*scored*): 50mg (168); 100mg (84)

Generic (POM)
Tablet: 50mg (56); 100mg (84)

Indications
- Prostate cancer:
  - to suppress 'flare' with initial gonadorelin therapy
  - long-term palliative treatment where gonadorelin analogues or orchidectomy are contraindicated or not tolerated, or where oral therapy preferred
  - treatment of hot flushes in patients receiving gonadorelin therapy or after orchidectomy.

Contraindications and precautions

- Hepatic toxicity has been reported in patients treated with cyproterone acetate 200–300mg PO daily, usually after several months. LFTs should be performed before and regularly during treatment. If symptoms of hepatotoxicity occur and are believed to be caused by cyproterone, it should normally be withdrawn.

- Use with caution in the following:
  - depression (condition may deteriorate)
  - hepatic impairment (see above)
  - history of thromboembolic disease (may recur with cyproterone)
  - diabetes (cyproterone can affect carbohydrate metabolism; also increased risk of thromboembolic events)
  - sickle cell anaemia.
- Regular blood counts (as well as LFTs) should be performed because of the risk of anaemia.
- Cyproterone may modify reactions and patients should be advised not to drive (or operate machinery) if affected.

☺ Undesirable effects
The frequency is not defined, but reported undesirable effects include:
- Depression
- Dry skin
- Dyspnoea
- Fatigue
- Galactorrhoea
- Gynaecomastia
- Hepatotoxicity (jaundice/ hepatitis)
- Hypochromic anaemia (long-term treatment)
- Osteoporosis
- Restlessness
- Sexual dysfunction (loss or reduction of sexual drive and potency)
- Thromboembolic events
- Weight gain (long-term treatment)

Drug interactions

Pharmacokinetic

- Cyproterone is metabolized by CYP3A4; at high doses it may inhibit CYP2C8, CYP2C9, CYP2C19, CYP2D6, and CYP3A4.
- The clinical significance of co-administration with CYP3A4 inhibitors or inducers (📖 end cover) is unknown. The prescriber should be aware of the potential for interactions and that dosage adjustments may be necessary.
- The clinical significance of co-administration with substrates of CYP2C8, CYP2C9, CYP2C19, CYP2D6, and CYP3A4 (📖 end cover) is unknown. The prescriber should be aware of the potential for interactions and that dosage adjustments may be necessary.

Pharmacodynamic

- None known

⚗ Dose

Suppression of 'flare'

- 300mg PO in 2–3 divided doses after meals for several days before and several weeks after gonadorelin therapy. The dose may be reduced to 200mg PO in 2–3 divided doses if the higher dose is not tolerated.

Long-term palliative treatment

- 200–300mg PO daily in 2–3 divided doses after meals.

Hot flushes

- Initial dose 50mg PO OD, increasing if necessary to 50mg PO BD–TDS.

⚗ Dose adjustments

Elderly

- Usual adult doses recommended.

Hepatic/renal impairment

- No specific guidance is available for use in hepatic impairment. The manufacturer advises caution.
- No specific guidance is available for use in renal impairment, although accumulation is unlikely given the hepatic clearance of the drug.

Additional information

- Although tablets may be crushed and dispersed in water prior to administration, this is not recommended because of the risk of exposure.

⟩ Pharmacology

Cyproterone is an anti-androgen that antagonizes the actions of testo-sterone and its metabolite, dihydrotestosterone. It also has progestogenic activity, which exerts a negative feedback effect on the hypothalamus, causing a reduction in gonadotrophin release and subsequent diminished production of testicular androgens. It is completely absorbed orally and undergoes extensive metabolism by various pathways. The main metabolite has similar anti-androgen properties but little progestogenic activity.

Dalteparin

Fragmin® (POM)

Injection (single-dose syringe for SC use): dalteparin sodium 12,500 units/mL, 2500 units (0.2mL syringe); 25,000 units/mL, 5000 units (0.2mL syringe); 7500 units (0.3mL syringe); 10,000 units (0.4mL syringe); 12,500 units (0.5mL syringe); 15,000 units (0.6mL syringe); 18,000 units (0.72mL syringe).

Injection (for SC or IV use): dalteparin sodium 2500 units/mL, 10,000 units (4mL ampoule); 10,000 units/mL, 10,000 units (1mL ampoule)

Injection (for SC use): 25,000 units/mL, 100,000 units (4mL multi-dose vial).

Injection (graduated syringe for SC use): dalteparin sodium 10,000 units/mL, 10,000 units (1mL syringe).

Indications
- Treatment and prophylaxis of deep vein thrombosis (DVT) and pulmonary embolism (PE)
- Prophylaxis of DVT
- Other indications apply but are not normally relevant in palliative care

Contraindications and precautions
- Dalteparin is contraindicated for use in:
  - acute gastroduodenal ulcer
  - cerebral haemorrhage
  - known haemorrhagic diathesis
  - subacute endocarditis.
- Use with caution in patients with an increased risk of bleeding complications:
  - brain tumours (increased risk of intracranial bleeding)
  - concurrent use of anticoagulant/antiplatelet agents/NSAIDs (see 📖 *Drug interactions*, p.126)
  - haemorrhagic stroke
  - retinopathy (hypertensive or diabetic)
  - surgery
  - severe hepatic impairment
  - severe renal impairment
  - trauma
  - thrombocytopenia
  - uncontrolled hypertension.
- A baseline platelet count should be taken prior to initiating treatment and monitored closely during the first 3 weeks (e.g. every 2–4 days) and regularly thereafter.
- Not for IM use.
- Advice should be sought from anaesthetist colleagues if considering an epidural intervention in a patient receiving dalteparin because of the risk of spinal haematoma.
- LMWH can inhibit aldosterone secretion, which can cause hyperkalaemia. Patients with pre-existing renal impairment are more at risk. Potassium should be measured in patients at risk prior to starting

a LMWH and monitored regularly thereafter, especially if treatment is prolonged beyond 7 days
- *Prophylactic doses of dalteparin are not sufficient to prevent valve thrombosis in patients with prosthetic heart valves.*

☹ Undesirable effects

Common
- Bleeding (at any site)
- Haematoma at injection site
- Transient changes to liver transaminase levels—clinical significance unknown
- Thrombocytopenia

Uncommon
- Hyperkalaemia
- Osteoporosis with long-term treatment
- Pruritus
- Urticaria

Rare
- Skin necrosis

Unknown
- Hypoaldosteronism
- Intracranial bleeds
- Prosthetic cardiac valve thrombosis (see *Contraindications and precautions*)
- Spinal or epidural haematoma

Drug interactions

Pharmacokinetic
- None recognized

Pharmacodynamic
- Drugs with anticoagulant or anti-platelet effect may enhance the effect of dalteparin:
  - aspirin
  - clopidogrel
  - dipyridamole
  - NSAIDs.
- *ACEIs*—increased risk of hyperkalaemia
- *Amiloride*—increased risk of hyperkalaemia
- *Antihistamines*—possibly reduce anticoagulant effect
- *Ascorbic acid*—possibly reduces anticoagulant effect
- *Corticosteroids*—increased risk of GI bleeding
- *Spironolactone*—increased risk of hyperkalaemia
- *SSRIs*—increased risk of bleeding

Dose

Treatment of DVT and PE

- The dose is weight dependent and is administered once daily subcutaneously (Table 3.3)
- Alternatively, a dose of 200 units/kg (max 18,000 units) can be given
- Patients at a high risk of bleeding should have the daily dose divided and administered twice daily

Table 3.3 Dalteparin dosage for treatment of DVT and PE

Weight (kg)	Dose (units)
<46	7500
46–56	10,000
57–68	12,500
69–82	15,000
≥83	18,000

- Patients usually start oral anticoagulation at the same time and continue both until the INR is within the target range. This generally takes 5 days. However, cancer patients unsuitable for oral anticoagulation may require long-term treatment with LMWH. Treatment is occasionally continued indefinitely.

Prophylaxis of DVT

- For medical prophylaxis (including immobile cancer patients) 5000 units SC OD, usually for no more than 14 days. Graduated compression stockings should be considered if LMWH is contraindicated.
- For surgical prophylaxis:
  - moderate risk—2500 units before procedure and each day for 5–7 days or longer (until mobilized)
  - high risk—2500 units before procedure and 8–12hours later, then 5000 units SC OD for 5–7 days or longer (until mobilized).

Dose adjustments

Elderly

- Usual adult doses recommended.

Hepatic/renal impairment

- No specific guidance is available for patients with hepatic impairment. The manufacturer advices caution because of an increased risk of bleeding.
- In the case of significant renal impairment, defined as CrCl <30mL/min, the dose of dalteparin should be adjusted based on anti-Factor Xa activity. If the anti-Factor Xa level is below or above the desired range, the dose of dalteparin should be increased or reduced, respectively, and the anti-Factor Xa measurement should be repeated after 3–4 new doses. This dose adjustment should be repeated until the desired anti-Factor Xa level is achieved.

Additional information

- The risk of heparin-induced thrombocytopenia is low with LMWH but may occur after 5–10 days. If there is a 50% reduction in the platelet count, LMWH should be stopped.

⊹ Pharmacology

Dalteparin is a low molecular weight heparin produced from porcine-derived sodium heparin. It acts mainly through its potentiation of the inhibition of Factor Xa and thrombin by antithrombin. Dalteparin is eliminated primarily via the kidneys, hence the need for dose adjustments in renal impairment. Local protocols may help to indicate when treatment of palliative care patients with dalteparin is appropriate.

Demeclocycline

Ledermycin® (POM)
Capsule: 150mg (28)

Indications
- Treatment of chronic syndrome of inappropriate secretion of anti-diuretic hormone (SIADH)

Contraindications and precautions
- Use with caution in patients with liver or renal impairment, or in patients with concurrent use of potentially hepatotoxic or nephrotoxic drugs.
- May cause photosensitive skin reactions. Warn the patient to avoid direct exposure to sunlight or sunlamps and to discontinue at the first sign of skin discomfort.

☺ Undesirable effects
The frequency is not defined, but reported undesirable effects include:
- Diarrhoea
- Dizziness
- Headache
- Nausea
- Oesophagitis
- Photosensitivity (avoid direct exposure to sunlight or artificial ultra-violet light)
- Renal impairment
- Visual disturbances
- Vomiting

Drug interactions
Pharmacokinetic
- *Antacids*—absorption of demeclocycline is impaired by the concomitant administration of preparations containing calcium, magnesium, aluminium, or sodium bicarbonate.

Pharmacodynamic
- *NSAIDs*—increased risk of nephrotoxicity.
- *Warfarin*—plasma prothrombin activity may be depressed, so lower warfarin doses may be needed.

⚬ Dose
Demeclocycline capsules should be swallowed whole with plenty of fluid while sitting or standing. Doses should be taken 1 hour before or 2 hours after meals as absorption is impaired by milk and food.
- Initial dose 900–1200mg daily in 3–4 divided doses.
- If poorly tolerated, a lower initial dose may be used (e.g. 150mg BD–TDS), but time to effect may be delayed.
- Usual maintenance dose is 600–900mg daily in 3–4 divided doses.

⚚ Dose adjustments

Elderly
- No specific guidance is available. Use the lowest effective dose.

Hepatic/renal impairment
- No specific guidance is available, although the manufacturer recommends that patients with liver disease should not receive more than 1g daily and lower doses are indicated in cases of renal impairment to avoid excessive systemic accumulation.
- In both cases, regular blood tests (LFTs, U&Es) are advisable with prolonged therapy.

Additional information
- The effect in SIADH should be apparent within 3–5 days.
- The capsule should not be opened for oral administration because of the risk of developing oesophagitis or oesophageal ulceration.

✧ Pharmacology
Demeclocycline is a tetracycline antibiotic. The use in SIADH actually relies on the undesirable effect of nephrogenic diabetes insipidus through inhibition of antidiuretic hormone (ADH) on renal tubules. It undergoes minor hepatic metabolism; the majority of a dose is excreted renally as unchanged drug.

Dexamethasone

Generic (POM)
Tablet: 0.5mg (28); 2mg (100)
Oral solution (*sugar-free*): 2mg/5mL (150mL)
Injection: 8mg/2mL (10); 4mg/mL (10)

Indications
- Cerebral oedema
- ¥ Appetite stimulation
- ¥ Bowel obstruction
- ¥ Dyspnoea
- ¥ Nausea and vomiting
- ¥ Pain (e.g. bone pain, nerve compression)
- ¥ Spinal cord compression
- ¥ Superior vena caval obstruction
- For end-of-life care issues see 📖 *Use of drugs in end-of-life care*, p.53.

Contraindications and precautions
- In general, contraindications are relative in conditions where the use of dexamethasone may be life saving.
- The use of dexamethasone is contraindicated in systemic infection unless specific anti-infective therapy is employed.
- Patients without a definite history of chickenpox should be advised to avoid close personal contact with chickenpox or herpes zoster.
- Caution is advised when considering the use of systemic corticosteroids in patients with the following conditions:
  - concurrent use of NSAIDs (see 📖 *Drug interactions*, p.133–4)
  - congestive heart failure
  - diabetes mellitus (risk of hyperglycaemia—close monitoring of blood glucose recommended)
  - epilepsy (see 📖 *Drug interactions*, p.133–4)
  - glaucoma
  - hypertension
  - hypokalaemia (correct before starting dexamethasone)
  - liver or renal impairment (see 📖 *Dose adjustments*, p.135)
  - osteoporosis
  - peptic ulceration
  - psychotic illness (symptoms can emerge within a few days or weeks of starting the treatment).

Dexamethasone withdrawal

In patients who have received more than physiological doses of systemic corticosteroids (i.e. >1mg dexamethasone) for >3 weeks, withdrawal should be gradual in order to avoid acute adrenal insufficiency. Abrupt withdrawal of doses of up to 6mg daily of dexamethasone for 3 weeks is unlikely to lead to clinically relevant hypothalamopituitary axis suppression in the majority of patients. In the following cases, withdrawal may need to be more gradual.

- Patients who have had repeated courses of systemic corticosteroids, particularly if taken for >3 weeks.
- Patients receiving doses of systemic corticosteroid >6mg dexamethasone daily.
- Patients repeatedly taking doses in the evening.

There is no evidence as to the best way to withdraw corticosteroids and it is often performed with close monitoring of the patient's condition. The dose may initially be reduced rapidly (e.g. by halving the dose daily) to physiological doses (approximately 1mg dexamethasone) and then more slowly (e.g. 500mcg per week for 1–2 weeks).

A 'withdrawal syndrome' may also occur including fever, myalgia, arthralgia, rhinitis, conjunctivitis, painful itchy skin nodules, and loss of weight.

In dying patients, once the decision is made to withdraw corticosteroids, they can be discontinued abruptly. Patients with brain tumours may require additional analgesia as raised intracranial pressure can develop and may manifest as worsening headache or terminal restlessness.

☻ Undesirable effects

The frequency is not defined. Undesirable effects are generally predictable and related to dosage, timing of administration, and the duration of treatment. They include the following.

- Endocrine:
  - diabetes mellitus
  - hirsutism
  - hyperlipidaemia
  - weight gain.
- Fluid and electrolyte disturbances:
  - congestive heart failure
  - hypertension
  - hypokalaemia.
  - sodium and water retention.
- Gastrointestinal:
  - acute pancreatitis
  - dyspepsia peptic ulceration with perforation
  - haemorrhage.

- Musculoskeletal:
  - aseptic necrosis of femoral head
  - avascular necrosis
  - loss of muscle mass
  - osteoporosis
  - proximal myopathy
  - tendon rupture.
- Neurological:
  - aggravation of epilepsy
  - anxiety
  - confusion
  - depression
  - insomnia
  - mood elevation
  - psychotic reactions.
- Other:
  - glaucoma
  - impaired wound healing
  - increased susceptibility and severity of infections (signs can be masked)
  - sweating.

Corticosteroid-induced osteoporosis

- Patients aged over 65 years and with prior or current exposure to oral corticosteroids are at increased risk of osteoporosis and bone fracture. Treatment with corticosteroids for periods as short as 3 months may result in increased risk. Three or more courses of corticosteroids taken in the previous 12 months are considered to be equivalent to at least 3 months of continuous treatment.
- Prophylactic treatment (e.g. bisphosphonate, calcium and vitamin D supplements, hormone replacement therapy) should be considered for all patients who may take an oral corticosteroid for 3 months or longer.

Drug interactions

Pharmacokinetic

- Dexamethasone is metabolized by CYP3A4. It is also a moderate inducer of CYP3A4.
- Note that low activity of CYP3A4 (e.g. through inhibition) can contribute to the development of osteonecrosis of the femoral head.
- *Carbamazepine*—effect of dexamethasone likely to be reduced; consider doubling the dexamethasone dose and monitor the response.
- *Colestyramine*—may decrease the absorption of dexamethasone.
- *Erythromycin*—may increase the effects of dexamethasone through inhibition of CYP3A4.
- *Phenytoin*—effect of dexamethasone likely to be reduced; consider doubling the dexamethasone dose and monitor the response.
- The clinical significance of co-administration with other inducers or inhibitors of CYP3A4 (📕 end cover) is unknown. The prescriber

should be aware of the potential for interactions and that dosage adjustments may be necessary.

- The clinical significance of co-administration with substrates of CYP3A4 (📖 end cover) is unknown. Caution is advised if dexamethasone is co-administered with drugs that are predominantly metabolized by CYP3A4. The prescriber should be aware of the potential for interactions and that dosage adjustments may be necessary, particularly for drugs with a narrow therapeutic index.
- Avoid excessive amounts of grapefruit juice as it may increase the bio-availability of dexamethasone through inhibition of intestinal CYP3A4.

Pharmacodynamic

- *Anticoagulants*—increased risk of bleeding.
- *Anti-hypertensives*—effect antagonized by dexamethasone.
- *Ciclosporin*—additive immunosuppressive effect; convulsions reported with combination.
- *Diuretics*—effect antagonized by dexamethasone; increased risk of hypokalaemia and hyperglycaemia.
- *Hypoglycaemic drugs*—effect antagonized by dexamethasone.
- *NSAIDs*—increased risk of GI toxicity.
- *SSRIs*—increased risk of bleeding.
- *Thalidomide* –toxic epidermal necrolysis reported with concurrent use.

⚙ Dose

Cerebral oedema

- Initial dose 8–16mg IV, followed by 4mg IV every 6 hours. Review after 2–4 days and consider stopping over 5–7 days.
- ¥ Alternatively, 8–16mg via CSCI over 24 hours or 8–16mg PO OM (or 8mg PO BD, last dose 2p.m.).

¥ Appetite

- Initial dose 2–6mg PO OM. Dose reduction should be guided by symptom response.

¥ Bowel obstruction, spinal cord compression, superior vena caval obstruction

- Initial dose 8–16mg via CSCI over 24 hours or 8–16mg PO OM (or 8mg PO BD, last dose 2p.m.). Review after 2–4 days. Dose reduction should be guided by symptom response.

¥ Dyspnoea, pain

- Initial dose 4–8mg PO OM. Dose reduction should be guided by symptom response.

¥ Nausea and vomiting

- Initial dose 4–16mg PO OM. Alternatively, 4–16mg via CSCI over 24 hours. Dose reduction should be guided by symptom response.

⚖ Dose adjustments

Elderly

- No specific dose adjustments are necessary. Use the lowest dose for the shortest duration possible since the elderly are more susceptible to undesirable effects.

Hepatic/renal impairment

- No specific guidance available. The lowest effective dose should be used for the shortest possible duration.

Additional information

- Consider oral hygiene with dexamethasone use. The patient may develop oral thrush and may need a course of nystatin.
- Oral anti-inflammatory corticosteroid equivalences are:
  - dexamethasone 750mcg = hydrocortisone 20mg = prednisolone 5mg
- Dexamethasone should be administered alone via CSCI unless specific compatibility data are available.
- Low-dose dexamethasone (0.5–1mg) is occasionally added to CSCIs in some centres to reduce site reactions. Unless specific compatibility is available, this practice cannot be recommended.

⟴ Pharmacology

Dexamethasone is a highly potent and long-acting glucocorticoid with negligible mineralocorticoid effects. Like other glucocorticoids, dexamethasone also has anti-allergic, antipyretic, and immunosuppressive properties. It is metabolized mainly in the liver, with some metabolism occurring in the kidney. Dexamethasone and its metabolites are excreted in the urine.

Diamorphine

Generic (CD POM)
Injection: 5mg (5), 10mg (5), 30mg (5), 100mg (5), 500mg (5)
Tablet: 10mg (rarely used)

Diamorphine is a Schedule 2 controlled drug (see Legal categories for medicine, p.23 for further information). Oral and parenteral products **can** be prescribed by nurse independent prescribers (Independent prescribing: palliative care issues, p.25).

Indications
- Relief of severe pain
- ✗ Painful skin lesions (topical)
- ✗ Mucositis (topical)
- ✗ Dyspnoea
- For end-of-life care issues see Use of drugs in end-of-life care, p.53.

Contraindications and precautions
- If the dose of an opioid is titrated correctly, it is generally accepted that there are no absolute contraindications to the use of such drugs in palliative care, although there may be circumstances where one opioid is favoured over another (e.g. renal impairment, constipation). Nonetheless, manufacturers state that diamorphine is contraindicated for use in patients with:
  - biliary colic
  - concurrent administration of MAOIs or within 2 weeks of discontinuation of their use (*NB: initial low doses, careful titration, and close monitoring may permit safe combination*)
  - obstructive airways disease (morphine may release histamine)
  - phaeochromocytoma (due to the risk of pressor response to histamine release)
  - respiratory depression.
- Use with caution in the following instances:
  - acute alcoholism
  - Addison's disease (adrenocortical insufficiency)
  - asthma (morphine may release histamine)
  - constipation
  - delirium tremens
  - diarrhoea (may mask underlying severe constipation)
  - diseases of the biliary tract
  - elderly patients
  - head injury
  - hepatic impairment (see above)
  - history of alcohol and drug abuse
  - hypotension associated with hypovolaemia (diamorphine may result in severe hypotension)
  - hypothyroidism
  - inflammatory bowel disorders
  - pancreatitis

- prostatic hypertrophy
- raised intracranial pressure
- significantly impaired hepatic and renal function.

☺ Undesirable effects

Strong opioids tend to cause similar undesirable effects, albeit to varying degrees. The frequency is not defined, but reported undesirable effects include:

- Anorexia
- Asthenia
- Biliary pain
- Confusion
- Constipation
- Drowsiness
- Dry mouth
- Dyspepsia
- Exacerbation of pancreatitis
- Euphoria
- Insomnia
- Headache

- Hyperhidrosis
- Myoclonus
- Nausea
- Pruritus
- Sexual dysfunction (e.g. amenorrhea, decreased libido, erectile dysfunction)
- Urinary retention
- Vertigo
- Visual disturbance
- Vomiting

The following can occur with excessive dose:
- Agitation
- Exacerbation of pain
- Hallucinations
- Miosis
- Paraesthesia
- Respiratory depression
- Restlessness

Drug interactions

Pharmacokinetic
- No clinically significant pharmacokinetic interactions reported.

Pharmacodynamic
- *Antihypertensives*—increased risk of hypotension.
- *CNS depressants*—risk of excessive sedation.
- *Haloperidol*—may be an additive hypotensive effect.
- *Ketamine*—there is a potential opioid-sparing effect with ketamine and the dose of morphine may need reducing.
- *Levomepromazine*—may be an additive hypotensive effect.

♔ Dose

Pain
- The initial dose of diamorphine depends upon the patient's previous opioid requirements. Refer to ▢ Opioid substitution, p.33 for information regarding opioid dose equivalences and ▢ Breakthrough cancer pain, p.35 for guidance relating to BTcP.
- Initial dose in opioid-naive patients is 2.5mg SC 4 hourly PRN. Alternatively, 10mg via CSCI over 24 hours and increase as necessary.
- Diamorphine is very soluble in water; 1g dissolves in 1.6mL of water, permitting high doses via SC injections.

¥ *Painful skin lesions (topical)*

- As with morphine, often use 0.1% or 0.125% w/w gels initially. These can be prepared immediately prior to administration by adding 10mg diamorphine injection (diluted with 0.5mL WFI) to 8g Intrasite® gel (making a 0.125% w/w gel). Higher-strength gels, typically up to 0.5%, can be made if necessary.
- Initial dose: 5–10mg diamorphine in Intrasite® gel applied to affected area at dressing changes (up to twice daily).
- Use within 1 hour of preparation and discard any remaining product.

¥ *Mucositis*

- As with morphine, often use 0.1% w/v initially. Preparations should be prepared immediately prior to administration by adding 10mg diamorphine injection (diluted with 0.5mL WFI) to 10mL of a suitable carrier (e.g. Gelclair®, Oralbalance Gel®).
- Higher-strength preparations (up to 0.5% w/v) can be used if required.
- Initial dose: 10mg applied to the affected area BD–TDS.
- Use within 1 hour of preparation and discard any remaining product.

¥ *Dyspnoea*

- For opioid naive patients, initial dose is 1.25mg SC PRN. If patients require more than two doses daily, CSCI should be considered.
- In patients established on opioids, a dose that is equivalent to 25% of the current PRN rescue analgesic dose may be effective. This can be increased up to 100% of the rescue dose in a graduated fashion.

⚓ Dose adjustments

Elderly

- No specific guidance is available, although lower starting doses in opioid-naive patients may be preferable. Dose requirements should be individually titrated.

Hepatic/renal impairment

- No specific guidance is available, although in patients with hepatic impairment the plasma concentration is expected to be increased. In view of its eventual hepatic metabolism. Caution is advised when giving diamorphine to patients with hepatic impairment. Lower starting doses in opioid-naive patients may be preferable and dose requirements should be individually titrated.
- No specific guidance is available for patients with renal impairment. However, in view of the fact that the active metabolite (morphine-6-glucuronide) is renally excreted, lower starting doses in opioid-naive patients may be preferable and dose requirements should be individually titrated. Alternatively, a different opioid may be more appropriate (e.g. alfentanil).

Additional information

- The United Kingdom is one of the few places where diamorphine is used medicinally. Its use developed in palliative care mainly because its high solubility in water enables large doses to be included in the contents of a syringe driver. Many of the listed side-effects are normally only seen when the dose of diamorphine is too high. When the dose is titrated accurately to manage pain, many of these should be absent.
- If other analgesic measures are introduced, pharmacological or otherwise (e.g. radiotherapy), the dose of diamorphine may need to be reduced.
- Diamorphine via CSCI is reportedly compatible with clonazepam, dexamethasone, glycopyrronium, haloperidol, hyoscine butylbromide, hyoscine hydrobromide, ketamine, ketorolac, levomepromazine, metoclopramide, midazolam, octreotide, ondansetron, and ranitidine. Refer to Dickman A et al., *The Syringe Driver* (2nd edn), Oxford University Press, 2005, for further information.
- Diamorphine displays concentration-dependent incompatibility with cyclizine. Mixtures are chemically and physically stable in WFI up to concentrations of 20mg/mL over 24 hours. If the diamorphine concentration exceeds 20mg/mL, crystallization may occur unless the concentration of cyclizine is ≤10mg/mL. Similarly, if the concentration of cyclizine exceeds 20mg/mL, crystallization may occur unless the concentration of diamorphine is ≤15mg/mL.

⤳ Pharmacology

Diamorphine is a synthetic opioid agonist with about 1.5 times the potency of morphine when both are given parenterally. Given orally, both diamorphine and morphine are considered equianalgesic. Diamorphine interacts predominantly with the μ-opioid receptor. It is rapidly de-acetylated to an active metabolite, 6-mono-acetylmorphine (6-MAM), which is also rapidly de-acetylated to morphine. Metabolism is then as for morphine.

Diazepam

Generic (CD Benz POM)
Tablet: 2mg (28); 5mg (28); 10mg (28)
Oral solution: 2mg/5mL (100mL)
Strong oral solution: 5mg/5mL (100mL)
Injection (emulsion): 5mg/mL (10)
Injection (solution): 5mg/mL (10)
Rectal solution: 2.5mg/1.25mL (2; 5); 5mg/2.5mL (2; 5); 10mg/5mL (2; 5)
Suppository: 10mg (6)

Note: Independent prescribers are authorized to prescribe diazepam
(☐ Independent prescribing: palliative care issues, p.25)

Indications
- Anxiety (short-term use only)
- Insomnia (short-term use only)
- Status epilepticus
- Muscle spasm

Contraindications and precautions
- Contraindicated for use in patients with
  - acute pulmonary insufficiency
  - myasthenia gravis
  - severe hepatic insufficiency
  - sleep apnoea syndrome.
- Diazepam should not be used alone in the treatment of depression or anxiety associated with depression because of the risk of precipitation of suicide.
- Use with caution if there is a history of drug or alcohol abuse.
- Diazepam should be used with caution in patients with chronic respiratory disease, renal impairment, or moderate hepatic impairment.
- Dose reductions may be necessary in the elderly (see below).
- Avoid abrupt withdrawal, even if short-duration treatment. Prolonged use of benzodiazepines may result in the development of dependence with subsequent withdrawal symptoms on cessation of use, e.g. agitation, anxiety, confusion, headaches, restlessness, sleep disturbances, sweating, and tremor. The risk of dependence increases with dose and duration of treatment. Gradual withdrawal is advised.
- Diazepam may modify reactions and patients should be advised not to drive (or operate machinery) if affected.

☹ Undesirable effects
The frequency is not defined, but reported undesirable effects include:
- Anterograde amnesia
- Ataxia
- Confusion
- Depression
- Dizziness
- Drowsiness

- Fatigue
- Hallucinations
- Headache
- Muscle weakness
- Nightmares
- Paradoxical events such as agitation, irritability and restlessness
- Respiratory depression
- Sexual dysfunction
- Sleep disturbance
- Visual disturbances

Drug interactions

Pharmacokinetic

- Diazepam is metabolized by CYP2C19 and CYP3A4. Unexpected effects may be explained by the fact that up to 5% of the Caucasian population are CYP2C19 poor metabolizers.
- *Carbamazepine*—may reduce the effect of diazepam.
- *Erythromycin*—may increase the effect of diazepam.
- *Fluconazole*—may increase the effect of diazepam.
- *Omeprazole*—may increase the effect of diazepam (inhibits CYP2C19 and CYP3A4).
- *Sodium valproate*—may increase the effect of diazepam.
- The clinical significance of co-administration with other inducers or inhibitors of CYP2C19 or CYP3A4 (📖 end cover) is unknown. The prescriber should be aware of the potential for interactions and that dosage adjustments may be necessary.
- Avoid excessive amounts of grapefruit juice as it may increase the bio-availability of diazepam through inhibition of intestinal CYP3A4.

Pharmacodynamic

- *Alcohol*—may precipitate seizures.
- *Antidepressants*—reduced seizure threshold.
- *Antipsychotics*—reduced seizure threshold.
- *Baclofen*—increased risk of sedation.
- *CNS depressants*—additive sedative effect.

🎵 Dose

Anxiety

- Patients may require lower than licensed doses. Initial dose 2mg PO at bedtime, increasing gradually as required to 2mg TDS. The dose can then be increased as necessary to a maximum of 30mg daily in divided doses.
- Although available, other alternatives such as SC midazolam are preferred to the use of rectal diazepam. Typical dose is 10–30mg PR daily (suppository) or 0.5mg/kg, repeated 12 hourly (rectal solution).

Insomnia

- Patients may require lower than licensed doses. Initial dose 2mg PO at bedtime, increasing gradually as necessary to 15mg PO at bedtime.
- Note that patients with insomnia related to anxiety may benefit from a single dose at bedtime (e.g. 10–15mg PO ON).

Status epilepticus
- 0.5mg/kg PR, repeated after 15 minutes if necessary (rectal solution)
- 10mg IV at a rate of 1mL/min (5mg/min), repeated if necessary after 10 minutes (injection).

Muscle spasm
- Patients may require lower than licensed doses. Initial dose 2mg PO at bedtime, increasing gradually as required to 2mg PO TDS. The dose can then be increased as necessary to a maximum of 30mg PO daily in divided doses.

Dose adjustments
Elderly
- Generally adopt half the normal adult dose.

Hepatic/renal impairment
- No specific guidance available. Patients with liver or renal impairment may be particularly susceptible to undesirable effects and lower initial doses should be used.

Additional information
- Diazepam has a long duration of action due to several active metabolites. The formation of these is highly variable and therefore treatment must be individualized. Some patients may be able to take diazepam once daily because of the presence of an active metabolite with a long half-life.
- If there are unexpected responses, such as excessive sedation, consider drug interactions, which could be additive.

Pharmacology
The exact mechanism of action is unknown, but it is believed to act via enhancement of GABA-ergic transmission in the CNS. Diazepam undergoes first-pass metabolism via cytochromes CYP2C19 and CYP3A4. Numerous active metabolites are formed, one of which can have a prolonged half-life.

Diclofenac

Standard release

Diclofenac sodium

Voltarol® (POM)
Tablet (*enteric-coated*): 25mg (84); 50mg (84)
Dispersible tablet (*sugar-free*): 50mg (21)
Injection: 75mg/3mL (10)
Suppository: 12.5mg (10); 25mg (10); 50mg (10); 100mg (10)

Generic (POM)
Tablet (*enteric-coated*): 25mg (84); 50mg (84)
Suppository: 100mg (10)

With misoprostol (📖 Misoprostol, p.336)

Arthrotec® 50 (POM)
Tablet: diclofenac sodium 50mg, misoprostol 200mcg (60)

Arthrotec® 75 (POM)
Tablet: diclofenac sodium 75mg, misoprostol 200mcg (60)

Modified release

Diclofenac sodium
Diclomax SR® (POM)
Capsule: 75mg (56)
Diclomax Retard® (POM)
Capsule: 100mg (28)
Motifene® 75mg (POM)
Capsule: 75mg (56)

Voltarol® 75mg SR (POM)
Tablet: 75mg (28; 56)
Voltarol® Retard (POM)
Tablet: 100mg (28)
Generic (POM)
Tablet: 100mg (28)

Diclofenac potassium

Voltarol® Rapid (POM)
Tablet: 25mg (30); 50mg (30)

Note: 12.5mg tablets are available for sale in pharmacies for the treatment of headache, dental pain, period pain, rheumatic and muscular pain, backache, and the symptoms of cold and flu (including fever). Patients must be aged over 14 years and the maximum daily dose is 75mg. Treatment should not exceed 3 days.

Indications

- Relief of pain and inflammation in several conditions:
  - acute gout
  - arthritic conditions
  - musculoskeletal disorders
  - pain resulting from trauma.

Contraindications and precautions

- Contraindicated for use in patients with:
  - a history of, or active, peptic ulceration
  - hypersensitivity reactions to ibuprofen, aspirin, or other NSAIDs
  - severe heart, hepatic, or renal impairment.
- Discontinue diclofenac at the first sign of skin rash, mucosal lesions, or any other signs of hypersensitivity.
- Use the minimum effective dose for the shortest duration necessary in order to reduce the risk of cardiac and GI events.
- Elderly patients are more at risk of developing undesirable effects.
- Use with caution in the following circumstances:
  - concurrent use of diuretics, corticosteroids, and NSAIDs (see 📖 Drug interactions, p.145)
  - congestive heart failure and/or left ventricular dysfunction
  - diabetes mellitus
  - established ischaemic heart disease, peripheral arterial disease, and/ or cerebrovascular disease need careful consideration because of the increased risk of thrombotic events
  - hepatic impairment
  - hyperlipidaemia
  - hypertension (particularly uncontrolled)
  - recovery from surgery
  - renal impairment
  - smoking.
- Patients undergoing long-term therapy need regular monitoring of renal and liver function.
- Abnormal LFTs can occur; discontinue NSAID if this persists.
- Patients with systemic lupus erythematosus (SLE) and mixed connective tissue disorders may be at risk of developing aseptic meningitis.
- Diclofenac may prevent the development of signs and symptoms of inflammation/infection (e.g. fever).
- Consider co-prescription of misoprostol or a proton pump inhibitor if:
  - long-term NSAID therapy
  - concurrent use of drugs that increase the risk of GI toxicity (see 📖 Drug interactions, p.145)
- For further information, including selection, see 📖 Selection of an NSAID, p.31.
- Diclofenac may modify reactions and patients should be advised not to drive (or operate machinery) if affected.

☹ Undesirable effects

Common

- Abdominal cramps
- Anorexia
- Diarrhoea
- Dizziness
- Dyspepsia
- Elevated LFTs (discontinue if this persists)
- Flatulence

- Headache
- Nausea
- Rashes
- Vomiting

Rare
- Gastritis
- GI bleeding
- GI ulcers
- Drowsiness
- Hepatitis
- Jaundice
- Oedema

Very rare
- Acute renal insufficiency
- Agranulocytosis
- Anaemia (aplastic; haemolytic)
- Congestive heart failure
- Erythema multiforme
- Hypertension
- Leucopenia
- Stevens–Johnson syndrome
- Thrombocytopenia

Drug interactions

Pharmacokinetic
- Diclofenac is metabolized by several cytochrome P450 isoenzymes and therefore enzyme inhibition is unlikely to be clinically significant. It is a substrate of CYP1A2, CYP2B6, CYP2C8, CYP2C9 (major), CYP2C19, CYP2D6 and CYP3A4. Diclofenac may have a clinically significant inhibitory action on CYP3A4 and CYP1A2.
- *Antacids*—avoid giving within 1 hour of enteric coated tablets
- *Methotrexate*—reduced excretion of methotrexate
- The clinical significance of co-administration with CYP2C9 inducers (📖 end cover) is unknown. The prescriber should be aware of the potential for interactions and that dosage adjustments may be necessary.
- The clinical significance of co-administration with CYP1A2 or CYP3A4 substrates (📖 end cover) is unknown. The prescriber should be aware of the potential for interactions and that dosage adjustments may be necessary.

Pharmacodynamic
- *Anticoagulants*—increased risk of bleeding
- *Antihypertensives*—reduced hypotensive effect
- *Antiplatelet drugs*—increased risk of bleeding
- *Corticosteroids*—increased risk of GI toxicity
- *Ciclosporin*—increased risk of nephrotoxicity
- *Diuretics*—reduced diuretic effect; nephrotoxicity of diclofenac may be increased

- *Rosiglitazone*—increased risk of oedema
- *SSRIs*—increased risk of GI bleeding

♣ Dose
Standard release
- Initial dose 50mg PO BD increasing to 50mg PO TDS as necessary.
- The rectal route is generally avoided in palliative care. Nonetheless, it may be preferable to a CSCI. The usual dose is 75–150mg daily in divided doses.
- * Alternatively, 100–150mg via CSCI over 24 hours. Note diclofenac should not be mixed with other drugs and a separate CSCI will be needed.

Modified release
- Dose 100mg OD or 75mg BD

♣ Dose adjustments
Elderly
- The elderly are at an increased risk of undesirable effects. Use the lowest effective dose for the shortest duration possible

Hepatic/renal impairment
- Diclofenac is contraindicated for use in patients with severe hepatic or renal impairment.
- In patients with mild to moderate liver impairment, no specific dose recommendations are available and the metabolism of diclofenac is stated to be unaffected. However, the lowest dose possible should be used for the shortest duration possible and the patient should be closely monitored. If abnormal LFTs develop and persist or deteriorate further, diclofenac must be discontinued.
- The use of diclofenac may result in deterioration of renal function. The lowest effective dose should be used and renal function monitored.

Additional information
- If *Arthrotec*® is used, ensure a PPI is not co-prescribed.
- Diclofenac via CSCI is incompatible with the majority of drugs likely to be encountered. Therefore it should be administered via a separate CSCI.

♦ Pharmacology
Diclofenac is an NSAID with analgesic, anti-inflammatory, and antipyretic properties. The potassium salt of diclofenac is more rapidly absorbed. The mechanism of action of diclofenac, like that of other NSAIDs, is not completely understood but may be related to inhibition of COX-1 and COX-2. Diclofenac is believed to be more selective for COX-2 and indeed has been shown to have a cardiovascular profile similar to the COX-2 inhibitors.

Diclofenac is rapidly and completely absorbed after oral administration, although the bioavailability is slightly less with the dispersible tablets. It is highly protein bound to albumin (about 99%) and extensively metabolized in the liver by a variety of isoenzymes (including CYP1A2, CYP2B6, CYP2C8, CYP2C9 (major), CYP2C19, CYP2D6, and CYP3A4) to inactive (or weakly active) metabolites; glucuronidation of the parent molecule also occurs to a lesser extent. The metabolites are glucuronidated and excreted via the kidney and faeces.

Diethylstilbestrol

Generic (POM)
Tablet: 1mg (28); 5mg (28)

Indications
- Palliation of prostate cancer
- Palliation of breast cancer in post menopausal women (uncommon)

Contraindications and precautions

There is a significant increase in risk of deep vein thrombosis with diethylstilbestrol treatment and patients should be reviewed for the need for concurrent antiplatelet/anticoagulant therapy.

- Diethylstilbestrol is contraindicated for use in patients with:
  - cardiovascular or cerebrovascular disorder or a history of thromboembolism
  - hyperlipoproteinaemia
  - moderate to severe hypertension
  - oestrogen-dependent neoplasms
  - porphyria
  - pre-menopausal carcinoma of the breast
  - severe or active liver disease
  - undiagnosed vaginal bleeding.
- It should be used with caution in patients with:
  - cardiac failure
  - cholelithiasis
  - cholestatic jaundice (or history of)
  - contact lenses
  - depression
  - diabetes (glucose tolerance may be lowered)
  - epilepsy
  - hepatic impairment
  - hypertension
  - migraine
  - renal impairment.
- Thyroid function tests may be difficult to interpret, as diethylstilbestrol may increase thyroid hormone binding globulin leading to increased circulating total thyroid hormone.

☺ Undesirable effects
The frequency is not defined, but reported undesirable effects include:
- Cholelithiasis
- Cholestatic jaundice
- Corneal discomfort (in contact lens wearers)
- Glucose tolerance reduced
- Gynaecomastia
- Hypercalcaemia and bone pain may occur in breast cancer

- Hypertension
- Impotence
- Nausea
- Sodium and water retention
- Thromboembolism
- Weight gain

Drug interactions

Pharmacokinetic
- Despite extensive hepatic metabolism, there are no recognized pharmacokinetic interactions.

Pharmacodynamic
- *Antihypertensives*—effect may be antagonized by diethylstilbestrol.
- *Diuretics*—effect may be antagonized by diethylstilbestrol.
- *Tamoxifen*—potential antagonism.

Dose

Prostate cancer
- Initial dose 1mg PO OD; dose can be increased, as determined by a specialist, to 3mg PO OD.
- Higher doses were previously used, but are no longer recommended.

Breast cancer
- Initial dose 10mg PO OD, increased as determined by a specialist to 20mg PO OD.

Dose adjustments

Elderly
- The recommended adult dose is appropriate.

Hepatic/renal impairment
- Diethylstilbestrol should not be used in patients with active liver disease.
- There are no specific dose recommendations for patients with renal impairment. The lowest effective dose should be used.

Additional information
- Ideally, blood pressure should be checked before initiating diethylstilbestrol and should be monitored at regular intervals. If hypertension develops, treatment should be stopped.

⊘ Pharmacology

Diethylstilbestrol is a synthetic oestrogen and it binds to an intracellular receptor protein within the cytoplasm when it is transported to the nucleus of the cell. It then has an action on mRNA and associated protein synthesis. Its action in palliative treatment is not completely understood.

Diethylstilbestrol is readily absorbed from the GI tract. It is slowly metabolized in the liver to three metabolites; CYP2A6 may be involved in this process. Further metabolism to glucuronides occurs. Excretion is mainly via the kidneys and gall bladder (enterohepatic circulation may occur).

Dihydrocodeine

Standard release
DF118 Forte® (CD Inv POM)
Tablet: 40mg (100)

Generic (CD Inv POM)
Tablet: 30mg (28)
Oral solution: 10mg/5mL (150mL)
Injection: 50mg/mL *(CD POM)*

Modified release
DHC Continus® (CD Inv POM)
Tablet: 60mg (56); 90mg (56); 120mg (56)

Combination products
Certain products containing less than 10mg dihydrocodeine and para-cetamol are available OTC.

Remedeine® (CD Inv POM)
Tablet: dihydrocodeine 20mg/paracetamol 500mg (112)

Remedeine Forte® (CD Inv POM)
Tablet: dihydrocodeine 30mg/paracetamol 500mg (112)

Generic (CD Inv POM)
Tablet *(scored)*: co-dydramol 10/500 (dihydrocodeine 10mg/paracetamol 500mg) (30)

Note: Independent prescribers are **NOT** authorized to prescribe parenteral dihydrocodeine (📖 Independent prescribing: palliative care issues, p.25)

Indications
• Management of moderate to severe pain

Contraindications and precautions
• Dihydrocodeine is contraindicated for use in:
  • acute alcoholism
  • head injury
  • obstructive airways disease
  • paralytic ileus
  • raised intracranial pressure
  • respiratory depression.
• Use with caution in the following instances:
  • asthma (can release histamine)
  • bowel obstruction
  • diseases of the biliary tract
  • elderly
  • hepatic impairment
  • pancreatitis

- prostatic hypertrophy
- renal impairment
- Dihydrocodeine may modify reactions and patients should be advised not to drive (or operate machinery) if affected.

☹ Undesirable effects

The frequency is not defined, but commonly reported undesirable effects include:

- Constipation
- Drowsiness
- Headache
- Nausea and/or vomiting
- Pruritus
- Rash

Less commonly reported undesirable effects include:

- Abdominal pain
- Biliary spasm
- Confusion
- Decreased libido
- Dizziness
- Dry mouth
- Flushing
- Hallucinations
- Hypotension
- Paraesthesia
- Paralytic ileus
- Respiratory depression
- Sweating
- Ureteric spasm
- Urinary retention
- Visual disturbances

Drug interactions

Pharmacokinetic

- Dihydrocodeine is metabolized by CYP2D6 to an active metabolite.
- The clinical significance of co-administration with CYP2D6 inhibitors (🕮 end cover) is unknown. The prescriber should be aware of the potential for interactions and that dosage adjustments may be necessary.
- Note that, unlike codeine, interactions between CYP2D6 inhibitors and dihydrocodeine do not appear to reduce analgesic benefit significantly.

Pharmacodynamic

- *Antihypertensives*—increased risk of hypotension.
- *CNS depressants*—risk of excessive sedation.
- *Haloperidol*—may be an additive hypotensive effect.
- *Ketamine*—there is a potential opioid-sparing effect with ketamine and the dose of dihydrocodeine may need reducing.
- *Levomepromazine*—may be an additive hypotensive effect.

♉ Dose

Oral

Standard release

- 30–60mg PO every 4–6 hours when required. Maximum daily dose 240mg.
- Using *DF118 Forte*®, 40–80mg PO TDS PRN. Maximum daily dose 240mg.

Modified release
• 60–120mg PO every 12 hours

Parenteral
• 50mg by SC or deep IM injection repeated every 4–6 hours.
• ¥ Alternatively, 100–200mg via CSCI over 24 hours. Higher doses have been used.

⚕ Dose adjustments

Elderly
• No specific guidance is available, although lower starting doses may be preferable. Dose requirements should be individually titrated.

Hepatic/renal impairment
• No specific guidance is available, although the plasma concentration is expected to be increased in patients with hepatic impairment. In view of its hepatic metabolism, caution is advised when giving dihydrocodeine to patients with hepatic impairment. Lower starting doses may be preferable and dose requirements should be individually titrated.
• No specific guidance is available for patients with renal impairment. However, in view of the fact that metabolites are renally excreted, lower starting doses may be preferable and dose requirements should be individually titrated.

Additional information

• Dihydrocodeine and codeine have traditionally been used instead of morphine (or alternative) for the headache associated with brain metastases. There is no evidence to support this use.
• *DHC Continus*® tablets must be swallowed whole and not be broken, crushed, or chewed.
• Nausea and vomiting are relatively common, limiting side-effects to the use of regular dihydrocodeine alone. This can be overcome by using lower doses more frequently (e.g. 30mg PO 4 hourly), or using a modified-release preparation.
• In the absence of a liquid formulation, oral standard-release tablets can be crushed and dispersed in water immediately prior to use.
• Via CSCI, dihydrocodeine has been shown to be compatible with cyclizine, glycopyrronium, haloperidol, levomepromazine, and midazolam.

➔ Pharmacology

Dihydrocodeine is a potent synthetic opioid analgesic with a low oral bio-availability, presumably due to first-pass metabolism. By mouth, it is of similar potency as codeine; parenterally it is considered to be twice as potent as codeine. Dihydrocodeine is metabolized in the liver by CYP2D6 to dihydromorphine, which adds to its analgesic effect. Unchanged drug plus metabolites are renally excreted.

Docusate sodium

Dioctyl® (P)
Capsule: 100mg (30; 100)

Docusol® (P)
Oral solution (*sugar-free*): 12.5mg/5mL (300mL); 50mg/5mL (300mL)

Norgalax Micro-enema® (P)
Enema: 120mg in 10g (1 × 10g)

Indications
- Chronic constipation
- ¥ Partial bowel obstruction

Contraindications and precautions
- Manufacturer advises that docusate should not be administered to patients with abdominal pain, nausea, vomiting, or intestinal obstruction.

☺ Undesirable effects
The frequency is not defined, but reported undesirable effects include:
- Abdominal cramps
- Diarrhoea
- Nausea
- Skin rash

Drug interactions
Pharmacokinetic
- *Mineral oils (e.g. liquid paraffin)*—increased risk of toxicity through enhanced absorption.

Pharmacodynamic
- *Anticholinergics*—antagonizes the laxative effect.
- *Cyclizine*—antagonizes the laxative effect.
- *Opioids*—antagonizes the laxative effect.
- *5-HT$_3$ antagonists*—antagonizes the laxative effect.
- *Tricyclic antidepressants*—antagonizes the laxative effect.

♪ Dose
Oral
- ¥ Initial dose 100mg PO BD, increased as necessary according to response, to a usual maximum of 200mg PO TDS.
- Licensed maximum dose is 500mg/day in divided doses.

Rectal
- Usual dose 120mg OD (one enema). It can be repeated on the same or the next day.

↕ Dose adjustments

Elderly
- No specific recommendations.

Hepatic/renal impairment
- No specific recommendations

Additional information
- Oral preparation can take up to 72 hours to work; enema usually works within 20 minutes

↔ Pharmacology
Docusate sodium is a surfactant and used as a faecal softening agent. It works by allowing water to penetrate faeces, allowing them to soften. It is believed to have a mild stimulant action, particularly at the higher doses.

Domperidone

Motilium® (POM)
Tablet: 10mg (30; 100)
Suspension: 5mg/5mL (200mL)
Suppository: 30mg (10)

Generic (POM)
Tablet: 10mg (30; 100)

Note: Tablets may be sold in pharmacies for the relief of post-prandial symptoms of excessive fullness, nausea, epigastric bloating, and belching, occasionally accompanied by epigastric discomfort and heartburn, at a maximum daily dose of 40mg.

Indications
- Nausea and vomiting
- Gastro-oesophageal reflux
- Dyspepsia

Contraindications and precautions
- Contraindicated for use in patients with:
  - bowel obstruction or perforation
  - GI haemorrhage
  - prolactinoma.
- Caution in renal impairment (see 📖 *Dose adjustments*).
- Manufacturer advises avoid in liver impairment.
- Avoid concurrent use of CYP3A4 inhibitors (see 📖 *Drug interactions,* p.155).

☹ Undesirable effects
Common
- Dry mouth
- Headache

Rare
- Hyperprolactinaemia (with associated symptoms, e.g. galactorrhoea, gynaecomastia, and amenorrhoea)
- Intestinal cramps

Very rare
- Extrapyramidal effects
- Urticaria

Drug interactions
Pharmacokinetic
- Domperidone is metabolized by CYP3A4, CYP1A2, and CYP2E1. The main metabolic pathway involves CYP3A4.
- Co-administration with CYP3A4 inhibitors (📖 end cover) can increase peak plasma concentrations of domperidone and can also lead to increases in the QT interval. The clinical significance is unknown, but the prescriber should be aware of the potential for interactions and the need to avoid concurrent use (see *Contraindications and precautions*).

Pharmacodynamic
- *Anticholinergics*—may antagonize the prokinetic effect.
- *Cyclizine*—may antagonize the prokinetic effect.
- *Opioids*—antagonize the prokinetic effect.
- *5-HT$_3$ antagonists*—antagonize the prokinetic effect.
- *Tricyclic antidepressants*—may antagonize the prokinetic effect.

Dose
- For all indications
  - PO 10–20mg TDS–QDS. Maximum daily dose 80mg.
  - PR 60mg BD

Dose adjustments
Elderly
- No specific guidance is available, but the dose should be carefully adjusted to individual requirements

Hepatic/renal impairment
- The manufacturer recommends that domperidone is avoided in patients with liver impairment because of extensive metabolism.
- In patients with severe renal impairment (i.e. SeCr >600μmol/L), the dosing frequency should be reduced to once or twice daily with repeated use. Dose adjustments are unnecessary for single administration

Additional information
- Domperidone is likely to be better tolerated than metoclopramide (i.e. less frequent and less severe undesirable effects).
- It is a suitable first-line choice for the management of nausea and vomiting associated with Parkinson's disease therapy.
- If necessary, the tablets can be crushed before administration if the suspension is unavailable.

Pharmacology
Domperidone is a peripheral D2 receptor antagonist and does not usually cross the blood–brain barrier. It undergoes extensive first-pass metabolism (CYP3A4) and metabolites are inactive. Its anti-emetic effect is due to two distinct effects: a prokinetic effect and dopamine blockade in the chemoreceptor trigger zone (CTZ), which lies outside the blood–brain barrier.

Donepezil

Aricept® (POM)
Tablet: 5mg (28); 10mg (28)

Aricept Evess® (POM)
Orodispersible tablet: 5mg (28); 10mg (28)

Indications
- Symptomatic treatment of mild to moderately severe Alzheimer's dementia
- * Mild to moderate dementia not associated with Alzheimer's disease

Contraindications and precautions
- Donepezil should be used with caution with the following:
  - asthma
  - chronic obstructive pulmonary disease
  - severe hepatic impairment
  - supraventricular conduction abnormalities (may cause bradycardia)
  - susceptibility to peptic ulcers (increase in gastric acid secretion).
- All patients receiving donepezil should have their ability to continue driving or operating complex machines evaluated.

☺ Undesirable effects
Very common
- Diarrhoea
- Headache
- Nausea

Common
- Agitation
- Dizziness
- Fatigue
- Hallucinations
- Insomnia
- Muscle cramps
- Sweating
- Urinary incontinence

Uncommon
- Bradycardia
- GI haemorrhage
- Peptic ulcer

Rare
- Extrapyramidal reactions

Drug interactions

Pharmacokinetic

- Metabolized by CYP3A4 and CYP2D6.
- The clinical significance of co-administration with CYP3A4 inhibitors/ inducers or inhibitors of CYP2D6 (🔲 end cover) is unknown. The prescriber should be aware of the potential for interactions and that dosage adjustments may be necessary.
- Avoid excessive amounts of grapefruit juice as it may increase the bioavailability of donepezil through inhibition of intestinal CYP3A4.

Pharmacodynamic

- *Anticholinergics*—may antagonize the effects

🎗 Dose

- Initial dose 5mg PO ON, increased if necessary after 1 month to maximum 10mg PO ON

🎗 Dose adjustments

Elderly

- Usual adult doses can be used.

Hepatic/renal impairment

- For patients with mild to moderate hepatic impairment, dose escalation should be performed according to individual tolerability. There is no recommendation for use in severe hepatic disease.
- Usual adult doses can be used in renal impairment.

Additional information

- Tablet can be dispersed in water immediately prior to administration if the orodispersible product is unavailable.

⊙ Pharmacology

Donepezil is a centrally acting, specific, and reversible inhibitor of acetyl-cholinesterase. Its therapeutic effect is through enhancement of cholin-ergic function. It is well absorbed with a relative oral bioavailability of 100%. It is metabolized by CYP3A4 and CYP2D6, as well as undergoing glucuronidation. The main metabolite has similar activity to donepezil. Approximately 17% of the dose is excreted unchanged in the urine.

Duloxetine

Cymbalta® (POM)
Capsule: 30mg (28); 60mg (28)

Yentreve® (POM) (licensed for stress incontinence in women and not discussed further).

Indications
- Major depressive episodes.
- Generalized anxiety disorder
- Diabetic peripheral neuropathic pain in adults.

Contraindications and precautions
- Duloxetine is contraindicated in the following conditions:
  - uncontrolled hypertension
  - moderate to severe hepatic impairment
  - severe renal impairment (CrCl <30mL/min)
- Co-administration with potent CYP1A2 inhibitors (see 📖 *Drug interactions, p.161*) must be avoided.
- Do not use with an irreversible MAOI, or within 14 days of stopping one. At least 5 days should be allowed after stopping duloxetine before starting an irreversible MAOI.
- Use with caution in:
  - elderly (greater risk of hyponatraemia)
  - epilepsy (lowers seizure threshold)
  - glaucoma (may cause mydriasis).
- The combination with selective reversible MAOIs (e.g. linezolid, moclobemide) is not recommended and the manufacturer offers no specific advice.
- Hyponatraemia should be considered in all patients who develop drowsiness, confusion, or convulsions while taking an antidepressant. Hyponatraemia has been associated with all types of antidepressants, although it is reportedly more common with SSRIs.
- Depression is associated with an increased risk of suicidal thoughts, self-harm, and suicide, which persists until remission. Note that that the risk of suicide may increase during initial treatment.
- Abrupt discontinuation should be avoided because of the risk of withdrawal reactions, e.g. agitation, anxiety, diarrhoea, dizziness, fatigue, headache, hyperhidrosis, nausea and/or vomiting, sensory disturbances (including paraesthesia), and sleep disturbances. When stopping treatment, the dose should be reduced gradually over at least 1–2 weeks. See 📖 Discontinuing and/or switching antidepressants, p.45 for information about switching or stopping antidepressants.
- May precipitate psychomotor restlessness, which usually appears during early treatment. The use of duloxetine should be reviewed.
- Duloxetine may modify reactions and patients should be advised not to drive (or operate machinery) if affected.

☻ Undesirable effects

Very common
- Dizziness
- Drowsiness
- Dry mouth
- Headache
- Nausea

Common
- Agitation
- Altered taste
- Anxiety
- Appetite reduced
- Blurred vision
- Constipation
- Diarrhoea
- Dyspepsia
- Hyperhidrosis
- Fatigue
- Insomnia
- Palpitations
- Sexual dysfunction
- Sleep disturbances (including abnormal dreams)
- Tremor
- Vomiting
- Weight loss

Uncommon
- Abnormal bleeding (bruising, epistaxis)
- Ear pain
- Hyperglycaemia (especially in diabetics)
- Myoclonus
- Restless legs syndrome
- Tachycardia
- Vertigo
- Visual disturbances

Rare
- Atrial fibrillation
- Convulsions
- Glaucoma
- Hallucinations
- SIADH/hyponatraemia

Unknown
- Hypertensive crisis
- Jaundice
- Psychomotor restlessness
- Serotonin syndrome (see 📖 *Drug interactions*, p.161)
- Stevens–Johnson syndrome
- Suicidal ideation

Drug interactions

Pharmacokinetic

- Duloxetine is a moderate inhibitor of CYP2D6; it is metabolized by CYP1A2 and CYP2D6.
- Smokers may have almost 50% lower plasma concentrations of duloxetine (CYP1A2 induction) compared with non-smokers. Dosage adjustments may be necessary upon smoking cessation (📖 Box 1.9, p.17) Co-administration of CYP1A2 inducers (📖 end cover) may lead to reduced duloxetine concentrations, although the clinical significance is unknown. The prescriber should be aware of the potential for interactions and that dosage adjustments may be necessary.
- Co-administration of duloxetine with potent inhibitors of CYP1A2, e.g. amiodarone, ciprofloxacin, fluvoxamine (📖 end cover), is likely to result in higher concentrations of duloxetine (see *Contraindications and precautions*).
- The clinical significance of co-administration with substrates of CYP2D6 (📖 end cover) is unknown. Caution is advised if duloxetine is co-administered with drugs that are predominantly metabolized by CYP2D6 (e.g. haloperidol, risperidone, tricyclic antidepressants). The prescriber should be aware of the potential for interactions and that dosage adjustments may be necessary, particularly of drugs with a narrow therapeutic index.
- The clinical significance of co-administration with prodrug substrates of CYP2D6 (e.g. codeine, tramadol) is unknown. The prescriber should be aware of the potential for interactions and that dosage adjustments may be necessary.
- The clinical significance of co-administration with inhibitors of CYP2D6 (📖 end cover) is unknown, but plasma concentrations of duloxetine may increase. The prescriber should be aware of the potential for interactions and that dosage adjustments may be necessary.

Pharmacodynamic

- *Anticoagulants*—potential increased risk of bleeding.
- *CNS depressants*—additive sedative effect.
- *Cyproheptadine*—may inhibit the effects of duloxetine.
- *Diuretics*—increased risk of hyponatraemia.
- *MAOIs*—risk of serotonin syndrome (see *Contraindications and precautions*).
- *NSAIDs*—increased risk of GI bleeding.
- *Serotonergic drugs*—caution is advisable if duloxetine is co-administered with serotonergic drugs (e.g. methadone, mirtazapine, SSRIs, tricyclic antidepressants, tramadol, trazodone) because of the risk of serotonin syndrome (📖 Box 1.10, p.19).
- *SSRIs*—increased risk of seizures and serotonin syndrome.
- *Tramadol*—increased risk of seizures and serotonin syndrome.

⬗ Dose

Major depressive episodes

- Initial and maintenance dose 60mg PO OD with or without food. There is no evidence to suggest that 120mg PO daily offers any therapeutic advantage.

Generalized anxiety disorder

- Initial dose 30mg PO OD with or without food. Doses can be increased as necessary to a usual maintenance dose of 60mg PO OD with or without food. Further dose increases up to 90mg or 120mg may be considered, based upon clinical response.

Diabetic peripheral neuropathic pain

- Initial dose 60mg PO OD with or without food. Doses can be increased as necessary to 60mg PO BD.

⬗ Dose adjustments

Elderly

- Dosage reductions not necessary

Hepatic/renal impairment

- Duloxetine is not recommended for use in patients with moderate to severe hepatic impairment
- No dosage adjustment is necessary for patients with mild or moderate renal impairment (CrCl ≥30mL/min). Duloxetine is contraindicated in patients with severe renal impairment (CrCl <30mL/min).

Additional information

- Antidepressant therapeutic response is usually seen after 2–4 weeks of treatment.
- In the treatment of anxiety, duloxetine should be continued for several months after therapeutic response in order to prevent relapse.
- For neuropathic pain, response to treatment should be evaluated after 2 months. If the patient has not responded after this time, benefit is unlikely and duloxetine should be gradually withdrawn. Patients who respond should be reassessed regularly (at least every 3 months).

⬥ Pharmacology

Although the exact mechanisms of the antidepressant and analgesic actions of duloxetine are unknown, they are believed to be related to its potentiation of serotonergic and noradrenergic activity in the CNS. Duloxetine is a combined serotonin and noradrenaline reuptake inhibitor, with a weak inhibition of dopamine reuptake.

Duloxetine is extensively metabolized by the cytochrome P450 isoenzymes CYP1A2 and CYP2D6; two major, but inactive, metabolites are formed which are mainly excreted renally.

Enoxaparin

Clexane® (POM)

Injection (*single-dose syringe for SC use*): 20mg (0.2mL, 2000 units); 40mg (0.4mL, 4000 units); 60mg (0.6mL, 6000 units); 80mg (0.8mL, 8000 units); 100mg (1mL, 10,000 units).

Clexane® Forte (POM)

Injection (*single-dose syringe for SC use*): 120mg (0.8mL, 12,000 units); 150mg (1mL, 15,000 units).

Clexane® Multidose (POM)

Injection (*multi-dose vial*): 300mg (3mL, 30,000 units).

Indications

- Treatment and prophylaxis of deep vein thrombosis (DVT) and pulmonary embolism (PE).
- Other indications apply but are not normally relevant in palliative care.

Contraindications and precautions

- Enoxaparin is contraindicated for use in patients with:
  - acute bacterial endocarditis
  - recent haemorrhagic stroke
  - thrombocytopenia
  - active gastric or duodenal ulceration
  - spinal anaesthesia.
- Use with caution in patients with an increased risk of bleeding complications:
  - brain tumours (increased risk of intracranial bleeding)
  - concurrent use of anticoagulant/antiplatelet agents/NSAIDs (see 🕮 *Drug interactions, p.164*)
  - haemorrhagic stroke
  - retinopathy (hypertensive or diabetic)
  - surgery
  - severe hepatic impairment
  - severe renal impairment
  - trauma
  - thrombocytopenia
  - uncontrolled hypertension.
- A baseline platelet count should be taken prior to initiating treatment and monitored closely during the first 3 weeks (e.g. every 2–4 days) and regularly thereafter.
- Not for IM use.
- Advice should be sought from anaesthetist colleagues if considering an epidural intervention in a patient receiving enoxaparin because of the risk of spinal haematoma.
- LMWH can inhibit aldosterone secretion, which can cause hyperkalaemia. Patients with pre-existing renal impairment are more at risk. Potassium should be measured in patients at risk prior to starting

LMWH and monitored regularly thereafter, especially if treatment is prolonged beyond 7 days.

- ***Prophylactic doses of enoxaparin are not sufficient to prevent valve thrombosis in patients with prosthetic heart valves***.
- Not for IM use.

☹ Undesirable effects

The frequency is not defined, but reported undesirable effects include:

- Bleeding (at any site)
- Haematoma at injection site
- Hyperkalaemia
- Hypoaldosteronism
- Intracranial bleeds
- Osteoporosis with long-term treatment
- Prosthetic cardiac valve thrombosis (see *Contraindications and precautions*)
- Skin necrosis
- Spinal or epidural haematoma
- Transient changes to liver transaminase levels—clinical significance unknown
- Thrombocytopenia

Drug interactions

Pharmacokinetic

- None recognized

Pharmacodynamic

- Drugs with anticoagulant or anti-platelet effect may enhance the effect of enoxaparin:
  - aspirin
  - clopidogrel
  - dipyridamole
  - NSAIDs.
- *ACEIs*—increased risk of hyperkalaemia.
- *Amiloride*—increased risk of hyperkalaemia.
- *Antihistamines*—possibly reduce anticoagulant effect.
- *Ascorbic acid*—possibly reduces anticoagulant effect.
- *Corticosteroids*—increased risk of GI bleeding.
- *Spironolactone*—increased risk of hyperkalaemia.
- *SSRIs*—increased risk of bleeding.

⚖ Dose

Treatment of DVT and PE

- Usual dose 1.5mg/kg (or 150 units/kg) daily, administered by SC injection.
- Patients usually start oral anticoagulation at the same time and continue both until INR is within the target range. This generally takes 5 days. However, cancer patients unsuitable for oral anticoagulation may require long-term treatment with LMWH. Treatment is occasionally continued indefinitely.

Prophylaxis of DVT and PE

- For medical prophylaxis (including immobile cancer patients), 40mg (4000 units) SC OD, usually for no more than 14 days. Graduated compression stockings should be considered if LMWH is contraindicated.
- For surgical prophylaxis:
  - moderate risk—20mg (2000 units) before procedure and each day for 7–10 days or longer (until mobilized)
  - high risk—40mg (4000 units) before procedure and each day for 7–10 days or longer (until mobilized).

⸫ Dose adjustments

Elderly

- Usual adult doses recommended.

Hepatic/renal impairment

- No specific guidance is available for patients with hepatic impairment. The manufacturer advices caution because of an increased risk of bleeding.
- No dosage adjustments are recommended in patients with moderate renal impairment (CrCl 30–50mL/min) or mild renal impairment (CrCl 50–80mL/min), although careful monitoring is recommended. Dosage adjustments are recommended in patients with severe renal impairment (CrCl <30mL/min). In severe renal impairment where 1.5mg/kg is indicated as a treatment dose, this should be reduced to 1mg/kg, and in prophylaxis, 40mg once daily should be reduced to 20mg once daily.

Additional information

- The risk of heparin-induced thrombocytopenia is low with LMWH but may occur after 5–10 days. If there is a 50% reduction of the platelet count, LMWH should be stopped.

⊕ Pharmacology

Enoxaparin is a low molecular weight heparin produced from porcine-derived sodium heparin. It acts mainly through its potentiation of the inhibition of Factor Xa and thrombin by antithrombin. Enoxaparin is eliminated primarily via the kidneys, hence the need for dose adjustments in renal impairment. Local protocols may help to indicate when treatment of palliative care patients with enoxaparin is appropriate.

Erlotinib

Tarceva® (POM)
Tablet: 25mg (30); 100mg (30); 150mg (30)

Indications
- Non-small-cell lung cancer
- Pancreatic cancer (in combination with gemcitabine)

Contraindications and precautions
- Avoid erlotinib in patients with severe hepatic and renal impairment (CrCl <15mL/min)
- Avoid concurrent use of the following drugs (see 📖 *Drug interactions*, p.167)
  - PPIs and H$_2$ antagonists
  - CYP3A4 inducers/inhibitors.
- There is an increased risk of GI perforation associated with erlotinib. Use with caution in patients with a history of peptic ulcer disease, or concurrent use of NSAIDs or corticosteroids.
- Patients with Gilbert's syndrome (a genetic glucuronidation disorder) may develop increased unconjugated bilirubin plasma concentrations because erlotinib is a potent inhibitor of UGT1A1 (a UDP glucurono-syltransferase isoenzyme).
- Use cautiously in patients with pre-existing liver disease or concomitant hepatotoxic drugs (periodic LFTs recommended).
- Smokers should be encouraged to discontinue smoking since the metabolism of erlotinib is increased (CYP1A2 induction) and plasma concentrations will be reduced.

☹ Undesirable effects
Very common
- Abdominal pain
- Alopecia
- Anorexia
- Conjunctivitis
- Cough
- Depression
- Diarrhoea
- Dry skin
- Dyspepsia
- Dyspnoea
- Fatigue
- Flatulence
- Headache
- Infection
- Nausea
- Peripheral neuropathy
- Rash
- Stomatitis
- Vomiting

Common
- Epistaxis
- GI bleeding (often associated with NSAID or warfarin co-administration)
- Keratitis
- Raised LFTs

Moderate or severe diarrhoea should be treated with loperamide and a dose reduction in steps of 50mg should be considered. Erlotinib treatment should be interrupted if severe or persistent diarrhoea, nausea, anorexia, or vomiting associated with dehydration develops.

Patients who develop a rash should use an emollient regularly. Consider the use of topical hydrocortisone 1% if the rash persists. Patients can develop a pustular rash, but topical antibiotic or acne formulations are not recommended, unless on the advice of a microbiologist. The rash may worsen on exposure to direct sunlight. Patients should use sunscreen or protective clothing in sunny weather. Patients who develop a rash may have a longer overall survival compared with patients who do not develop a rash. Patients who do not develop a rash after 4–8 weeks of treatment should be reviewed.

Drug interactions
Pharmacokinetic
- Erlotinib is metabolized mainly by CYP3A4, although CYP1A2 is also involved. Erlotinib is a moderate inhibitor of CYP3A4 and CYP2C8; it is also a potent inhibitor of UGT1A1 and a substrate of P-gp, although the clinical significance of this is unknown.
- *Antacids*—take at least 4 hours before or 2 hours after erlotinib.
- *Ciprofloxacin*—plasma concentration of erlotinib may increase (dose may need reducing if undesirable effects develop).
- H_2 *antagonists*—take erlotinib at least 2 hours before or 10 hours after H_2 antagonist.
- *PPIs*—avoid combination as bioavailability of erlotinib can be significantly reduced.
- Concomitant administration of CYP3A4 and CYP2C8 substrates is unlikely to cause significant interactions. However, concomitant administration of other inhibitors will be additive in effect and may cause problems with drugs that have a narrow therapeutic index.
- The clinical significance of co-administration with CYP3A4 inducers or inhibitors (📖 end cover) is unknown. The prescriber should be aware of the potential for interactions and that dose adjustments may be necessary.
- Avoid grapefruit juice as it may increase the bioavailability of erlotinib through inhibition of intestinal CYP3A4.

Pharmacodynamic
- None known

🥄 Dose
Non-small-cell lung cancer
- 150mg PO OD taken at least 1 hour before or 2 hours after the ingestion of food.

Pancreatic cancer
- 100mg PO OD taken at least 1 hour before or 2 hours after the ingestion of food.

,♌ Dose adjustments

Elderly
- No dose adjustments necessary.

Hepatic/renal impairment
- No specific guidance is available. Use with caution in patients with mild to moderate hepatic impairment; avoid in patients with severe hepatic impairment.
- No dose adjustments are necessary for patients with mild to moderate renal impairment; avoid in patients with severe renal impairment (CrCl <15mL/min).

⟳ Pharmacology

Erlotinib is a human epidermal growth factor receptor type 1/epidermal growth factor receptor (HER1/EGFR) tyrosine kinase inhibitor. It inhibits the intracellular phosphorylation of tyrosine kinase associated with EGFR which causes cell stasis and/or death. Erlotinib is metabolized mainly by CYP3A4, and to a lesser extent CYP1A2, to several active metabolites and it is predominantly excreted in the faeces.

Erythromycin

Erymax® (POM)
Capsule: 250mg (28; 112)

Erythrocin® (POM)
Tablet: 250mg (28); 500mg (28)

Erythroped® (POM)
Oral suspension (*as powder for reconstitution, sugar-free*): 125mg/5mL (140mL); 250mg/5mL (140mL); 500mg/5mL (140mL).

Erythroped A® (POM)
Tablet: 500mg (28)

Generic (POM)
Tablet: 250mg (28); 500mg (28)
Capsule: 250mg (28)
Oral suspension (*as powder for reconstitution*): 125mg/5mL (100mL); 250mg/5mL (100mL); 500mg/5mL (100mL)
Note: *Sugar-free formulations are available*
Injection: 1g

Indications
- Refer to local guidelines
- Broad-spectrum antibiotic indicated for the treatment of commonly occurring bacterial infections
- ¥ Pro-kinetic agent

Contraindications and precautions
- Because of the risk of QT prolongation and cardiac arrhythmias, concurrent use of the following drugs is contraindicated:
  - amisulpride
  - astemizole
  - ergotamine
  - mizolastine
  - pimozide
  - sertindole
  - simvastatin
  - terfenadine
  - tolterodine.
- Erythromycin should be avoided in patients with acute porphyria.
- Electrolyte disturbances (e.g. hypokalaemia) must be corrected because of the risk of QT prolongation.
- Erythromycin should be used with caution in patients with hepatic and/ or renal impairment (see 📖 *Dose adjustments,* p.171).
- Avoid grapefruit juice as it may increase the bioavailability of erythromycin through inhibition of intestinal CYP3A4.

☹ Undesirable effects

- Abdominal discomfort
- Abnormal LFTs
- Arrhythmias
- Cholestatic jaundice
- Confusion
- Diarrhoea (antibiotic-associated colitis reported)
- Nausea
- Pancreatitis
- Reversible hearing loss (reported after large doses by IV infusion)
- Urticaria
- Vomiting

Drug interactions

Pharmacokinetic

- Erythromycin is metabolized by CYP3A4; it is also a strong inhibitor of CYP3A4.
- It may raise the plasma concentration of many drugs through enzyme inhibition. Several interactions are listed below, but see 📖 end cover for a list of drugs that may potentially be affected.
- *Alfentanil*—increased risk of alfentanil toxicity; dose reduction may be necessary.
- *Carbamazepine*—risk of carbamazepine toxicity (avoid combination or monitor closely).
- *Fentanyl*—increased risk of fentanyl toxicity; dose reduction may be necessary.
- *Midazolam*—increased risk of midazolam toxicity; use lower initial doses. Dose adjustments may be necessary if erythromycin is added or discontinued.
- *Theophylline*—risk of theophylline toxicity; dose reduction may be necessary.
- *Warfarin*—risk of raised INR.
- *Zopiclone*—increased plasma concentration and effects of zopiclone.
- The clinical significance of co-administration with other substrates of CYP3A4 (📖 end cover) is unknown. Caution is advised if erythromycin is co-administered with drugs that are predominantly metabolized by this isoenzyme. The prescriber should be aware of the potential for interactions and that dosage adjustments may be necessary, particularly of drugs with a narrow therapeutic index.
- The clinical significance of co-administration with CYP3A4 inducers or inhibitors (📖 end cover) is unknown. The prescriber should be aware of the potential for interactions and that dosage adjustments may be necessary.

Pharmacodynamic

- Erythromycin has been associated with prolongation of the QT interval. There is a potential risk that co-administration with other drugs that also prolong the QT interval (e.g. amiodarone, amitriptyline, haloperidol, quinine) may result in ventricular arrhythmias.

Dose
Antimicrobial
- Standard doses are described here. Refer to local guidelines for specific advice.
- Usual dose 250–500mg PO QDS (6 hourly) or 0.5–1g BD (12 hourly).
- Maximum oral dose is 4g daily in divided doses.
- Administered by continuous IV infusion, 50mg/kg daily, or by intermittent infusion 6 hourly.

¥ *Prokinetic effect*
- Initial dose 250mg PO or IV infusion BD. The dose can be increased if necessary to achieve the desired response.

Dose adjustments
Elderly
- Usual adult doses can be used.

Hepatic/renal impairment
- No specific guidance available. In hepatic impairment, the manufacturer advises caution since erythromycin has been associated with increased liver enzymes and/or cholestatic hepatitis.
- No specific guidance is available for patients with renal impairment. In severe impairment, it is suggested that a dose reduction of up to 50% should be made.

Additional information
- Once reconstituted, the **oral solution** must be discarded after 7 days.
- To reconstitute the **injection**, add 20mL *WFI* to each 1g vial to give a solution of 50mg/mL. This solution must be further diluted prior to administration as follows:
  - dilute 20mL of the reconstituted erythromycin (50mg/mL) with at least 200mL NaCl 0.9% and administer over 20–60 minutes
  - for the prokinetic effect, dilute 5mL of the reconstituted erythromycin (250mg) to at least 50mL with NaCl 0.9% and infuse over 20 minutes

Pharmacology
Erythromycin is a broad-spectrum bacteriostatic macrolide antibiotic. It acts by penetrating the bacterial cell membrane and reversibly binding to ribosomes during cell division, resulting in suppression of protein synthesis. It diffuses readily into most body fluids. Erythromycin is extensively metabolized by CYP3A4, with only 5% being excreted unchanged in the urine.

Esomeprazole

Nexlum® (POM)
Tablet: 20mg (28); 40mg (28)
IV injection/infusion: 40mg

Indications
- Gastro-oesophageal reflux disease.
- Treatment and prophylaxis of NSAID-associated peptic ulcer disease.

Contraindications and precautions
- Do not administer with atazanavir or erlotinib.
- Treatment with esomeprazole may lead to a slightly increased risk of developing GI infections (e.g. *Clostridium difficile*). Therefore avoid unnecessary use or high doses.
- Rebound acid hypersecretion may occur on discontinuation if the patient has received more than 8 weeks treatment.

☺ Undesirable effects
Common
- Abdominal pain
- Constipation
- Diarrhoea
- Flatulence
- Headache
- Nausea/vomiting

Uncommon
- Dermatitis
- Dizziness
- Drowsiness
- Dry mouth
- Paraesthesia
- Peripheral oedema
- Pruritus
- Raised liver enzymes
- Rash
- Urticaria
- Vertigo

Rare
- Agitation
- Alopecia
- Arthralgia
- Bronchospasm
- Confusion
- Depression
- Hepatitis with or without jaundice
- Hyponatraemia
- Leukopenia
- Photosensitivity

- Taste disturbance
- Thrombocytopenia

Drug interactions

Pharmacokinetic

- Esomeprazole is metabolized by CYP2C19 (major) and CYP3A4 (minor). It may inhibit CYP2C19.
- Drugs with pH-dependent absorption can be affected:
  - *Atazanavir*—avoid combination due to substantially reduced absorption
  - *Digoxin*—increased plasma concentrations possible
  - *Erlotinib*—avoid combination as bioavailability of erlotinib can be significantly reduced
  - *Ketoconazole/Itraconazole*—risk of sub-therapeutic plasma concentrations
  - *Metronidazole suspension*—esomeprazole may reduce/prevent the absorption of metronidazole.
- *Azole antifungals*—fluconazole may cause increased esomeprazole concentrations (CYP2C19 inhibition).
- *Citalopram*—esomeprazole can increase the plasma concentration of citalopram through inhibition of CYP2C19.
- *Clarithromycin*—inhibition of CYP3A4 metabolism can lead to increased esomeprazole concentrations.
- *Clopidogrel*—antiplatelet action may be reduced (avoid combination).
- *Diazepam*—plasma concentrations of diazepam can be increased through inhibition of CYP2C19.
- The clinical significance of co-administration with CYP2C19 inducers or inhibitors (🕮 end cover) is unknown. The prescriber should be aware of the potential for interactions and that dosage adjustments may be necessary.
- The clinical significance of co-administration with CYP3A4 inducers or inhibitors (🕮 end cover) is unknown. The prescriber should be aware of the potential for interactions and that dosage adjustments may be necessary.
- The clinical significance of co-administration of CYP2C19 substrates (🕮 end cover) is unknown. Caution is advised if esomeprazole is co-administered with drugs that are predominantly metabolized by CYP2C19. The prescriber should be aware of the potential for interactions and that dosage adjustments may be necessary, particularly of drugs with a narrow therapeutic index.

Pharmacodynamic

- No clinically significant interactions noted.

⚕ Dose

Gastro-oesophageal reflux disease

- With oesophagitis, initial dose 40mg PO OD for 4 weeks. Continue for a further 4 weeks if not fully healed or symptoms persist.
- Alternatively, in patients unable to tolerate oral therapy, 40mg IV or IV infusion OD.
- Maintenance dose 20mg PO OD.

- In the absence of oesophagitis, initial dose 20mg PO OD for up to 4 weeks.
- Alternatively, in patients unable to tolerate oral therapy, 20mg IV or IV infusion OD.
- Maintenance dose 20mg PO OD PRN.

Treatment of NSAID-associated gastric ulcer
- Initial dose 20mg PO OD for 4–8 weeks.
- Alternatively, in patients unable to tolerate oral therapy, 20mg IV or IV infusion OD.

Prophylaxis of NSAID-associated peptic ulcer disease
- 20mg PO OD.
- Alternatively, in patients unable to tolerate oral therapy, 20mg IV or IV infusion OD.

Dose adjustments
Elderly
- Dose adjustments are not necessary in the elderly.

Hepatic/renal impairment
- In liver impairment, the dose should not exceed 20mg OD.
- Dosage adjustments are not required for patients with renal impairment.

Additional information
- The tablet can be dispersed in water to form a suspension of enteric-coated granules. The solution can be swallowed, or administered via a feeding tube.
- Injection should be administered over at least 3 minutes.
- IV infusion should be administered over a period of 10–30 minutes.

Pharmacology
Esomeprazole is the S-isomer of omeprazole. It is a proton pump inhibitor that suppresses gastric acid secretion in a dose-related manner by specific inhibition of the H^+/K^+-ATPase in the gastric parietal cell. Esomeprazole is rapidly absorbed orally, with a bioavailability of 89% after repeated dosing. It is completely metabolized by the liver, with CYP2C19 being involved in the major metabolic pathway. CYP3A4 is also involved in the metabolism of esomeprazole, but to a lesser extent. The major metabolites of esomeprazole are inactive.

Etamsylate

Dicynene® (POM)
Tablet: 500mg (100)

Indications
- ⚹ Prophylaxis and control of haemorrhages from small blood vessels.

Contraindications and precautions
- Contraindicated for use in patients with porphyria.
- Avoid in patients with wheat allergy (tablet contains wheat starch).
- Discontinue treatment if the patient develops a fever.

☺ Undesirable effects
The frequency is not defined, but reported undesirable effects include:
- Diarrhoea
- Fever
- Headaches
- Nausea
- Skin rashes
- Vomiting

Drug interactions
Pharmacokinetic
- No clinically important interactions.

Pharmacodynamic
- No clinically important interactions.

Dose
- 500mg PO QDS.
- Take after food if symptoms such as nausea and vomiting occur.

Dose adjustments
Elderly
- No specific dose reductions stated.

Hepatic/renal impairment
- No specific dose reductions stated.

Additional information
- Tablets can be dispersed in water prior to administration.

Pharmacology
Etamsylate is a non-hormonal agent which reduces capillary exudation and blood loss. It does not affect normal coagulation since it has no effect on prothrombin times, fibrinolysis, platelet count or function. Although the exact mechanism is unknown, etamsylate is believed to increase capillary vascular wall resistance, platelet adhesiveness through inhibition of the synthesis and action of prostaglandins that cause platelet disaggregation, vasodilation and increased capillary permeability.

Etamsylate is well absorbed orally and excreted via the kidneys unchanged.

Etoricoxib

Arcoxia® (POM)

Tablet: 30mg (28); 60mg (28); 90mg (28); 120mg (7)

Indications

- Pain and inflammation in osteoarthritis, rheumatoid arthritis, and anky-
  losing spondylitis.
- Acute gout.
- * Pain associated with cancer.

Contraindications and precautions

- Etoricoxib is contraindicated for use in patients with:
  - active peptic ulceration or GI bleeding
  - congestive heart failure (NYHA II–IV)
  - established ischaemic heart disease, peripheral arterial disease,
    and/or cerebrovascular disease
  - hypersensitivity reactions to ibuprofen, aspirin or other NSAIDs
    (including COX-2 inhibitors)
  - hypertension persistently elevated above 140/90mmHg which has
    not been adequately controlled
  - inflammatory bowel disease
  - severe hepatic dysfunction (serum albumin <25g/L or Child–Pugh
    score ≥10)
  - severe renal impairment (estimated renal CrCl <30mL/min).
- Use the minimum effective dose for the shortest duration necessary in
  order to reduce the risk of cardiac and GI events.
- Elderly patients are more at risk of developing undesirable effects.
- Treatment should be reviewed after **two weeks**. In the absence of
  benefit, other options should be considered.
- Use with caution in the following circumstances:
  - concurrent use of diuretics, corticosteroids and NSAIDs (see 📖
    Drug interactions, p.177)
  - congestive heart failure and/or left ventricular dysfunction
  - diabetes mellitus
  - established ischaemic heart disease, peripheral arterial disease,
    and/or cerebrovascular disease need careful consideration because
    of the increased risk of thrombotic events
  - hepatic impairment
  - hyperlipidaemia
  - hypertension (particularly uncontrolled)
  - prior history of GI disease
  - recovery from surgery
  - renal impairment
  - smoking.
- Etoricoxib may prevent the development of signs and symptoms of
  inflammation/infection (e.g. fever).
- Discontinue treatment at the first appearance of skin rash, mucosal
  lesions, or any other sign of hypersensitivity.

- Consider co-prescription of misoprostol or a proton pump inhibitor if:
  - long-term NSAID therapy
  - concurrent use of drugs that increase the risk of GI toxicity (see 📖 Drug interactions, p.177).
- For further information, including selection, refer to 📖 Selection of an NSAID, p.31.
- Etoricoxib may modify reactions and patients should be advised not to drive (or operate machinery) if affected.

☺ Undesirable effects

Common

- Abdominal pain
- Altered liver enzymes (raised ALT/AST)
- Diarrhoea
- Dizziness
- Dyspepsia
- Ecchymosis
- Flatulence
- Headache
- Heartburn
- Nausea
- Oedema
- Palpitations

Uncommon

- Anxiety
- Cerebrovascular accident
- Congestive heart failure
- Cough
- Depression
- Drowsiness
- Dry mouth
- Dysgeusia
- Dyspnoea
- Gastroduodenal ulcer
- Infection (e.g. gastroenteritis, upper respiratory infection, urinary tract infection)
- Insomnia
- Myocardial infarction
- Pruritus
- Transient ischaemic attack
- Visual disturbances

Drug interactions

Pharmacokinetic

- Metabolized primarily by CYP3A4.
- The clinical significance of co-administration with CYP3A4 inducers or inhibitors (📖 end cover) is unknown. The prescriber should be aware of the potential for interactions and that dosage adjustments may be necessary.
- Avoid excessive amounts of grapefruit juice as it may increase the bio-availability of etoricoxib through inhibition of intestinal CYP3A4.

Pharmacodynamic

- *Anticoagulants*—increased risk of bleeding
- *Antihypertensives*—reduced hypotensive effect
- *Antiplatelet drugs*—increased risk of bleeding
- *Ciclosporin*—increased risk of nephrotoxicity
- *Corticosteroids*—increased risk of GI toxicity
- *Diuretics*—reduced diuretic effect
- *Rosiglitazone*—increased risk of oedema
- *SSRIs*—increased risk of GI bleeding.

₅ Dose

Osteoarthritis
- 30mg PO OD increased to 60mg PO OD as necessary.

Rheumatoid arthritis/ankylosing spondylitis
- 90mg PO OD.

Acute gout
- 120mg PO OD for 8 days.

¥ *Pain associated with cancer:*
- Initial dose 60mg PO OD, increased as necessary to 120mg PO OD (NB: risk of serious events increases with dose and duration). If no benefit after **two weeks** discontinue treatment and review.

₅ Dose adjustments

Elderly
- Usual adult doses recommended. Note that the elderly are particularly susceptible to undesirable effects. Use the lowest effective dose for the shortest duration possible.

Hepatic/renal impairment
- In patients with mild hepatic impairment (Child–Pugh score 5–6) 60mg PO OD should not be exceeded. In patients with moderate hepatic impairment (Child–Pugh score 7–9), 60mg on alternate days should not be exceeded; administration of 30mg PO OD can also be considered. Etoricoxib is contraindicated in patients with severe hepatic impairment.
- Use of etoricoxib in patients with severe renal impairment is contraindicated. No dosage adjustment is necessary for patients with CrCl ≥30mL/min.

Additional information

- Etoricoxib tablets may be dispersed in water prior to administration.

⊕ Pharmacology

Like traditional NSAIDs, the mechanism of action of etoricoxib is believed to be due to inhibition of prostaglandin synthesis. However, unlike most NSAIDs, etoricoxib is a selective non-competitive inhibitor of COX-2. It has no effect on platelet aggregation. Etoricoxib is well absorbed orally, with an absolute bioavailability of 100%. It is extensively metabolized, with CYP3A4 being the major isoenzyme involved. Some of the metabolites are weakly active COX-2 inhibitors, the rest have no appreciable action. Less than 1% of the total dose is excreted unchanged in the urine.

Exemestane

Aromasin® (POM)
Tablet: 25mg (30; 90)

Indications
- Adjuvant treatment of oestrogen-receptor-positive early breast cancer in postmenopausal women following 2–3 years of tamoxifen therapy.
- Advanced breast cancer in postmenopausal women in whom anti-oestrogen therapy has failed.

Contraindications and precautions
- Not to be used in premenopausal women.
- Use with caution in patients with hepatic or renal impairment.
- May cause reduction in bone mineral density and an increased fracture rate. Women with osteoporosis or at risk of osteoporosis should have their bone mineral density formally assessed and treatment should be initiated in at-risk patients.
- Exemestane may modify reactions and patients should be advised not to drive (or operate machinery) if affected.

☺ Undesirable effects
Very common
- Fatigue
- Headache
- Hot flushes
- Increased sweating
- Insomnia
- Musculoskeletal pain
- Nausea

Common
- Anorexia
- Carpal tunnel syndrome
- Depression
- Dizziness
- Dyspepsia
- Fracture
- Osteoporosis
- Peripheral oedema

Uncommon
- Asthenia
- Drowsiness

Drug interactions

Pharmacokinetic

- Metabolized by CYP3A4.
- The clinical significance of co-administration with CYP3A4 inhibitors or inducers (📖 end cover) is unknown. The prescriber should be aware of the potential for interactions and that dosage adjustments may be necessary.
- The effect of grapefruit juice on the absorption of exemestane is unknown.

Pharmacodynamic

- *Oestrogens*—may antagonize the effect of exemestane.

🦴 Dose

- 25mg PO OD, after food.

🦴 Dose adjustments

Elderly

- Dose adjustments are unnecessary.

Hepatic/renal impairment

- No dose adjustments are required for patients with liver or renal impairment.

Additional information

- In patients with early breast cancer, treatment should continue until completion of 5 years of combined sequential adjuvant hormonal therapy (tamoxifen followed by exemestane), or earlier if tumour relapse occurs.
- In patients with advanced breast cancer, treatment should continue until tumour progression is evident.

⟿ Pharmacology

Exemestane is an irreversible steroidal aromatase inhibitor which does not possess any progestogenic, androgenic, or oestrogenic activity. It reduces oestrogen levels by blocking the action of aromatase in the adrenal glands.

Fentanyl

It is not possible to ensure the interchangeability of different makes of fentanyl transdermal patches in individual patients. Also note that the transmucosal tablet formulations are not identical, and changing from one product to another will require a new dose titration. Therefore it is recommended that patients should remain on the same product once treatment has been stabilized. Inclusion of the brand name on the prescription is suggested.

Standard release

Abstral® (CD POM)
Sublingual tablet: 100mcg (10; 30); 200mcg (10; 30); 300mcg (10; 30); 400mcg (10; 30); 600mcg (30); 800mcg (30).

Actiq® (CD POM)
Lozenge: 200mcg (3; 30); 400mcg (3; 30); 600mcg (3; 30); 800mcg (3; 30); 1200mcg; 1600mcg (3; 30).

Effentora® (CD POM)
Buccal tablet: 100mcg (4); 200mcg (4); 400mcg (4); 600mcg (4); 800mcg (4).

Instanyl® (CD POM)
Nasal spray: 50mcg per spray (10; 20); 100mcg per spray (10; 20); 200mcg per spray (10; 20).

Sublimaze® (CD POM)
Injection: 100mcg/2mL (10); 500mcg/10mL (5).

Modified release

Durogesic DTrans® (CD POM)
Patch *(matrix)*:
12mcg/hr (5)
25mcg/hr (5)
50mcg/hr (5)
75mcg/hr (5)
100mcg/hr (5)

Matrifen® (CD POM)
Patch *(matrix)*:
12mcg/hr (5)
25mcg/hr (5)
50mcg/hr (5)
75mcg/hr (5)
100mcg/hr (5)

Mezolar® (CD POM)
Patch *(matrix)*:
12mcg/hr (5)
25mcg/hr (5)
50mcg/hr (5)
75mcg/hr (5)
100mcg/hr (5)

Fentalis® (CD POM)
Patch *(reservoir)*:
25mcg/hr (5)
50mcg/hr (5)
75mcg/hr (5)
100mcg/hr (5)

Fentanyl is a Schedule 2 controlled drug (see 📖 Legal categories for medicines, p.23 for further information). Independent prescribers are **NOT** authorized to prescribe parenteral or transmucosal fentanyl (📖 Independent prescribing: palliative care issues, p.25).

Indications
- Severe chronic pain (*transdermal*).
- BTcP (*transmucosal*). For guidance relating to BTcP see 📖 Breakthrough cancer pain, p.35.
- * Treatment of severe pain via subcutaneous administration (*parenteral*).
- For end-of-life care issues see 📖 Use of drugs in end-of-life care, p.53.

Contraindications and precautions
- If the dose of an opioid is titrated correctly, it is generally accepted that there are no absolute contraindications to the use of such drugs in palliative care, although there may be circumstances where one opioid is favoured over another (e.g. renal impairment, constipation).
- Nonetheless, manufacturers' contraindications and precautions are described below.
- Fentanyl may modify reactions and patients should be advised not to drive (or operate machinery) if affected.

Transdermal
- Should not be used in opioid-naive patients, or for the treatment of acute or intermittent pain.
- Not recommended for use if the patient has received an MAOI within the previous 2 weeks.
- Use with caution in patients with:
  - severe respiratory disease
  - concurrent CYP3A4 inhibitors (see 📖 *Drug interactions*, p.184)
  - bradyarrhythmias
  - hepatic impairment—empirical dose adjustment may be necessary (see 📖 *Dose adjustments*)
  - pyrexia (increased fentanyl delivery rate).
- Patients should be advised to avoid exposing the patch application site to direct heat sources such as hot-water bottles, electric blankets, heat lamps, saunas, or baths because of the risk of increased fentanyl absorption.
- Patients who experience serious adverse events should have the patches removed immediately and should be monitored for up to 24 hours after patch removal.

Transmucosal
- Contraindicated for use in:
  - opioid-naive patients
  - previous facial radiotherapy (Instanyl®)
  - recurrent episodes of epistaxis (Instanyl®)
  - severe respiratory disease.
- Not recommended for use if the patient has received an MAOI within the previous 2 weeks.

- Patient's background analgesia must be stabilized before use (otherwise the patient does not have BTcP).
- Avoid concomitant use of a nasal vasoconstrictor with Instanyl® (see 📖 *Drug interactions*, p.184).
- Avoid concomitant use of other nasally administered medicinal products (effect on Instanyl® unknown).
- Use with caution in the following:
  - concurrent use of CYP3A4 inhibitors (see 📖 *Drug interactions*, p.184)
  - diabetic patients (Actiq® lozenges contain 1.89g glucose per dose)
  - elderly (see *Dose adjustments*)
  - head injury and/or raised intracranial pressure
  - hepatic impairment
  - oral lesions (absorption of fentanyl may be affected from oral formulations)
  - recurrent episodes of epistaxis or nasal discomfort (Instanyl®).
- Ensure good oral hygiene in order to prevent tooth damage (Actiq®).
- *Effentora*® 100mcg tablets contain 8mg of sodium (0.3mmol); the 200, 400, 600, and 800mcg tablets each contain 16mg of sodium (0.6mmol).

Parenteral
- No specific contraindications if being used for end-of-life care via CSCI.
- Dose adjustments may be necessary if CYP3A4 inducers or inhibitors are used concurrently.

☺ Undesirable effects
- Strong opioids tend to cause similar undesirable effects, albeit to varying degrees. See also 📖 Morphine, p.340.

Very common
- Constipation
- Drowsiness
- Dizziness
- Fatigue (*transmucosal*)
- Headache
- Insomnia
- Mouth ulcers (*transmucosal*)
- Nausea
- Pruritus
- Sweating
- Vomiting

Common
- Anorexia (*transdermal*)
- Anxiety
- Application site skin reactions (*transderma—consider alternative patch*)
- Confusion
- Depression
- Dry mouth
- Dyspepsia
- Dysphagia (*transmucosal*)
- Hallucinations
- Myoclonus

- Reduced appetite
- Stomatitis (*transmucosal*)

Uncommon
- Agitation
- Amnesia
- Bradycardia
- Diarrhoea
- Dyspnoea
- Euphoria
- Paraesthesia
- Speech disturbances
- Tremor
- Urinary retention

Rare
- Arrhythmia
- Hiccups
- Vasodilatation

Drug interactions

Pharmacokinetic
- Fentanyl is metabolized by CYP3A4.
- Fentanyl should be used with caution if CYP3A4 inhibitors are co-prescribed because of the increased risk of extended therapeutic effects and undesirable effects. Alterations in intestinal CYP3A4 activity (induction or inhibition) appear to have little influence on *transmucosal* fentanyl absorption, or onset of effect. Nonetheless, since a significant proportion (approximately 75%) is swallowed and its systemic clearance may be decreased by CYP3A4 inhibitors, caution is required with co-administration.
- *Carbamazepine*—patient may need higher doses of fentanyl if carbamazepine is introduced to treatment

The clinical significance of co-administration with other CYP3A4 inducers (📖 end cover) is unknown. The prescriber should be aware of the potential for interactions and that dosage adjustments may be necessary.

Pharmacodynamic
- *Antihypertensives*—increased risk of hypotension.
- *CNS depressants*—risk of excessive sedation.
- *Haloperidol*—may be an additive hypotensive effect.
- *Ketamine*—there is a potential opioid-sparing effect with ketamine and concurrent transdermal fentanyl use is not recommended; however, an empirical fentanyl dose reduction of 25–50% at least 12 hours *before* starting ketamine is suggested (additional opioid requirements can be treated using PRN analgesia).
- *Levomepromazine*—may be an additive hypotensive effect.
- *Nasal vasoconstrictors*—can reduce effect of Instanyl®.

⏛ Dose

Transdermal

- Initial dosage of fentanyl is based upon previous opioid requirements. Refer to ⏛ Opioid substitution, p.33 for information regarding opioid dose equivalences. Table 3.4 serves as a suggestion and differs from the guidance advised by the manufacturers.

Table 3.4 Suggested oral opioid dose equivalences

Morphine (mg/day)	Oxycodone (mg/day)	Transdermal fentanyl (mcg/hr)
30	20	12
60	40	25
120	80	50
180	120	75
240	160	100
300	200	125
360	240	150
400	260	162–175
490	320	200
540	340	225
600	400	250
660	440	275
720	480	300
840	560	350*
960	640	400*
1080	720	450*

*Manufacturer recommends that above doses of 300mcg/hr, alternative or additional method analgesia should be used.

Transmucosal

Products are licensed for use in patients taking at least 60mg oral morphine per day, or equivalent (see ⏛ Opioid substitution, p.33 for information regarding opioid dose equivalences), for a week or longer. The effective dose of transmucosal formulations for BTcP is not predictable from the daily maintenance dose of opioid, and titration to an effective dose is necessary.

Abstral®

- No more than two sublingual tablets should be used for a single episode of BTcP.

Table 3.5 Titration schedule for Abstral®

Dose of first Abstral® tablet per episode of BTcP (mcg)	Dose of additional Abstral® tablet to be taken 15–30min after first tablet, if required (mcg)
100	100
200	100
300	100
400	200
600	200
800	–

- During titration, if adequate analgesia is not obtained within 15–30 minutes of using the first sublingual tablet, a second tablet may be used as shown in Table 3.5.
- Doses above 800mcg have not been evaluated.
- Maintain the patient on the dose established during titration. This may be more than one tablet per BTcP incident.
- Abstral® is licensed to be given for **four** episodes of BTcP per day. If more than four episodes of BTcP occur in a day for more than four consecutive days, review background analgesia and consider re-evaluating the dosing schedule.
- May discontinue abruptly if no longer required and the patient continues to receive chronic opioid treatment.

Actiq®

- During titration, if adequate analgesia is not obtained within 15 minutes of using the first lozenge, a second lozenge of the same strength may be used.
- If signs of excessive opioid effects appear before the lozenge is fully consumed, it should be removed immediately and the dose should be reviewed.
- No more than two lozenges should be used to treat a single episode of BTcP.
- Table 3.6 illustrates the titration schedule. At 1600mcg, a second dose is only likely to be required by a minority of patients.
- Maintain the patient on the dose established during titration.
- Actiq® is licensed to be given for **four** episodes of BTcP per day. If more than four episodes of BTcP occur in a day for more than four consecutive days, review background analgesia and consider re-evaluating the dosing schedule.
- May discontinue abruptly if no longer required and the patient continues to receive chronic opioid treatment.

Table 3.6 Titration schedule for Actiq®

Dose of first Actiq® lozenge per episode of BTcP (mcg)	Dose of additional Actiq® lozenge to be taken 15min after first lozenge, if required (mcg)
200	200
400	400
600	600
800	800
1200	1200
1600	1600

Effentora®

- During titration, if adequate analgesia is not obtained within 30 minutes of using the first buccal tablet, a second tablet of the same strength may be used.
- No more than two tablets should be used to treat any individual BTcP episode, **except** during titration as described below.
- The manufacturer recommends using up to **four** 100 or 200 mcg tablets to treat a single episode of BTcP during titration.
- Table 3.7 illustrates the titration schedule.
- Doses above 800mcg have not been evaluated.
- Patients should wait at least 4 hours before treating another BTcP episode with Effentora® during titration or maintenance therapy. If more than four episodes of BTcP occur in a day for more than four consecutive days, review background analgesia and consider re-evaluating the dosing schedule.
- May discontinue abruptly if no longer required and the patient continues to receive chronic opioid treatment.

Table 3.7 Titration schedule for Effentora®

Dose of first Effentora® buccal tablet per episode of BTcP (mcg)	Dose of additional Effentora® buccal tablet to be taken 30min after first tablet, if required (mcg)
100	100
200	200
400	200
600	200
800	–

Instanyl®

- During titration, if adequate analgesia is not obtained after 10 minutes, an additional dose of the same strength can be administered.
- No more than two doses should be used to treat any individual BTcP episode.

- Patients should wait at least 4 hours before treating another break-through pain episode with Instanyl® during both titration and maintenance therapy.
- Table 3.8 illustrates the titration schedule.

Table 3.8 Titration schedule for Instanyl®

Dose of first Instanyl® nasal spray per episode of BTcP (mcg)	Dose of additional Instanyl® nasal spray to be used 10min after first dose, if required (mcg)
50	50
100	100
200	200
400	–

- Instanyl® is licensed to be given for **four** episodes of BTcP per day. If more than four episodes of BTcP occur in a day for more than four consecutive days, review background analgesia and consider re-evaluating the dosing schedule.
- May discontinue abruptly if no longer required and the patient continues to receive chronic opioid treatment.

Parenteral
- ✱ For CSCI, dose is based on previous opioid requirements (see 📖 Opioid substitution, p.33 for information regarding opioid dose equivalences).
- Given the volume of injection, fentanyl is unlikely to be administered by SC injection and use in CSCI will be uncommon.

🔧 Dose adjustments
Elderly
- No specific guidance available. Dose requirements should be individually titrated.

Hepatic/renal impairment
- No specific guidance available. Dose requirements should be individually titrated.

Additional information
- Opioid withdrawal symptoms (e.g. nausea, vomiting, diarrhoea, anxiety, and shivering) can occur in patients after switching from previously prescribed opioids to a fentanyl patch. This is because the majority of the opioid dose is entering the CNS, creating a withdrawal situation in the periphery. Patients can be administered immediate-release morphine or oxycodone to treat these symptoms if warranted.

Transdermal
- The analgesic effect should not be evaluated until the patch has been worn for at least 24 hours (to allow for the gradual increase in

plasma-fentanyl concentration). Steady-state plasma concentrations of fentanyl are generally achieved in 36–48h, and the patient should be encouraged to use PRN doses during the initial 72 hours (to ameliorate potential withdrawal symptoms). If necessary, the dose should be adjusted at 72-hour intervals in steps of 12–25mcg/hr.

- The following is a guide on how to initiate the patch in relation to previous opioid therapy:
  - 4-hourly hydromorphone/morphine/oxycodone—give regular 4-hourly doses for the first 12 hours after applying the patch
  - 12-hourly hydromorphone/morphine/oxycodone—give the final oral dose at the same time as applying the first patch
  - 24-hourly morphine—apply the patch 12 hours after the final oral dose
  - CSCI—continue the syringe driver for the first 12 hours after applying the patch
- When converting from hydromorphone, morphine, or oxycodone to fentanyl, the dose of any laxative should be halved and subsequently adjusted according to need.
- High quantities of fentanyl remain in the transdermal patches after a 72-hour period. Used transdermal patches should be folded with the adhesive surfaces inwards, covering the release membrane.
- If a CSCI is needed, treatment should continue with the patch and additional analgesic requirements should be managed with suitable doses of rescue medication. Refer to 📖 Opioid substitution, p.33 for information regarding opioid dose equivalences.
- Ensure that patients and caregivers are aware of the signs and symptoms of fentanyl overdose, i.e. sedation, confusion, and feeling faint, dizzy, or confused. Patients and caregivers should be advised to seek medical attention immediately if overdose is suspected.

Transmucosal

- Abstral® sublingual tablets should be administered directly under the tongue and at the deepest part. The patient must not swallow, suck, or chew the tablet, and should not eat or drink anything until the tablet has completely dissolved (happens within less than a minute). Water may be used to moisten the buccal mucosa in patients with a dry mouth.
- Actiq® lozenges should be rubbed against the cheek or sucked, but not chewed. Water may be used to moisten the buccal mucosa in patients with a dry mouth. The lozenge should be consumed within 15 minutes.
- Effentora® buccal tablets should be placed in the upper portion of the buccal cavity (above an upper rear molar between the cheek and gum). The tablet should not be sucked, chewed, or swallowed, and the patient should not eat or drink anything while the tablet is in the mouth. The tablet usually disintegrates within 14–25 minutes; after 30 minutes, the mouth can be rinsed to remove the remnants. Water may be used to moisten the buccal mucosa in patients with a dry mouth.
- Effentora® buccal tablets can be placed sublingually if necessary.
- Fentanyl exposure from Instanyl® is unaffected by the common cold (provided that nasal vasoconstrictors are not co-administered).

- Before using Instanyl® for the first time, the nasal spray must be primed until a fine mist appears; 3–4 actuations of the nasal spray are usually required.
- If the product has not been used for a period of more than 7 days, the nasal spray must be actuated once before the next dose is taken.

Parenteral

- Fentanyl via CSCI is reportedly compatible with dexamethasone, haloperidol, hyoscine hydrobromide, ketorolac, levomepromazine, metoclopramide, midazolam, and ondansetron.

Pharmacology

Fentanyl is a synthetic opioid, chemically related to pethidine, with an action primarily at the μ-receptor. The main route of elimination is hepatic metabolism via CYP3A4 to inactive compounds, which are mainly excreted in the urine. The metabolites of fentanyl are non-toxic and inactive. Fentanyl is a suitable opioid for use in patients with renal failure.

Finasteride

Proscar® (POM)
Tablet: 5mg (28)

Indications
• Benign prostatic hyperplasia (BPH)

Contraindications and precautions
• Finasteride causes a decrease in serum prostate-specific antigen concentrations by approximately 50% in patients with BPH even in the presence of prostate cancer. Reference values may need adjustment.

☺ Undesirable effects
The frequency is not defined, but reported undesirable effects include:
• Decreased libido
• Dizziness
• Gynaecomastia
• Impotence
• Postural hypotension
• Testicular pain
• Weakness

Drug interactions
• Metabolized by CYP3A4, but no clinically important drug interactions have been identified

♪ Dose
• 5mg PO OD.

♪ Dose adjustments
Elderly
• No dosage adjustments necessary.

Hepatic/renal impairment
• There are no specific dose recommendations for use in liver impairment; the manufacturer states there are no data available in patients with hepatic insufficiency.
• Dosage adjustments are unnecessary in patients with renal impairment.

Additional information
• Although tablets may be crushed and dispersed in water prior to administration, this is not recommended because of the risk of exposure.

♦ Pharmacology
Finasteride is a competitive and specific inhibitor of 5 α-reductase, an intracellular enzyme that converts testosterone into the more potent dihydrotestosterone (DHT). Inhibition results in significant decreases in serum and tissue DHT concentrations.

Flucloxacillin

Generic (POM)
Capsule: 250mg (28); 500mg (28)
Oral suspension: (as powder for reconstitution): 125mg/5mL (100mL); 250mg/5mL (100mL)
Injection (as powder for reconstitution): 250mg (10); 500mg (10); 1g (10)

Indications
- Refer to local guidelines.
- Antibiotic indicated for the treatment of infections due to sensitive Gram-positive organisms.

Contraindications and precautions
- Contraindicated for use in patients with penicillin hypersensitivity and with a previous history of flucloxacillin-associated jaundice/hepatic dysfunction.
- Use with caution if:
  - hepatic impairment (greater risk of severe hepatic reaction)
  - patients >50years old
  - renal impairment (see 📖 Dose adjustments, p.193).
- Cholestatic jaundice and hepatitis may occur up to several weeks after treatment with flucloxacillin has been discontinued. Administration for more than 2 weeks and increasing age are risk factors.
- With prolonged treatment, regular monitoring of hepatic and renal function is recommended.

☻ Undesirable effects
Common
- Minor gastrointestinal disturbances

Uncommon
- Rash
- Urticaria

Very rare
- Cholestatic jaundice
- Hepatitis
- Interstitial nephritis
- Pseudomembranous colitis

Drug interactions
Pharmacokinetic
- Oral contraceptives—reduced efficacy

Pharmacodynamic
- None known

₰ Dose

Standard doses are described here. Refer to local guidelines for specific advice.

- 250–500mg PO QDS, at least 30 minutes before food.
- 250mg–1g IV injection or infusion QDS.

₰ Dose adjustments

Elderly

- No dose adjustment necessary.

Hepatic/renal impairment

- No specific guidance is available for use in hepatic impairment. Use the lowest effective dose.
- Patients in severe renal impairment (CrCl <10mL/min) may need dose adjustments. The manufacturer suggests that a reduction in dose or extension of the dose interval should be considered. Standard adult doses should be tolerated; only the high doses for severe infections may need reducing.

Additional information

- Once reconstituted, the **oral solution** must be discarded after 14 days.
- To reconstitute the **injection**, add 5mL WFI to 250mg vial, 10mL WFI to 500mg vial, or 15–20mL WFI to 1g vial.
- Administer IV **injection** over 3–4 minutes; administer IV **infusion** in 50–100mL NaCl 0.9% (or glucose 5%) over 30–60 minutes.

⟴ Pharmacology

Flucloxacillin is a β-lactam antibiotic active against Gram-positive bacteria. It is bactericidal in that it interferes with the synthesis of the bacterial cell wall. As a result, the cell wall is weakened and the bacterium swells and then ruptures. Flucloxacillin is stable against hydrolysis by a variety of β-lactamases.

Fluconazole

Diflucan® (POM)
Capsule: 50mg (7); 150mg (1); 200mg (7)
Suspension: 50mg/5mL (35mL); 200mg/5mL (35mL) (*both supplied as powder for reconstitution with 24mL water*).

Generic (POM)
Capsule: 50mg (7); 150mg (1); 200mg (7).
Note: Capsules may be sold in pharmacies for genital candidiasis in those aged 16–60 years of age at a maximum dose of 150mg.

Indications
- Mucosal candidiasis (including oropharyngeal and oesophageal).
- Genital candidiasis.
- For other fungal infections, seek local microbiological advice.

Contraindications and precautions
- Patients may develop abnormal LFTs during fluconazole therapy. Fluconazole should be discontinued if clinical signs or symptoms consistent with liver disease develop.
- Fluconazole is tenuously associated with prolongation of the QT interval and it should be used with caution in the following circumstances:
  - electrolyte disturbances, e.g. hypokalaemia
  - co-administration drugs that prolong the QT interval (see 🕮 *Drug interactions*, p.194).

☺ Undesirable effects
The frequency is not defined, but commonly reported undesirable effects include:
- Diarrhoea
- Elevated LFTs
- Headache
- Nausea
- Rash

Other reported undesirable effects include:
- Dizziness
- Hepatitis
- Jaundice
- QT prolongation
- Skin reactions (Stevens–Johnson syndrome has been reported)

Drug interactions
Pharmacokinetic
- Fluconazole is a potent inhibitor of both CYP2C9 and CYP2C19; at higher doses (>200mg/day) it inhibits CYP3A4. Interactions are less likely to be clinically relevant with a single-dose course of treatment (e.g. 150mg for genital candidiasis).

- *Alfentanil*—increased opioid effect due to CYP3A4 inhibition.
- *Amitriptyline*—increased risk of adverse effects due to inhibition of metabolism; other factors may be necessary before this interaction becomes significant (e.g. co-administration of other interacting drugs).
- *Calcium-channel blockers*—increased risk of adverse effects due to inhibition of CYP3A4; dose adjustments may be necessary.
- *Carbamazepine*—increase in adverse effects possible due to inhibition of CYP3A4.
- *Celecoxib*—increased plasma levels due to inhibition of CYP2C9; half celecoxib dose if combination necessary.
- *Cyclophosphamide*—possible reduced effect due to a decrease in the formation of active metabolite via CYP2C9.
- *Midazolam*—increased sedative effects due to CYP3A4 inhibition.
- *Rifampicin*—reduces the plasma concentration of fluconazole.
- *Phenytoin*—increases the plasma concentrations of phenytoin; consider alternative treatment or closely monitor phenytoin plasma concentration.
- *Warfarin*—anticoagulant effect potentiated in dose-related manner; patient should be closely monitored and the warfarin dose adjusted accordingly.
- The clinical significance of co-administration with other CYP2C19, CYP2C9, and CYP3A4 substrates (📖 end cover) is unknown but dosage adjustments may be necessary.

Pharmacodynamic

- Fluconazole has been associated with prolongation of the QT interval. There is a potential risk that co-administration with other drugs that also prolong the QT interval (e.g. amiodarone, amitriptyline, erythromycin, quinine) may result in ventricular arrhythmias.

Dose
Mucosal candidiasis

- 50mg PO OD for 7–14 days.
- Dose may be increased as appropriate to 100mg PO OD in difficult cases.
- In oesophagitis, duration of treatment may need to be up to 30 days.

Genital candidiasis

- 150mg PO as a single dose

Dose adjustments
Elderly

- No dose adjustments necessary.

Hepatic/renal impairment

- Adjustments to single-dose therapy are not necessary.

Table 3.9 Fluconazole dose for patients with impaired renal function

Creatinine clearance	Percentage of recommended dose
>50mL/min	100%
≤50mL/min (no dialysis)	50%
Regular dialysis	100% after each dialysis

- In patients with impaired renal function, the normal dose should be used on day 1; subsequent doses are based on the degree of renal impairment as shown in Table 3.9.

Additional information
- In general, the treatment of choice for oral candidiasis is nystatin.
- Resistance to fluconazole is a problem and should be borne in mind in apparent cases of treatment failure.
- Be aware of the potential for drug interactions with fluconazole.

◑ Pharmacology
Fluconazole is fungistatic and its mechanism of action is believed to be through an increase in the permeability of the cellular membrane. The resulting damage leads to leakage of cellular contents and the prevention of uptake of essential molecules.

Fluconazole is not greatly affected by enzyme induction/inhibition since the majority of the dose is excreted unchanged in the urine.

Flumazenil

Anexate® (POM)
Injection: 500mcg/5mL

Generic (POM)
Injection: 500mcg/5mL

Indications
- Reversal of sedative effects of benzodiazepines.

Contraindications and precautions
- Flumazenil is contraindicated in patients receiving a benzodiazepine for control of a potentially life-threatening condition (e.g. control of intracranial pressure or status epilepticus).
- Use with caution in epileptic patients receiving benzodiazepines as the abrupt cessation of effect may precipitate a seizure.
- Use with caution in patients with hepatic impairment (see 📖 *Dose adjustments*, p.198).

☻ Undesirable effects
The frequency is not defined, but reported undesirable effects include:
- Agitation/anxiety (if given too rapidly)
- Flushing
- Nausea
- Seizures (in patients with epilepsy or severe hepatic impairment)
- Vomiting

Drug interactions
Pharmacokinetic
- None known

Pharmacodynamic
- *Benzodiazepines*—reversal of effect
- *Zolpidem/zopiclone*—reversal of effect

♣ Dose
- 200mcg slow IV injection over 15 seconds.
- If desired level of consciousness is not obtained within 60 seconds, a further 100mcg IV should be given and repeated at 60-second intervals to a maximum dose of 1mg IV (or 2mg IV if in intensive care).
- Usual dose needed is 300–600mcg.

🔁 Dose adjustments

Elderly
- No specific guidance available. Titrate dose to effect.

Hepatic/renal impairment
- No specific guidance is available for use in hepatic impairment. However, the manufacturer advises caution in hepatic impairment because of the hepatic metabolism of flumazenil. In any event, the dose is titrated to effect.
- No dose adjustments are necessary in renal impairment.

Additional information
- If drowsiness recurs, an infusion of 100–400mcg per hour may be used. The rate of infusion is individually determined

⟳ Pharmacology
Flumazenil antagonizes the actions of drugs that act via benzodiazepine receptors in the central nervous system.

Fluoxetine

Prozac® (POM)
Capsule: 20mg (30)
Liquid: 20mg/5mL (70mL)

Generic (POM)
Capsule: 20mg (30); 60mg (30)
Liquid: 20mg/5mL (70mL)

Indications
- Depression
- ¥ Anxiety

Contraindications and precautions
- Do not use with an irreversible MAOI, or within 14 days of stopping one, or at least 24 hours after discontinuation of a reversible MAOI (e.g. moclobemide, linezolid). At least 5 weeks should elapse after discontinuing fluoxetine treatment before starting an MAOI. Note that in exceptional circumstances linezolid may be given with paroxetine, but the patient must be closely monitored for symptoms of serotonin syndrome (📖 Box 1.10, p.19).
- Depression is associated with an increased risk of suicidal thoughts, self-harm, and suicide which persists until remission. Note that that the risk of suicide may increase during initial treatment.
- Hyponatraemia should be considered in all patients who develop drowsiness, confusion, or convulsions while taking an antidepressant. Hyponatraemia has been associated with all types of antidepressants, although it is reportedly more common with SSRIs.
- Use with caution in
  - diabetes (alters glycaemic control)
  - elderly (greater risk of hyponatraemia)
  - epilepsy (lowers seizure threshold)
  - hepatic impairment.
- May precipitate psychomotor restlessness, which usually appears during early treatment.
- Withdrawal symptoms can occur. Agitation, anxiety, asthenia, dizziness, headache, nausea and vomiting, sensory disturbances (e.g. paraesthesia), sleep disturbances (e.g. insomnia, intense dreams), and tremor are the most commonly reported reactions. They usually occur within the first few days of discontinuing treatment. Generally, these symptoms are self-limiting and usually resolve within 2 weeks, although some may persist for up to 3 months or longer. While it is advised that fluoxetine is gradually tapered over 1–2 weeks, it has a longer plasma half-life than other SSRIs and seems to be associated with a lower incidence of withdrawal symptoms; discontinuation without tapering can be considered. See 📖 Discontinuing and/or switching antidepressants, p.45 for information about switching or stopping antidepressants.

- Fluoxetine may increase the risk of haemorrhage (see 📖 *Drug interactions* (below))
- It may modify reactions and patients should be advised not to drive (or operate machinery) if affected.

☺ Undesirable effects

The frequency is not defined, but reported undesirable effects include:
- Abnormal bleeding
- Anorexia
- Anxiety
- Diarrhoea
- Drowsiness
- Dry mouth
- Dyspepsia
- Headache
- Hypoglycaemia
- Insomnia
- Nausea
- Pharyngitis
- Sexual dysfunction
- Tremor
- Yawning

Drug interactions

The long elimination half-lives (plasma concentrations detectable for up to 5–6 weeks after withdrawal) of both fluoxetine and its metabolite norfluoxetine should be borne in mind when considering pharmacokinetic and/or pharmacodynamic drug interactions.

Pharmacokinetic
- Fluoxetine is a strong inhibitor of CYP2D6 and moderately inhibits CYP1A2 and CYP2C19. It is metabolized by CYP2C9 and CYP2D6.
- *Carbamazepine*—potential risk of carbamazepine toxicity possibly due to CYP2C19 inhibition. Possible reduction in effect of fluoxetine due to CYP2C9 induction.
- *Codeine*—reduced analgesic benefit due to CYP2D6 inhibition.
- *Fluconazole*—risk of fluoxetine toxicity due to inhibition of CYP2C9.
- *Haloperidol*—increased risk of adverse effects from both drugs due to CYP2D6 inhibition.
- *Risperidone*—increased risk of adverse effects due to CYP2D6 inhibition.
- *Tramadol*—reduced analgesic benefit due to CYP2D6 inhibition.
- *Tricyclic antidepressants*—metabolism may be inhibited by fluoxetine.
- The clinical significance of co-administration with other substrates or inhibitors of CYP2D6 (📖 end cover) is unknown. Caution is advised if fluoxetine is co-administered with drugs that are predominantly metabolized by CYP2D6. The prescriber should be aware of the potential for interactions and that dosage adjustments may be necessary, particularly for drugs with a narrow therapeutic index.

- The clinical significance of co-administration with substrates of CYP1A2 or CYP2C19 (□ end cover) is unknown. The prescriber should be aware of the potential for interactions and that dosage reductions may be necessary, particularly for drugs with a narrow therapeutic index.
- The clinical significance of co-administration with other inducers or inhibitors of CYP2C9 is unknown.

Pharmacodynamic
- *Antidiabetics*—increased risk of hypoglycaemia.
- *Anticoagulants*—potential increased risk of bleeding.
- *Carbamazepine*—increased risk of hyponatraemia.
- *Cyproheptadine*—may inhibit the effects of fluoxetine.
- *Diuretics*—increased risk of hyponatraemia.
- *MAOIs*—risk of serotonin syndrome (see *Contraindications and precautions*).
- *NSAIDs*—increased risk of GI bleeding.
- *Serotonergic drugs*, e.g. duloxetine, methadone, mirtazapine, tricyclic antidepressants, tramadol, and trazodone—risk of serotonin syndrome (□ Box 1.10, p.19).

Dose
Depression
- Initial dose 20mg PO OD, increased if necessary after 3–4 weeks of initiation of treatment and subsequently as judged clinically appropriate to a maximum of 60mg PO OD.

¥ *Anxiety*
- Initial dose 10mg PO OD. After a week, the dose can be increased to 20mg PO OD if necessary. The dose can be increased after several weeks if no clinical improvement is observed. The maximum dose is 60mg PO OD.

Dose adjustments
Elderly
- No specific dose reductions are necessary, but the elderly may tolerate lower doses better. Generally, 40mg PO OD should not be exceeded.

Hepatic/renal impairment
- In significant liver impairment, a lower dose or alternate-day dosing is recommended.
- A dose reduction is considered unnecessary in patients with impaired renal function.

Additional information
- Fluoxetine and norfluoxetine have long half-lives that may minimize the risk of withdrawal symptoms after sudden cessation of treatment. Gradual reduction of the dose is generally unnecessary. However, if withdrawal symptoms are apparent, resuming the previous dose and instigating a more gradual withdrawal is advised.
- Fluoxetine should be administered as a single dose during or between meals. If adverse effects are troublesome, the dose can be divided.
- The oral liquid formulations contain sucrose.

❧ Pharmacology

Fluoxetine is a selective inhibitor of serotonin reuptake. It has almost no affinity for adrenergic, dopaminergic, histaminergic, muscarinic, or serotonergic receptors. Fluoxetine is well absorbed from the GI tract after oral administration. It is extensively metabolized by the polymorphic enzymes CYP2D6 and CYP2C8/9, with minor metabolic pathways involving several other isoenzymes (including CYP3A4). Fluoxetine also significantly inhibits CYP2D6, and moderately inhibits CYP1A2 and CYP2C19. There is one active metabolite, norfluoxetine, which contributes to the overall pharmacodynamic profile of fluoxetine.

The elimination half-lives of fluoxetine norfluoxetine are 4–6 days and 4–16 days, respectively. These long half-lives are responsible for persistence of the drug for 5–6 weeks after discontinuation. Excretion is mainly (about 60%) via the kidney.

Flutamide

Generic (POM)
Tablet: 250mg (84)

Indications
• Advanced prostate cancer.

Contraindications and precautions
• Use with caution in hepatic impairment—flutamide is associated with hepatic toxicity.
• Must not be used in patients with serum transaminase levels exceeding 2–3 times the upper limit of normal.
• LFTs should be checked monthly for first 4 months of treatment and periodically thereafter.
• Patient should be advised to seek medical attention at the first sign or symptom of liver impairment (e.g. pruritus, dark urine, jaundice).
• Avoid excessive alcohol consumption.
• Avoid combination with CYP1A2 inhibitors (see ☐ *Drug interactions*, p.203).

☺ Undesirable effects
Very common
• Galactorrhoea
• Gynaecomastia

Common
• Diarrhoea
• Drowsiness
• Increased appetite
• Insomnia
• Nausea
• Vomiting

Rare
• Anxiety
• Depression
• Dizziness
• Lymphoedema
• Oedema
• Visual disturbance

Drug interactions
Pharmacokinetic
• Metabolized by CYP1A2. May display competitive inhibition of CYP1A2.
• Theophylline—cases of theophylline toxicity reported.

- Co-administration of CYP1A2 inducers, including smoking (📖 Box 1.9, p.17) can lead to more rapid production of an active metabolite. The clinical significance is unknown.
- The clinical significance of co-administration with CYP1A2 inhibitors (📖 end cover) is unknown. The prescriber should be aware of the potential for toxicity and that dose adjustments may be necessary.

Pharmacodynamic
- None known

Dose
- 250mg PO TDS.

Dose adjustments
Elderly
- No dose adjustments are necessary.

Hepatic/renal impairment
- No specific guidance is available for use in hepatic impairment. The manufacturer advises that flutamide should only be administered after careful assessment of the individual benefits and risks.
- No specific guidance is available for use in renal impairment. The manufacturer does not make a recommendation for dose adjustments. It is highly protein bound and unlikely to be removed by dialysis.

Additional information
Although tablets may be crushed and dispersed in water prior to administration, this is not recommended because of the risk of exposure.

Pharmacology
Flutamide is a non-steroidal anti-androgen which blocks the action of androgens of adrenal and testicular origin that stimulate the growth of normal and malignant prostatic tissue. It is completely absorbed following oral administration and is highly protein bound. Flutamide is extensively metabolized by CYP1A2 to an active metabolite. The metabolites are eliminated via the kidneys and bile.

Furosemide

Lasix® (POM)
Injection: 20mg/2mL (10)

Generic (POM)
Tablet: 20mg (8); 40mg (28); 500mg (28)
Oral solution (*sugar-free*): 20mg/5mL (150mL); 40mg/5mL (150mL); 50mg/5mL (150mL).
Injection: 20mg/2mL; 50mg/5mL; 250mg/25mL

Indications
- Management of oedema associated with congestive heart failure and hepatic or renal disease.
- Resistant hypertension.
- For end-of-life care issues see 📖 Use of drugs in end-of-life care, p.53.

Contraindications and precautions
- Furosemide is contraindicated for use in the following conditions:
  - anuria
  - dehydration
  - drug-induced renal failure
  - hypersensitivity to sulphonamides
  - hypovolaemia
  - severe hypokalaemia or hyponatraemia.
- Use with caution in the following:
  - bladder outflow obstruction (risk of urinary retention)
  - diabetes (may cause hyperglycaemia)
  - gout
  - hepatorenal syndrome
  - hypotension
  - nephrotic syndrome (the effect of furosemide may be reduced and its ototoxicity potentiated)
  - patients at risk of electrolyte imbalance
  - prostatic hypertrophy (risk of urinary retention).
- Oral solutions may contain up to 10% v/v of alcohol.
- Avoid combination of risperidone and furosemide. Treatment with this combination is associated with a higher mortality than with either drug alone.

☺ Undesirable effects
The frequency is not defined, but reported undesirable effects include:
- Arrhythmias
- Confusion
- Diarrhoea
- Dizziness
- Electrolyte disturbances (e.g. hyponatraemia, hypokalaemia, hypomagnesaemia, hypocalcaemia)
- Headache
- Hyperglycaemia (less common than with thiazides)

- Hyperuricaemia (and gout)
- Hypotension
- Muscle cramps
- Muscle weakness
- Nausea
- Tetany
- Thirst
- Vomiting

Other reported rare undesirable effects include:
- Aplastic anaemia
- Bone marrow depression
- Hypersensitivity manifested as skin reactions, dermatitis
- Pancreatitis
- Paraesthesia
- Tinnitus and deafness (especially associated with over-rapid IV injection/infusion)

Drug interactions
Pharmacokinetic
- *Phenytoin*—effect of furosemide reduced, possibly through an unknown effect on absorption.
- *Sucralfate*—reduced absorption of furosemide; not be taken within 2 hours of each other.

Pharmacodynamic
- *ACEIs*—increased risk of hypotension.
- *Aminoglycosides*—furosemide may increase nephrotoxicity.
- *Antihypertensives*—increased risk of hypotension.
- *β₂-agonists*—increased risk of hypokalaemia.
- *Bisphosphonates*—risk of hypocalcaemia and dehydration.
- *Corticosteroids*—increased risk of hypokalaemia; diuretic effect reduced.
- *Digoxin*—hypokalaemia increases toxicity.
- *NSAIDs*—reduced diuretic effect; risk of renal impairment increased.
- *Reboxetine*—increased risk of hypokalaemia.
- *Risperidone*—increased risk of mortality associated with combination.
- *Theophylline*—increased risk of hypokalaemia.

Dose
Oral
Oral doses should be administered in the morning to avoid nocturnal diuresis.

Oedema
- Initial dose 40mg PO OM. Typical maintenance doses range from 20 to 40mg PO OD. In resistant cases, this may be increased to 80–120mg PO OM. Higher doses may be required.
- ⁎ Alternatively, 20–40mg SL OM (using tablet formulation) may be used.

Resistant hypertension
- 40–80mg PO OM. Higher doses may be required.

Parenteral

IV furosemide must be injected or infused slowly; a rate of 4mg/min must not be exceeded.

Oedema

- By IM or slow IV injection 20–50mg increased if necessary in steps of 20mg, not more frequently than every 2 hours. Doses >50mg should be administered via slow IV infusion. Maximum 1.5g daily.
- ✳ Alternatively, 20–140mg via CSCI over 24 hours can be used for management of endstage congestive heart failure.

↓♭ Dose adjustments

Elderly

- No specific guidance is available, but the dose should be titrated until the required response is achieved.

Hepatic/renal impairment

- Patients with hepatic impairment are more at risk of encephalopathy due to hypokalaemia so other diuretics may be more appropriate.
- Patients with renal impairment may require higher doses (furosemide must be excreted in order to exert its effect).

Additional information

- Diuresis normally starts within 1 hour of oral administration and is regarded as complete after 6 hours.
- The kidney appears to develop tolerance to furosemide for 6 hours post-diuresis. Therefore it should be given as a single daily dose in the morning *unless* the patient has an indwelling urinary catheter, when it can be given twice daily (12 hours apart).
- Furosemide injection has an alkaline pH, so it is unlikely to be compatible with many drugs. It is advisable to use a separate CSCI. However, furosemide is compatible with dexamethasone via CSCI.

↪ Pharmacology

Furosemide is a loop diuretic which acts by inhibiting reabsorption of sodium and chloride in the ascending limb of the loop of Henle, leading to an increased excretion of water and sodium. Its mechanism of action involves the inhibition of a Na/K/Cl co-transport system. Potassium secretion from the distal convoluted tubule is also increased because of the exchange of potassium for sodium. Furosemide also increases the excretion of bicarbonate, calcium, hydrogen, magnesium, and phosphate.

Gabapentin

Neurontin® (POM)
Capsule: 100mg (100); 300mg (100); 400mg (100)
Tablet (scored): 600mg (100); 800mg (100)

Generic (POM)
Capsule: 100mg (100); 300mg (100); 400mg (100)
Tablet: 600mg (100); 800mg (100)

Indications
- Monotherapy and adjunctive treatment of partial seizures with or without secondary generalization.
- Peripheral neuropathic pain.
- ¥ Malignant bone pain.
- ¥ Restless legs syndrome.

Contraindications and precautions
- Avoid sudden withdrawal. Independent of indication. Discontinue gradually over at least a week in order to avoid undesirable effects such as nausea, vomiting, flu syndrome, anxiety, and insomnia. These withdrawal effects have been reported even after short-term use.
- Caution in elderly and renal impairment—dosage adjustments may be necessary (see 📖 *Dosage adjustments*).
- Use with caution in patients with congestive heart failure.
- Diabetic patients may need to adjust hypoglycaemic treatment as weight gain occurs.
- If affected by drowsiness and dizziness, patients should be warned about driving.

☺ Undesirable effects

Very common
- Ataxia
- Dizziness
- Fatigue
- Somnolence

Common
- Abnormal thoughts
- Amnesia
- Confusion
- Diarrhoea
- Dry mouth
- Erectile dysfunction
- Headache
- Hostility
- Increased appetite
- Infection (chest, urinary tract)
- Leucopenia
- Nausea and vomiting
- Peripheral oedema
- Tremor
- Weight gain

Rare
- Allergic reactions (urticaria)
- Hallucinations
- Movement disorders

- Pancreatitis (withdraw treatment)
- Tinnitus

Drug interactions

Pharmacokinetic
- Avoid taking antacid medication within 2 hours of gabapentin (may reduce bioavailability by 20% or more).
- Morphine and other opioids may increase the absorption of gabapentin.
- The clinical significance of these interactions is unknown but the prescriber should be aware of the potential for interactions and that dosage adjustments may be necessary.

Pharmacodynamic
- *CNS depressants*—increased risk of undesirable CNS effects.
- *Opioids*—possible opioid-sparing affect, necessitating opioid dose review.

.ᢃ Dose

- The licensed schedule is shown in Table 3.10. This may be poorly tolerated by elderly patients or those with cancer, and a more cautious titration is suggested for these patients. Whichever strategy is adopted, undesirable effects are more common around the time of dose escalation but usually resolve in a few weeks. The slower titration may be preferred in the elderly or cancer population, although it may take longer to appreciate the therapeutic benefit.
- ⁑ This approach can be used for restless legs syndrome. The usual maximum dose is 1.8g daily in divided doses.

Table 3.10 Titration of gabapentin

	Licensed dose		Suggested dose
Day 1	300mg PO ON	Day 1	100mg PO ON
Day 2	300mg PO BD	Day 2	100mg PO BD
Day 3	300mg PO TDS	Day 3	100mg PO TDS
Increase by 300mg PO OD according to response up to a maximum of 1.2g PO TDS		Increase by 100mg PO TDS every 2 days as needed to a maximum of 1.2g PO TDS	

.ᢃ Dose adjustments

Elderly
- May require a more cautious titration as described above, or may need a dose reduction due to renal impairment (Table 3.11).

Table 3.11 Dosage for patients with renal impairment

Creatinine clearance (mL/min)	Maximum dose
≥80	1200mg PO TDS
50–79	600mg PO TDS
30–49	300mg PO TDS
15–29	300mg PO OD
<15	300mg PO ALT DIE, OD

Renal impairment
- Dose adjustments are necessary for patients in renal failure or undergoing haemodialysis.
- Adjust the starting dose as necessary.

Patients undergoing haemodialysis
- Anuric patients—initial loading dose 300–400mg, then 200–300mg of gabapentin after each 4 hours of haemodialysis. On dialysis-free days, there should be no treatment with gabapentin.
- Renally impaired patients—dose as per Table 3.11 based on creatinine clearance. An additional 200–300mg dose following each 4-hour haemodialysis treatment is recommended.

Additional information
- Gabapentin capsules can be opened and the contents dispersed in water or fruit juice immediately prior to use.
- Neuropathic pain should improve within a week.
- There may be a reduction in anxiety within a few weeks, although the effect is not as pronounced as with pregabalin.
- Some patients may respond to a BD regime.
- With high doses, increasing the dosing frequency can improve tolerance
- There may be an improvement in sleep, but the effect does not appear as pronounced as with pregabalin.

✦ Pharmacology
Gabapentin was originally developed as an agonist of the $GABA_A$ receptor, but it is actually devoid of GABA effects. The analgesic benefit of gabapentin is due to its affinity for the $\alpha_2\delta$ subunit of N and P/Q voltage-dependent calcium channels. Gabapentin binds to the $\alpha_2\delta$ subunit, effectively closing the channel and preventing the release of neurotransmitters and modulators. It is readily absorbed after oral administration, although the mechanism of absorption is saturable within the normal dosing range. Therefore increasing the dose does not proportionally increase the amount absorbed. Gabapentin is largely excreted unchanged in the urine, so dose adjustment is needed in renal impairment.

Gliclazide

Standard release
Diamicron® *(POM)*
Tablet (*scored*): 80mg (60)

Generic (POM)
Tablet (*scored*): 80mg (28)

Modified release

Diamicron® MR
Tablet: 30mg (28; 56)

Indications
- Type 2 diabetes mellitus.

Contraindications and precautions
- Gliclazide is contraindicated for use in the following:
  - concurrent use of miconazole (see 📖 *Drug interactions*, p.212)
  - diabetic ketoacidosis
  - diabetic pre-coma and coma
  - hypersensitivity to sulphonylurea or sulphonamides
  - severe hepatic impairment (see 📖 *Dose adjustments*, p.212)
  - severe renal impairment (see 📖 *Dose adjustments*, p.212)
  - type 1 diabetes.
- Use with caution in patients with hepatic and/or renal impairment (see 📖 *Dose adjustments*, p.212).
- The risk of hypoglycaemia increases with:
  - adrenal insufficiency
  - hepatic impairment
  - hypopituitarism
  - renal impairment.
- Patients must have a regular carbohydrate intake, avoid skipping meals, and ensure a balance between physical exercise and carbohydrate intake.
- Patients should be aware of the symptoms of hypoglycaemia and be careful when driving and using machinery.

☺ Undesirable effects
The frequency is not defined, but reported undesirable effects include:
- Diarrhoea
- Dizziness
- Headache
- Hepatitis
- Hypoglycaemia (especially if meals skipped; dose dependent)
- Hyponatraemia
- Jaundice
- Nausea

- Nervousness
- Transient visual disturbances
- Vomiting

Drug interactions
Pharmacokinetic
- The metabolism of gliclazide appears to be mediated mainly via CYP2C9.
- *Miconazole*—contraindicated for use (enhanced hypoglycaemic effect, presumably CYP2C9 inhibition).
- The clinical significance of co-administration with CYP2C9 inducers or inhibitors (🕮 end cover) is unknown. The prescriber should be aware of the potential for interactions and that dosage adjustments may be necessary.

Pharmacodynamic
- *ACEIs*—increased risk of hypoglycaemia.
- *β_2-agonists*—hypoglycaemic effect may be antagonized.
- *Corticosteroids*—hypoglycaemic effect antagonized.
- *Diuretics*—hypoglycaemic effect may be antagonized.
- *Fluoxetine*—increased risk of hypoglycaemia.
- *Warfarin*—increased anticoagulant effect.

💊 Dose
Standard release
- Initial dose, 40–80mg PO OD. Can be increased as necessary up to 160mg as a single daily dose with breakfast. Higher doses must be administered in divided doses. Maximum dose 320mg daily.

Modified release
- Initial dose 30mg PO OD with breakfast. Dose can be adjusted according to response every 4 weeks, or after 2 weeks if no decrease in blood glucose. Maximum dose 120mg daily.

Note: Diamicron® MR 30mg may be considered to be approximately equivalent in therapeutic effect to standard formulation Diamicron® 80mg.

💊 Dose adjustments
Elderly
- Usual adult doses can be used. Dose should be titrated to effect.

Hepatic/renal impairment
- Care should be exercised in patients with hepatic and/or renal impairment and a smaller initial dose should be used with careful patient monitoring. Dose should be titrated to effect.
- Patients with mild to moderate renal impairment may use the usual dosing regimen for Diamicron® MR with careful patient monitoring.
- In severe hepatic and renal impairment, insulin therapy should be used.

Additional information

- Standard-release tablets can be crushed and dispersed in water immediately prior to use.

⟳ Pharmacology

Gliclazide is a sulphonylurea which stimulates β-cells of the islet of Langerhans in the pancreas to release insulin. It also enhances peripheral insulin sensitivity. It restores the first peak of insulin secretion in response to glucose and increases the second phase of insulin secretion. The metabolism of many sulphonylureas is catalysed by CYP2C9. While this has not been categorically shown for gliclazide, drug interactions would suggest that this is the case.

Glimepiride

Amaryl® (POM)
Tablet (scored): 1mg (30); 2mg (30); 3mg (30); 4mg (30)

Generic (POM)
Tablet: 1mg (30); 2mg (30); 3mg (30); 4mg (30)

Indications
• Type 2 diabetes mellitus.

Contraindications and precautions
• Glimepiride is contraindicated for use in the following:
  • diabetic ketoacidosis
  • diabetic pre-coma and coma
  • hypersensitivity to sulphonylurea or sulphonamides
  • severe hepatic impairment (see 📖 *Dose adjustments*, p.215)
  • severe renal impairment (see 📖 *Dose adjustments*, p.215)
  • type 1 diabetes.
• Use with caution in patients with:
  • concomitant use of CYP2C9 inducers/inhibitors (see 📖 *Drug interactions*, p.215)
  • glucose 6-phosphate dehydrogenase (G6PD) deficiency
  • hepatic and/or renal impairment (see 📖 *Dose adjustments*, p.215).
• The risk of hypoglycaemia increases with:
  • adrenal insufficiency
  • hepatic impairment
  • hypopituitarism
  • renal impairment.
• Patients must have a regular carbohydrate intake, avoid skipping meals, and ensure a balance between physical exercise and carbohydrate intake.
• The manufacturer recommends regular hepatic and haematological monitoring (especially leucocytes and thrombocytes) during treatment.
• Patients should be aware of the symptoms of hypoglycaemia and be careful when driving and using machinery.

☺ Undesirable effects
The frequency is not defined, but reported undesirable effects include:
• Cholestatic jaundice
• Diarrhoea
• Dizziness
• Drowsiness
• Headache
• Hypoglycaemia (especially if meals skipped; dose dependent)
• Hyponatraemia
• Nausea
• Nervousness
• Transient visual disturbances
• Vomiting

Drug interactions

Pharmacokinetic

- Glimepiride is metabolized by CYP2C9.
- *Fluconazole*—increases plasma concentration of glimepiride
- The clinical significance of co-administration with CYP2C9 inducers or inhibitors (📖 end cover) is unknown. The prescriber should be aware of the potential for interactions and that dosage adjustments may be necessary.

Pharmacodynamic

- *ACEIs*—increased risk of hypoglycaemia.
- *β_2-agonists*—hypoglycaemic effect may be antagonized.
- *Corticosteroids*—hypoglycaemic effect antagonized.
- *Diuretics*—hypoglycaemic effect may be antagonized.
- *Fluoxetine*—increased risk of hypoglycaemia.
- *Warfarin*—increased anticoagulant effect.

⚕ Dose

- Initial dose 1mg PO OD taken shortly before or during the first main meal. The dose can be increased by 1mg daily every 1–2 weeks to a usual maximum of 4mg PO OD. A dose of 6mg PO OD can be used in exceptional cases.

⚕ Dose adjustments

Elderly

- Usual adult doses can be used. Dose should be titrated to effect.

Hepatic/renal impairment

- Care should be exercised in patients with hepatic and/or renal impairment. Dose should be titrated to effect.
- Glimepiride should be avoided in patients with severe hepatic and/or renal impairment, and insulin treatment should be initiated.

Additional information

- Tablets can be crushed and dispersed in water immediately prior to administration if necessary.

⊕ Pharmacology

Glimepiride is a sulphonylurea which stimulates β-cells of the islet of Langerhans in the pancreas to release insulin. It also enhances peripheral insulin sensitivity. It restores the first peak of insulin secretion in response to glucose and increases the second phase of insulin secretion. The metabolism of glimepiride is catalysed by CYP2C9.

Glipizide

Glibenese® (POM)
Tablet (*scored*): 5mg (56)

Minodiab® (POM)
Tablet: 5mg (*scored* – 28)

Generic (POM)
Tablet: 5mg (56)

Indications
- Type 2 diabetes mellitus.

Contraindications and precautions
- Glipizide is contraindicated for use in the following:
  - concurrent use of miconazole (see 📖 *Drug interactions*, p.217)
  - diabetic ketoacidosis
  - diabetic pre-coma and coma
  - hypersensitivity to sulphonylurea or sulphonamides
  - severe hepatic impairment (see 📖 *Dose adjustments*, p.217)
  - severe renal impairment (see 📖 *Dose adjustments*, p.217)
  - type 1 diabetes.
- Use with caution in patients with hepatic and/or renal impairment (see 📖 *Dose adjustments*, p.217).
- The risk of hypoglycaemia increases with:
  - adrenal insufficiency
  - hepatic impairment
  - hypopituitarism
  - renal impairment.
- Patients must have a regular carbohydrate intake, avoid skipping meals, and ensure a balance between physical exercise and carbohydrate intake.
- Patients should be aware of the symptoms of hypoglycaemia and be careful when driving and using machinery.

☺ Undesirable effects
The frequency is not defined, but reported undesirable effects include:
- Cholestatic jaundice
- Diarrhoea
- Dizziness
- Drowsiness
- Headache
- Hypoglycaemia (especially if meals skipped; dose dependent)
- Hyponatraemia
- Nausea
- Nervousness
- Transient visual disturbances
- Vomiting

Drug interactions

Pharmacokinetic
- Glipizide is metabolized by CYP2C9.
- *Miconazole*—contraindicated for use (enhanced hypoglycaemic effect, presumably CYP2C9 inhibition).
- The clinical significance of co-administration with CYP2C9 inducers or inhibitors (🕮 end cover) is unknown. The prescriber should be aware of the potential for interactions and that dosage adjustments may be necessary.

Pharmacodynamic
- *ACEIs*—increased risk of hypoglycaemia.
- *β_2-agonists*—hypoglycaemic effect may be antagonized.
- *Corticosteroids*—hypoglycaemic effect antagonized.
- *Diuretics*—hypoglycaemic effect may be antagonized.
- *Fluoxetine*—increased risk of hypoglycaemia.
- *Warfarin*—increased anticoagulant effect.

⚗ Dose
- Initial dose 2.5–5mg PO OD, taken before breakfast or lunch. The dose can be increased as necessary by 2.5–5mg PO OD over several days. The maximum recommended single dose is 15mg PO daily; doses above 15mg should be divided. The maximum daily dose is 20mg.

⚗ Dose adjustments
Elderly
- Usual adult doses can be used, although the elderly are more susceptible to undesirable effects. The initial dose should be 2.5mg PO OD and should be titrated to effect.

Hepatic/renal impairment
- Care should be exercised in patients with hepatic and/or renal impairment and a smaller initial dose should be used with careful patient monitoring. Dose should be titrated to effect.
- Glipizide should be avoided in patients with severe hepatic and/or renal impairment and insulin treatment should be initiated.

Additional information
- Tablets can be crushed and dispersed in water immediately prior to administration if necessary.

⊕ Pharmacology
Glipizide is a sulphonylurea which stimulates β-cells of the islet of Langerhans in the pancreas to release insulin. It also enhances peripheral insulin sensitivity. It restores the first peak of insulin secretion in response to glucose and increases the second phase of insulin secretion. The metabolism of many sulphonylureas is catalysed by CYP2C9.

Glyceryl trinitrate (GTN)

Rectogesic® (POM)
Rectal ointment: glyceryl trinitrate 0.4% (30g)

Unlicensed Special (POM)
Rectal ointment: glyceryl trinitrate 0.2% (20g)
See additional information below for supply issues.

Generic (P)
Sublingual tablet: 300mcg (100); 500mcg (100); 600mcg (100)
Note: Tablets should be stored in the original container and discarded 8 weeks from opening.
Aerosol spray: 400 mcg per metered dose (200)
Transdermal patch: 5mg/24 hours (28); 10mg/24 hours (28); 15mg/24 hours (28).
Various proprietary formulations are available (see current *BNF*).

Indications
- Anal fissure
- Angina (*not discussed*)
- * Smooth muscle spasm pain (e.g. anus, oesophagus, rectum)

Contraindications and precautions
- Contraindicated for use in the following:
  - aortic and/or mitral stenosis
  - closed-angle glaucoma
  - concomitant use with phosphodiesterase inhibitors (e.g. sildenafil, tadalafil, vardenafil)
  - constrictive pericarditis
  - extreme bradycardia
  - glucose-6-phosphate dehydrogenase deficiency
  - hypertrophic obstructive cardiomyopathy
  - hypotensive shock
  - migraine or recurrent headache
  - severe anaemia
  - severe hypotension (systolic BP <90mmHg)
- Use with caution in patients with:
  - hypothermia
  - hypothyroidism
  - malnutrition
  - recent history of myocardial infarction
  - severe hepatic impairment
  - severe renal impairment
  - susceptibility to angle-closure glaucoma.
- Note that transdermal patches that contain metal must be removed before an MRI (to avoid burns).

- Tolerance can rapidly develop with long-acting or transdermal nitrates with consequential loss of effect. This can be prevented by adopting a 'nitrate-free' period of 4–8 hours each day.
- Dry mouth may reduce the effectiveness of transmucosal GTN.
- Can exacerbate the hypotensive effects of other drugs (see 📖 *Drug interactions*, p.219).
- GTN may cause dizziness, light-headedness, and blurred vision especially on first use. Patients should be advised not to drive (or operate machinery) if affected.

☺ Undesirable effects

Very common
- Headache

Common
- Dizziness
- Facial flushing
- Nausea
- Weakness

Uncommon
- Diarrhoea (rectal formulation)
- Anal discomfort (rectal formulation)
- Vomiting (rectal formulation)
- Rectal bleeding (rectal formulation)
- Oral discomfort e.g. stinging, burning (oral formulations)

Rare
- Tachycardia

Drug interactions

Pharmacokinetic
- None known

Pharmacodynamic
- *Alcohol*—potentiates the hypotensive effect of GTN
- *Heparin*—the anticoagulant effect may be reduced by GTN; dose adjustment may be necessary
- The risk of hypotension is increased if GTN is taken concurrently with the following drugs:
  - β-blockers
  - calcium antagonists
  - diuretics
  - haloperidol
  - levomepromazine
  - opioids
  - phosphodiesterase inhibitors (e.g. sildenafil, tadalafil, or vardenafil)
  - tricyclic antidepressants.

♣ Dose

Anal fissure

- Apply a small amount (approximately 2.5cm) intra-anally BD until the pain improves or for a maximum of 8 weeks.

¥ *Oesophageal spasm*

- 400–500mcg SL 5–15mins before food.
- If the tablet is used, it can be removed once the pain has subsided.

¥ *Rectal pain*

- Apply a small amount (approximately 2.5cm) PR BD. Do not use for more than 8 weeks.

♣ Dose adjustments

Elderly

- No dose adjustment necessary.

Hepatic/renal impairment

- No specific guidance available. Manufacturers advise caution in patients with severe hepatic and/or renal impairment.

Additional information

- The rectal ointment should be applied using a finger covering, such as cling film.
- Rectal ointment 0.2% is an unlicensed special and is available from Queens Medical Centre, Nottingham (Tel 0115 875 4521).

♦ Pharmacology

GTN is converted to nitric oxide (NO) *in vivo* which causes a cascade of intracellular events resulting in the subsequent release of calcium ions and relaxation of smooth muscle cells.

Glycopyrronium

Robinul® (POM)
Injection: 200mcg/mL (10 × 1mL; 10 × 3mL)
Powder: 3g

Generic (POM)
Injection: 200mcg/mL (10 × 1mL; 10 × 3mL)

Unlicensed (POM)
Tablet (*scored*): 1mg; 2mg
Oral solution: Various strengths (prepared from injection, powder or tablets)
See *Additional information* for supply issues

Indications
- ⅍ Hypersalivation
- ⅍ Nausea and vomiting (associated with bowel obstruction)
- ⅍ Smooth muscle spasm (e.g. bowel colic)
- ⅍ Sweating associated with cancer
- ⅍ Terminal secretions
- For end-of-life care issues see 📖 Use of drugs in end-of-life care, p.53.

Contraindications and precautions
- No absolute contraindications. However, it has potent peripheral anti-cholinergic activity and can predispose to tachycardia.
- Use with caution in patients with:
  - bladder outflow obstruction
  - cardiac arrhythmias
  - congestive heart failure
  - coronary artery disease
  - hypertension
  - myasthenia gravis (particularly larger doses)
  - narrow-angle glaucoma
  - paralytic ileus
  - pyrexia (reduces sweating)
  - renal impairment (see 📖 Dose adjustments, p.222)
  - thyrotoxicosis
- Glycopyrronium may modify reactions and patients should be advised not to drive (or operate machinery) if affected.

☺ Undesirable effects
The frequency is not defined, but reported undesirable effects include:
- confusion
- difficulty in micturition
- dizziness
- drowsiness
- dry mouth
- inhibition of sweating
- palpitations
- tachycardia
- visual disturbances

Drug interactions

Pharmacokinetic

- Undergoes minimal hepatic metabolism; mostly excreted unchanged by the kidneys
- No recognized pharmacokinetic interactions

Pharmacodynamic

- β_2-agonists—increased risk of tachycardia.
- Cyclizine—increased risk of anticholinergic undesirable effects.
- Domperidone—may inhibit prokinetic effect.
- Metoclopramide—may inhibit prokinetic effect.
- Nefopam—increased risk of anticholinergic undesirable effects.
- TCAs—increased risk of anticholinergic undesirable effects.

Dose

¥ Hypersalivation

- Initial dose 200mcg PO TDS; increase every 2–3 days as necessary up to 1mg PO TDS. Higher doses have been used (e.g. 2mg PO TDS).

¥ Nausea and vomiting/smooth muscle spasm/sweating/terminal secretions

- Initial dose 200mcg SC PRN or 600mcg via CSCI over 24 hours.
- Dose can be increased to a maximum of 2.4mg via CSCI over 24 hours.

Dose adjustments

Elderly

- No specific guidance available. Use the lowest effective dose as the elderly may be more susceptible to the undesirable effects.

Hepatic/renal impairment

- No specific guidance available. However, glycopyrronium accumulates in renal impairment, so dosage adjustments will be necessary.

Additional information

- Glycopyrronium tablets can be imported as unlicensed products via IDIS (tel: 01932 824 000; www.idispharma.com).
- Glycopyrronium oral solution 1mg/5mL can be ordered as a special from the pharmacy manufacturing unit at Huddersfield (Tel: 01484 355388).
- Alternatively, an oral solution can be prepared in several ways. For immediate use, the contents of the ampoule can be administered orally, or via a PEG (using a filter needle). The tablets can also be dispersed in water prior to administration. Alternatively, a 1mg/10mL oral solution can be prepared from the powder (this can be stored in a refrigerator for 7 days).

- The stability of glycopyrronium is affected above pH 6 as ester hydrolysis can occur. There are incompatibility issues with dexamethasone, dimenhydrinate, and phenobarbital.
- Via CSCI, glycopyrronium is reportedly compatible with alfentanil, clonazepam, diamorphine, haloperidol, hydromorphone, levomepromazine, metoclopramide, midazolam, octreotide, ondansetron, oxycodone, promethazine, ranitidine, and tramadol.
- There may be concentration-dependent compatibility issues with cyclizine (but less so than with hyoscine butylbromide–cyclizine).

✷ Pharmacology

Glycopyrronium is a quaternary ammonium antimuscarinic that inhibits the peripheral actions of acetylcholine (e.g. smooth muscle, cardiac muscle, AV node, exocrine glands). At higher doses, it may also block nicotinic receptors. Because of the polarity of the quaternary compound, it does not readily cross the blood–brain barrier and is unlikely to produce symptoms such as sedation or paradoxical agitation (☐ Hyoscine hydrobromide, p.237). However, it does not have a direct anti-emetic action like hyoscine hydrobromide. Glycopyrronium is mainly excreted unchanged by the kidneys and lower doses may be required in renal impairment.

Granisetron

Kytril® (POM)
Tablet: 1mg (10); 2mg (5)
Injection: 1mg/mL (5); 3mg/3mL (5; 10)

Indications
- Nausea and vomiting (induced by chemotherapy or radiotherapy).
- * Nausea and vomiting (e.g. drug-induced, cancer-related, refractory).
- For end-of-life care issues see 📖 Use of drugs in end-of-life care, p.53.

Contraindications and precautions
- Since granisetron increases large bowel transit time, use with caution in patients with signs of subacute bowel obstruction.
- Use with caution in patients with:
  - cardiac rhythm or conduction disturbances
  - concurrent use of anti-arrhythmic agents or β-adrenergic blocking agents (see 📖 Drug interactions, p.225)
  - significant electrolyte disturbances
- Granisetron may modify reactions and patients should be advised not to drive (or operate machinery) if affected.

☺ Undesirable effects

Very common
- Headache

Common
- Agitation
- Anorexia
- Anxiety
- Asthenia
- Constipation
- Dizziness
- Hypertension
- Insomnia
- Somnolence
- Taste disorder

Uncommon
- Abnormal vision
- Skin rashes

Rare
- Abnormal LFTs (raised transaminases)
- Arrhythmias
- Dystonia and dyskinesia

Drug interactions
Pharmacokinetic
- Metabolized by CYP3A4.
- Carbamazepine and phenytoin can reduce granisetron serum concentrations and reduce the effect.
- The clinical significance of co-administration with other CYP3A4 inducers, or inhibitors (□ end cover) is unknown. The prescriber should be aware of the potential for interactions and that dosage adjustments may be necessary.
- *Paracetamol*—possible reduced analgesic benefit.
- *Tramadol*—reduced analgesic benefit.
- The effect of grapefruit juice on the absorption of granisetron is unknown.

Pharmacodynamic
- Granisetron may prolong the QT interval. There is a potential risk that co-administration with other drugs that also prolong the QT interval (e.g. amiodarone, erythromycin, haloperidol, quinine) may result in ventricular arrhythmias.
- Granisetron increases bowel transit time. This effect can be enhanced by drugs such as opioids, TCAs, and anticholinergics.
- *Domperidone/metoclopramide*—granisetron reduces the prokinetic effect.
- *SSRIs*—risk of serotonin syndrome.

⸬ Dose
Nausea and vomiting
- 1mg PO BD or 2mg PO OD. The dose can be increased if necessary up to a maximum of 9mg daily.
- Alternatively, the parenteral route may be used:
  - 1mg IV/SC(¥) BD, increased to 3mg IV/SC(¥) TDS if necessary.
  - ¥ 1–3mg via CSCI over 24 hours, increased to a maximum of 9mg daily.

⸬ Dose adjustments
Elderly
- No dosage adjustments are necessary.

Hepatic/renal impairment
- No dosage adjustments are necessary in liver or renal impairment. Nonetheless, since hepatic metabolism is important for the elimination of granisetron, the lowest effective dose should be used in patients with hepatic impairment.

Additional information

- 5-HT₃ antagonists differ in chemical structure, pharmacokinetics, and pharmacodynamics. There may be individual variation in response, and it may be worth considering an alternative 5-HT₃ antagonist if response to granisetron is not as expected.
- Treatment with granisetron should be used regularly for 3 days and then response assessed. Avoid using on a PRN basis.
- The compatibility of granisetron with other drugs via CSCI is unknown, although it is expected to be similar to ondansetron.

⊕ Pharmacology

Granisetron is a selective 5-HT₃ receptor antagonist, blocking serotonin peripherally on vagal nerve terminals and centrally in the chemoreceptor trigger zone. It is a particularly useful in the treatment of nausea and vomiting associated with serotonin release (e.g. damage to enterochromaffin cells due to bowel injury, chemotherapy, or radiotherapy). It has little or no affinity for other serotonin receptors (including 5-HT₂), dopamine D_2 receptors, α_1-, α_2-, or β-adrenoreceptors, and histamine H_1 receptors.

Haloperidol

Serenace® (POM)
Capsule: 500mcg (30)
Tablet: 1.5mg (30); 5mg (30); 10mg (30)
Oral liquid: 2mg/mL (500mL, *sugar-free*)

Haldol® (POM)
Tablet (*scored*): 5mg (20); 10mg (20)
Oral liquid: 2mg/mL (100mL, *sugar-free*)
Injection: 5mg/mL (1mL)

Dozic® (POM)
Oral liquid: 1mg/mL (100mL, *sugar-free*)

Generic (POM)
Tablet: 500mcg (28); 1.5mg (28); 5mg (28); 10mg (28); 20mg (28)

Indications
- Psychosis
- Intractable hiccup
- Restlessness and agitation in the elderly
- ¥ Delirium
- ¥ Nausea and vomiting
- For end-of-life care issues see ⬚ Use of drugs in end-of-life care, p.53.

Contraindications and precautions
- Must not be used in the following circumstances:
  - avoid using in patients with dementia unless patient at immediate risk of harm or severely distressed (increased mortality reported)
  - lesions of the basal ganglia
  - Parkinson's disease
  - recent acute myocardial infarction
- Haloperidol should be used with caution in the following circumstances:
  - co-administration of CYP2D6 and/or CYP3A4 inhibitors (see ⬚ Drug interactions, p.228)
  - diabetes (risk of hyperglycaemia in elderly)
  - elderly (see ⬚ Dose adjustments, p.230)
  - epilepsy
  - hepatic/renal impairment (see ⬚ Dose adjustments, p.230)
  - Lewy body dementia
  - poor metabolizers of CYP2D6 (if aware)
- Electrolyte disturbances must be corrected (e.g. hypokalaemia) because of the risk of QT prolongation.
- Rapid discontinuation may lead to a rebound worsening of symptoms. Withdraw gradually whenever possible.
- Haloperidol may modify reactions and patients should be advised not to drive (or operate machinery) if affected.

☹ Undesirable effects
Most frequent
- Akathisia
- Extrapyramidal symptoms
- Tardive dyskinesia
- Weight gain

Less frequent
- Dry mouth
- Fatigue
- Postural hypotension
- Sedation

Rare
- Neuroleptic malignant syndrome
- Prolonged QT interval

Drug interactions
Pharmacokinetic
- Haloperidol is metabolized by CYP2D6 and CYP3A4, with a minor pathway involving CYP1A2. It is an inhibitor of CYP2D6 and CYP3A4.
- *Carbamazepine*—increases the metabolism of haloperidol through CYP3A4 induction. Other CYP3A4 inducers may have the same effect. Therefore the haloperidol dose may need to be increased, according to the patient's response.
- *Fluoxetine*—increased risk of haloperidol undesirable effects through inhibition of CYP2D6.
- *Paroxetine*—increased risk of undesirable effects from both drugs due to inhibition of CYP2D6.
- *Venlafaxine*—increased risk of haloperidol undesirable effects through inhibition of CYP2D6.
- Other CYP2D6 inhibitors (📖 end cover) may also increase plasma concentrations of haloperidol. Consider using a lower dose.
- The clinical significance of co-administration with substrates of CYP2D6 or CYP3A4 (📖 end cover) is unknown. Caution is advised if haloperidol is co-administered with drugs that are predominantly metabolized by CYP2D6 or CYP3A4. The prescriber should be aware of the potential for interactions and that dosage adjustments may be necessary, particularly for drugs with a narrow therapeutic index.
- The clinical significance of co-administration with prodrug substrates of CYP2D6 (e.g. codeine, tramadol) is unknown. The prescriber should be aware of the potential for interactions and that dosage adjustments may be necessary.
- Inhibitors of CYP3A4 (📖 end cover) may increase plasma concentrations of haloperidol; other factors may be necessary before this interaction becomes significant (e.g. co-administration of other interacting drugs).
- Avoid grapefruit juice as it may increase the bioavailability of haloperidol through inhibition of intestinal CYP3A4.

Pharmacodynamic

- Haloperidol can cause dose-related prolongation of the QT interval. There is a potential risk that co-administration with other drugs that also prolong the QT interval (e.g. amiodarone, erythromycin, quinine) may result in ventricular arrhythmias.
- *Antiepileptics*—may need to be increased to take account of the lowered seizure threshold.
- *Antihypertensives*—increased risk of hypotension
- *CNS depressants*—additive sedative effect.
- *Levodopa and dopamine agonists*—effect antagonized by haloperidol.
- *Levomepromazine*—may be an additive hypotensive effect; increased risk of extrapyramidal symptoms.
- *Metoclopramide*—increased risk of extrapyramidal symptoms.
- *Opioids*—may be an additive hypotensive effect.
- *Trazodone*—may be an additive hypotensive effect.

℞ Dose

When prescribing haloperidol, the subcutaneous dose should be lower than the corresponding oral dose (which undergoes significant first-pass metabolism). There should be a separate prescription for each route, ensuring that the same dose cannot be given PO or by SC/CSCI.

Psychosis

- Initial dose 1.5mg PO BD–TDS. If severe, 3mg PO BD–TDS.
- Increase as necessary to a maximum of 30mg PO daily. Usual maintenance dose is 5–10mg PO daily.
- May be prescribed on a PRN basis (e.g. 1.5mg PO PRN, max BD–TDS).
- ¥ Alternatively, 3–5mg SC OD or via CSCI. Can increase to usual max 10mg SC daily, or via CSCI.
- ¥ May be prescribed on a PRN basis (e.g. 0.5–1.5mg SC PRN max TDS).

Intractable hiccup

- Initial dose 1.5mg PO TDS and adjust to response.
- Usual maintenance dose 1.5–3mg PO ON.
- May be prescribed on a PRN basis (e.g. 1.5mg PO PRN, max BD–TDS).
- ¥ Alternatively, 1.5–3mg SC OD, or via CSCI, and adjust to response.
- ¥ May be prescribed on a PRN basis (e.g. 0.5–1.5mg SC PRN max TDS).

Restlessness and agitation in the elderly

- Initial dose 1.5–3mg PO BD–TDS titrated as required to achieve maintenance dose (range 1.5–30mg PO daily).
- May be prescribed on a PRN basis (e.g. 1.5mg PO PRN, max BD–TDS).
- ¥ Alternatively, 1.5–3mg SC OD, or via CSCI. Can increase to usual max 10mg SC daily, or via CSCI.
- ¥ May be prescribed on a PRN basis (e.g. 0.5–1.5mg SC PRN max TDS).

¥ *Delirium*

- Initial dose 1.5–3mg PO OD. Titrated as required to achieve the maintenance dose (range 1.5–30mg daily).
- May be prescribed on a PRN basis (e.g. 1.5mg PO PRN, max BD–TDS).
- Alternatively 1.5–3mg SC OD, or via CSCI. Increase to usual max 10mg SC daily, or via CSCI.

¥ *Nausea and vomiting*

- Initial dose 1.5–3mg SC OD, or via CSCI. Increase to usual maximum of 10mg SC daily, or via CSCI.
- Oral route not usually appropriate, but 1.5–3mg PO ON–BD can be used. Can be increased to 5mg PO ON–BD as necessary.

♪ Dose adjustments

Elderly

- Wherever possible, lower doses should be used. The elderly are more susceptible to undesirable effects, particularly the anticholinergic effects. There may be an increased risk for cognitive decline and dementia.

Hepatic/renal impairment

- Wherever possible, lower doses should be used. Patients may be more susceptible to undesirable effects.

Additional information

- Haloperidol via CSCI is compatible with alfentanil, cyclizine, diamorphine, fentanyl, glycopyrronium, hydromorphone, ketamine, metoclopramide, midazolam, oxycodone, and tramadol.

⟡ Pharmacology

The pharmacology of haloperidol is complex and, as yet, has not been fully elucidated. It is a butyrophenone antipsychotic agent which selectively acts via dopamine D_2 receptors. It also has some effects at α_1-adrenoreceptors and muscarinic, H_1, and $5\text{-}HT_2$ receptors. The metabolism of haloperidol is complex, with a variety of metabolites being formed (including active metabolites). It is extensively metabolized by CYP2D6 and (at higher doses) by CYP3A4, with a minor pathway involving CYP1A2.

Hydromorphone

Standard release

Palladone® (CD POM)
Capsule: 1.3mg (*orange/clear*, 56); 2.6mg (*red/clear*, 56)
Unlicensed (CD POM)
Injection: 10mg/mL; 20mg/mL; 50mg/mL
See *Additional information* for supply issues

Modified release

Palladone SR® (CD POM)
Capsule: 2mg (*yellow/clear*, 56); 4mg (*pale blue/clear*, 56); 8mg (*pink/clear*, 56); 16mg (*brown/clear*, 56); 24mg (*dark blue/clear*, 56).

Hydromorphone is a Schedule 2 controlled drug (see ☐ Legal categories for medicines, p.23 for further information). Independent prescribers are **NOT** authorized to prescribe hydromorphone (☐ Independent prescribing: palliative care issues, p.25).

Indications
- Severe cancer pain
- For end-of-life care issues see ☐ Use of drugs in end-of-life care, p.53.

Contraindications and precautions
- If the dose of an opioid is titrated correctly, it is generally accepted that there are no absolute contraindications to the use of such drugs in palliative care, although there may be circumstances where one opioid is favoured over another (e.g. renal impairment, constipation). Nonetheless, the manufacturer states that hydromorphone is contraindicated for use in patients with:
  - acute abdomen
  - concurrent administration of MAOIs or within 2 weeks of discontinuation of their use
  - head injury
  - hepatic impairment
  - paralytic ileus
  - raised intracranial pressure.
- Use with caution in the following instances:
  - acute alcoholism
  - Addison's disease (adrenocortical insufficiency)
  - delirium tremens
  - diseases of the biliary tract
  - elderly patients
  - pancreatitis
  - prostatic hypertrophy
  - raised intracranial pressure
  - hepatic impairment (see above)
  - history of alcohol and drug abuse
  - hypotension
  - hypothyroidism
  - hypovolaemia
  - inflammatory bowel disorders
  - renal impairment
  - severe pulmonary disease
  - toxic psychosis.

- Hydromorphone may modify reactions and patients should be advised not to drive (or operate machinery) if affected.

☹ Undesirable effects

Strong opioids tend to cause similar undesirable effects, albeit to varying degrees. The frequency is not defined, but commonly reported undesirable effects include:

- Anorexia
- Asthenia
- Biliary pain
- Confusion
- Constipation
- Drowsiness
- Dry mouth
- Dyspepsia
- Exacerbation of pancreatitis
- Euphoria
- Insomnia
- Headache
- Hyperhidrosis
- Myoclonus
- Nausea
- Pruritus
- Sexual dysfunction (e.g. amenorrhea, decreased libido, erectile dysfunction)
- Urinary retention
- Vertigo
- Visual disturbance
- Vomiting

The following can occur with excessive dose:
- Agitation
- Exacerbation of pain
- Hallucinations
- Miosis
- Paraesthesia
- Respiratory depression
- Restlessness

Drug interactions

Pharmacokinetic
- CYP3A4 and CYP2C9 appear to have a minor role in the metabolism of hydromorphone.
- No clinically significant pharmacokinetic interactions reported.

Pharmacodynamic
- *Antihypertensives*—increased risk of hypotension.
- *CNS depressants*—risk of excessive sedation.
- *Haloperidol*—may be an additive hypotensive effect.
- *Ketamine*—there is a potential opioid sparing effect with ketamine and the dose of hydromorphone may need reducing.
- *Levomepromazine*—may be an additive hypotensive effect.

♏ Dose

The initial dose of morphine depends upon the patient's previous opioid requirements. Refer to 📖 Opioid substitution, p.33 for information regarding opioid dose equivalences and to 📖 Breakthrough cancer pain, p.35 for guidance relating to BTcP.

Oral
- Standard release
  - For opioid naive patients, initial dose is 1.3mg PO every 4–6 hours and PRN. The dose is then increased as necessary until a stable dose is attained. The patient should then be converted to a m/r formulation.
- Modified release
  - Patients should ideally be titrated using Palladone® before commencing Palladone SR®.
  - If necessary, for opioid-naive patients, initial dose is 2mg PO BD. The dose can then be titrated as necessary.

¥ *Subcutaneous*
- Initial dose in opioid-naive patients is 1–2mg via CSCI over 24 hours and increase as necessary.

♪ Dose adjustments
Elderly
- No specific guidance available, although lower starting doses in opioid-naive patients may be preferable. Dose requirements should be individually titrated.

Hepatic/renal impairment
- The manufacturer contraindicates the use of hydromorphone in patients with hepatic impairment. Nonetheless, hydromorphone is used in this group of patients and the dose should be titrated carefully to the patients need.
- No specific guidance is available for patients with renal impairment and dose requirements should be individually titrated. Alternatively, a different opioid may be more appropriate (e.g. oxycodone or fentanyl).
- By CSCI, hydromorphone is reportedly compatible with cyclizine, glycopyrronium, haloperidol, hyoscine hydrobromide, ketorolac, levomepromazine, metoclopramide, midazolam, octreotide, ondansetron, and phenobarbital.
- Hydromorphone shows concentration-dependent compatibility with dexamethasone.

Additional information
- The capsules can be swallowed whole or opened and their contents sprinkled on to cold soft food.
- The unlicensed injection is available from Martindale Pharma (Tel: 01277 266 600).

♦ Pharmacology
Hydromorphone is a synthetic analogue of morphine with analgesic activity at μ-opioid receptors. It is has an oral bioavailability of approximately 50% and is metabolized to conjugated hydromorphone, dihydroisomorphine and dihydromorphine.

Hyoscine butylbromide

Buscopan® (POM)
Tablet: 10mg (56)
Injection: 20mg/mL (10)

Note: Hyoscine butylbromide tablets can be sold to the public provided that a single dose is ≤20mg, the daily dose is ≤80mg, and the pack contains ≤240mg.

Indications
- Spasm of the genitourinary tract or GIract (tablet).
- Irritable bowel syndrome (tablet).
- ¥ Nausea and vomiting (associated with bowel obstruction).
- ¥ Smooth muscle spasm (e.g. bowel colic).
- ¥ Sweating.
- ¥ Terminal secretions.
- For end-of-life care issues see 📖 Use of drugs in end-of-life care, p.53.

Contraindications and precautions
- Note that for the management of terminal secretions, contraindications should be individually assessed.
- Manufacturer states that hyoscine butylbromide should be avoided in patients with:
  - mechanical stenoses in the region of the GI tract
  - megacolon
  - myasthenia gravis
  - narrow-angle glaucoma
  - paralytic ileus
  - prostatic enlargement with urinary retention
  - tachycardia.
- Hyoscine butylbromide possesses anticholinergic properties so it should be used with caution in the following:
  - bladder outflow obstruction
  - cardiac arrhythmias
  - congestive heart failure
  - coronary artery disease
  - diarrhoea (may be masking intestinal obstruction)
  - elderly (more susceptible to undesirable effects)
  - GI reflux disease
  - hypertension
  - hyperthyroidism
  - pyrexia (reduces sweating)
  - renal impairment (see 📖 *Dose adjustments*, p.235)
  - ulcerative colitis.
- Hyoscine butylbromide may modify reactions and patients should be advised not to drive (or operate machinery) if affected.

☺ Undesirable effects

The frequency is not defined, but reported undesirable effects include:
- confusion
- difficulty in micturition
- dizziness
- drowsiness
- dry mouth
- inhibition of sweating
- palpitations
- tachycardia
- visual disturbances.

☺ Drug interactions

Pharmacokinetic
- No recognized pharmacokinetic interactions.

Pharmacodynamic
- β$_2$-agonists—increased risk of tachycardia.
- Cyclizine—increased risk of anticholinergic undesirable effects.
- Domperidone—may inhibit prokinetic effect.
- Metoclopramide—may inhibit prokinetic effect.
- Nefopam—increased risk of anticholinergic undesirable effects.
- Tricyclic antidepressants—increased risk of anticholinergic undesirable effects.

♣ Dose

Spasm of the genito-urinary tract or GI tract
- 20mg PO QDS.
- ¥ Alternatively, 10–20mg SC and 60mg via CSCI.

Irritable bowel syndrome
- Initial dose 10mg PO TDS, increasing as necessary to 20mg PO QDS.

¥ Nausea and vomiting/smooth muscle spasm/sweating/terminal secretions
- Initial dose 20mg SC, or 60mg via CSCI over 24 hours.
- Dose can be increased as necessary to a usual maximum of 120mg.
- Higher doses (e.g. 300mg) have been reported, although treatment should be reviewed if 120mg is unsatisfactory.

♣ Dose adjustments

Elderly
- No specific guidance available. Use the lowest effective dose as the elderly may be more susceptible to the undesirable effects.

Hepatic/renal impairment
- No specific guidance available. Use the lowest effective dose.

Additional information

- Tablets may be crushed prior to administration if necessary.
- Hyoscine butylbromide is poorly absorbed orally, so the usefulness of this route of administration is questionable, apart from possible benefit in bowel colic.
- Via CSCI, hyoscine butylbromide is reportedly compatibility with alfentanil, clonazepam, diamorphine, fentanyl, levomepromazine, metoclopramide, midazolam, octreotide, ondansetron, oxycodone, ranitidine, and tramadol.
- There may be concentration-dependent incompatibility with cyclizine and haloperidol.

⊘ Pharmacology

Hyoscine butylbromide is a quaternary ammonium antimuscarinic that inhibits the peripheral actions of acetylcholine. Following both oral and parenteral administration, hyoscine butylbromide concentrates in the tissue of the GI tract, liver and kidneys. As it is a quaternary ammonium compound, it does not usually cross the blood–brain barrier; thus it is devoid of central activity such as drowsiness or a direct anti-emetic effect.

Hyoscine hydrobromide

Kwells® (P)
Tablet: 150mcg (12); 300mcg (12)

Joy-rides® (P)
Tablet: 150mcg

Scopoderm TTS® (POM)
Transdermal patch: 1.5mg (releasing 1mg over 72 hours)

Generic (POM)
Injection: 400mcg (10); 600mcg (10)

Indications
- Motion sickness (oral/transdermal)
- * Hypersalivation
- * Nausea and vomiting
- * Smooth muscle spasm (e.g. bowel colic)
- * Sweating
- * Terminal secretions
- For end-of-life care issues see 📖 Use of drugs in end-of-life care.

Contraindications and precautions
- Note that for the management of terminal secretions, contraindications and precautions should be individually assessed.
- Contraindicated for use in patients with narrow-angle glaucoma.
- The manufacturers state use with caution in the following:circumstances:

  - bladder outflow obstruction
  - cardiac arrhythmias
  - congestive heart failure
  - diarrhoea (may be masking intestinal obstruction)
  - Down's syndrome
  - elderly patients (see *Dose adjustments*)
  - epilepsy
  - GI reflux disease
  - hepatic impairment
  - hyperthyroidism
  - intestinal obstruction
  - myasthenia gravis
  - paralytic ileus
  - prostatic enlargement
  - pyrexia (reduces sweating)
  - renal impairment
  - ulcerative colitis.

- Idiosyncratic reactions may occur with ordinary therapeutic doses of hyoscine (e.g. agitation, hallucinations)
- Undesirable effects may persist for up to 24 hours or longer after patch removal
- Remove transdermal patch prior to MRI due to risk of burns.
- Hyoscine hydrobromide may modify reactions and patients should be advised not to drive (or operate machinery) if affected.

☺ Undesirable effects
The frequency is not defined, but reported undesirable effects include:
- Agitation (paradoxical)
- Amnesia

- Bradycardia (tachycardia with excessive dose)
- Confusion
- Difficulty in micturition
- Dizziness
- Drowsiness
- Dry mouth
- Hallucinations
- Inhibition of sweating (risk of hyperthermia in hot weather, or pyrexia)
- Seizures
- Visual disturbances (e.g. blurred vision).

Drug interactions

Pharmacokinetic

- No recognized pharmacokinetic interactions.

Pharmacodynamic

- *Donepezil*—effect may be antagonized
- *β₂-agonists*—increased risk of tachycardia
- *Cyclizine*—increased risk of anticholinergic undesirable effects
- *Domperidone*—may inhibit prokinetic effect
- *Galantamine*—effect may be antagonized
- *Metoclopramide*—may inhibit prokinetic effect
- *Nefopam*—increased risk of anticholinergic undesirable effects
- *Rivastigmine*—effect may be antagonized
- *Tricyclic antidepressantss*—increased risk of anticholinergic undesirable effects

⅀ Dose

¥ *Hypersalivation/sweating*

- 1mg every 72 hours via transdermal patch. Two patches may be used if necessary.
- Alternatively, 300mcg PO up to TDS can be tried.
- It may be more appropriate to use alternative treatments (e.g. glycopyrronium, propantheline).

¥ *Nausea and vomiting/smooth muscle spasm*

- Other options are usually used for these indications (e.g. hyoscine butylbromide).
- 1mg every 72 hours via transdermal patch. Two patches may be used if necessary.
- Alternatively, 300mcg PO up to TDS can be tried.
- Via CSCI, initially 400mcg over 24 hours increased as necessary up to 1.2mg.

¥ *Terminal secretions*

- Initial dose 400 mcg SC injection, followed by 1.2mg via CSCI over 24 hours.
- If necessary, the dose can be increased to 2.4mg over 24 hours.

♪ Dose adjustments

Elderly
• No specific guidance available. Use the lowest effective dose as the elderly may be more susceptible to the undesirable effects, particularly the anticholinergic effects. The patient may be at an increased risk for cognitive decline and dementia.

Hepatic/renal impairment
• No specific guidance available. Use the lowest effective dose.

Additional information

• Via CSCI, hyoscine hydrobromide is reportedly compatible with alfentanil, clonazepam, cyclizine, dexamethasone, diamorphine, fentanyl, haloperidol, hydromorphone, levomepromazine, metoclopramide, midazolam, morphine hydrochloride, morphine sulphate, morphine tartrate, octreotide, ondansetron, oxycodone, promethazine, and ranitidine.

♦ Pharmacology

Hyoscine is an anticholinergic drug which blocks the action of acetylcholine at post-ganglionic parasympathetic sites including smooth muscle, secretary glands, and CNS sites. It effectively reduces secretions (bowel, salivary and bronchial), has a direct anti-emetic effect (unlike glycopyrronium and hyoscine butylbromide), and reduces sweating. It may cause amnesia and, unlike glycopyrronium, it is more likely to cause bradycardia than tachycardia. It is extensively metabolized, although the exact details are unknown.

Ibuprofen

Standard release

Brufen® (POM)
Tablet: 200mg (100); 400mg (100); 600mg (100)
Effervescent Granules: 600mg (20) *(contains 9mmol Na$^+$ per sachet)*
Syrup: 100mg/5mL (500mL)

Generic (POM)

Tablet: 200mg; 400mg; 600mg (various pack sizes)
Oral Suspension: 100mg/5mL (100mL; 150mL; 500mL) *(sugar-free versions are available; specify on prescription).*

Modified release

Brufen Retard® (POM)
Tablet: 800mg (56)

Fenbid Spansule® (POM)
Capsule: 300mg (120)

Note: Ibuprofen is available over-the-counter in a variety of formulations (e.g. tablets, caplets, capsules, creams, gels) and strengths.

Indications

- Mild to moderate pain.
- Inflammatory conditions (e.g. rheumatoid and other musculoskeletal disorders).
- Fever.

Contraindications and precautions

- Contraindicated for use in patients with:
  - a history of, or active, peptic ulceration
  - hypersensitivity reactions to ibuprofen, aspirin, or other NSAIDs
  - severe heart failure.
- Use the minimum effective dose for the shortest duration necessary in order to reduce the risk of cardiac and GI events.
- Elderly patients are more at risk of developing undesirable effects.
- Use with caution in the following circumstances:
  - concurrent use of diuretics, corticosteroids, and NSAIDs (see 📖 *Drug interactions, p.241*)
  - congestive heart failure and/or left ventricular dysfunction
  - diabetes mellitus
  - established ischaemic heart disease, peripheral arterial disease, and/or cerebrovascular disease need careful consideration because of the increased risk of thrombotic events (especially at doses >1200mg/day)
  - hepatic impairment
  - hyperlipidaemia
  - hypertension (particularly uncontrolled)
  - recovery from surgery

- renal impairment
- smoking.
- Patients on long-term therapy need regular monitoring of renal and liver function.
- Abnormal LFTs can occur; discontinue NSAID if this persists.
- Ibuprofen may prevent the development of signs and symptoms of inflammation/infection (e.g. fever).
- Consider co-prescription of misoprostol or a proton pump inhibitor if:
  - long-term NSAID therapy
  - concurrent use of drugs that increase the risk of GI toxicity (see 📖 *Drug interactions, (below)*)
- Refer to 📖 Selection of an NSAID, p.31 for further information, including selection.

☺ Undesirable effects

The frequency is not defined, but reported undesirable effects include:
- Abdominal pain
- Cardiac failure
- Diarrhoea
- Dyspepsia
- Fatigue
- GI haemorrhage
- Headache
- Hypersensitivity reactions (e.g. anaphylaxis, asthma, dyspnoea, pruritus, rash, severe skin reactions)
- Hypertension
- Jaundice
- Melaena
- Nausea
- Oedema
- Peptic ulcer
- Renal failure
- Vomiting.

Drug interactions

Pharmacokinetic

- Ibuprofen is metabolized to some extent by CYP2C8/9 and CYP2C19 but it also undergoes glucuronidation. However, ibuprofen is an inhibitor of CYP2C8/9.
- *Methotrexate*—reduced excretion of methotrexate.
- *Warfarin*—possible increased risk of bleeding through inhibition of warfarin metabolism (5–11% of Caucasians have a variant of CYP2C9, requiring lower maintenance doses of warfarin; combination with ibuprofen may further reduce warfarin metabolism).
- The clinical significance of co-administration with CYP2C8/9 substrates (📖 end cover) is unknown. The prescriber should be aware of the potential for interactions and that dosage adjustments may be necessary.

Pharmacodynamic
- *Anticoagulants*—increased risk of bleeding.
- *Antihypertensives*—reduced hypotensive effect.
- *Antiplatelet drugs*—increased risk of bleeding.
- *Corticosteroids*—increased risk of GI toxicity.
- *Ciclosporin*—increased risk of nephrotoxcity.
- *Diuretics*—reduced diuretic effect; nephrotoxicity of ibuprofen may be increased.
- *Rosiglitazone*—increased risk of oedema.
- *SSRIs*—increased risk of GI bleeding.

Dose

To be taken with or after food.

Standard release
- Initial dose 400mg PO TDS, increasing if necessary to a maximum of 800mg PO TDS.

Modified release
Brufen Retard ®
- Initial dose 2 tablets (1600mg) PO OD, preferably in the early evening.
- Can be increased to 3 tablets (2400mg) PO daily in two divided doses.

Fenbid Spansule®
- Initial dose 2 capsules (600mg) PO BD.
- Can be increased in severe cases to 3 capsules (900mg) PO BD.

Dose adjustments

Elderly
- No special dosage modifications are required, but check hepatic/renal impairment.

Hepatic/renal impairment
- No specific dosage modifications are available. However, NSAIDs should be used cautiously in patients with liver and/or renal impairment because of the increased risks of undesirable effects. The lowest effective dose should be used for the shortest time permissible and regular monitoring of liver and/or renal function is advisable.

Additional information
- Ibuprofen at doses <1200mg/day appears not to increase the risk of thrombotic events
- It is considered to be the safest NSAID in terms of GI toxicity, especially at doses <1200mg/day.

Pharmacology

Ibuprofen is an NSAID that possesses anti-inflammatory, analgesic, and antipyretic activity. Its mode of action, like that of other NSAIDs, is not completely understood, but may be related to inhibition of COX-1 and COX-2. Ibuprofen is well-absorbed orally and is rapidly metabolized and eliminated in the urine.

Imatinib

Glivec® (POM)

Tablet: 100mg (*scored*, 60); 400mg (30)

Indications

- Acute lymphoblastic leukaemia.
- Advanced hypereosinophilic syndrome and chronic eosinophilic leukaemia.
- Chronic myeloid leukaemia (accelerated and chronic phase; blast crisis).
- Dermatofibrosarcoma protuberans.
- Gastrointestinal stromal tumours (GISTs).
- Myelodysplastic/myeloproliferative diseases.

Contraindications and precautions

- Use cautiously in the following:
  - cardiac disease (risk of fluid retention and subsequent cardiac failure)
  - concomitant use with drugs that inhibit CYP3A4 (see 📖 *Drug interactions*, p.244)
  - diabetes (can cause hyperglycaemia)
  - elderly patients
  - gout (can cause hyperuricaemia)
  - hepatic impairment (see 📖 *Dose adjustments*, p.245)
  - renal impairment (see 📖 *Dose adjustments*, p.245).
- Ideally, patients should not use high doses of paracetamol with imatinib since glucuronidation may be affected.
- Imatinib may cause dizziness and fatigue. Patients should be advised not to drive (or operate machinery) if affected.

☺ Undesirable effects

Very common

- Abdominal pain
- Anaemia
- Arthralgia
- Bone pain
- Dermatitis/eczema/rash
- Diarrhoea
- Dyspepsia
- Fatigue
- Fluid retention
- Headache
- Muscle spasm and cramps
- Myalgia
- Nausea
- Neutropenia
- Periorbital oedema
- Thrombocytopenia
- Vomiting
- Weight increase (probably fluid retention)

Common

- Anorexia
- Blurred vision
- Conjunctival haemorrhage
- Conjunctivitis
- Constipation
- Cough
- Dizziness
- Dry eye
- Dry mouth
- Dyspnoea
- Epistaxis
- Eyelid oedema

- Febrile neutropenia
- Flatulence
- Flushing
- Gastritis
- Gastro-oesophageal reflux
- Hypoaesthesia
- Insomnia
- Lacrimation increased

- Night sweats
- Pancytopenia
- Paraesthesia
- Photosensitivity reaction
- Pruritus
- Pyrexia
- Raised LFTs
- Taste disturbance
- Weight loss

Uncommon
- Acute renal failure
- Gastric ulcer
- Gout/hyperuricaemia
- Haematuria
- Hepatitis
- Hypercalcaemia
- Hyperglycaemia
- Hypertension
- Hypokalaemia
- Jaundice
- Oesophagitis
- Pleural effusion
- Sexual dysfunction
- Stomatitis

Drug interactions

Pharmacokinetic
- Imatinib is metabolized by CYP3A4; it is also an inhibitor of CYP3A4.
- *Paracetamol*—glucuronidation inhibited by imatinib; potential paracetamol toxicity with prolonged use.
- The clinical significance of co-administration with inducers, inhibitors, or substrates of CYP3A4 (end cover) is unknown. The prescriber should be aware of the potential for interactions and that dose adjustments may be necessary, particularly for those drugs with a narrow therapeutic index.
- Avoid grapefruit juice as it may increase the bioavailability of imatinib through inhibition of intestinal CYP3A4.

Pharmacodynamic
- None known.

Dose

Acute lymphoblastic leukaemia
- 600mg PO OD.

Advanced hypereosinophilic syndrome and chronic eosinophilic leukaemia
- 600mg PO OD, increased if necessary to maximum dose of 400mg PO BD

Chronic myeloid leukaemia
- Accelerated phase—600mg PO OD, increased if necessary to maximum dose 400mg PO BD.

- Blast crisis—600mg PO OD, increased if necessary to maximum dose 400mg PO BD.
- Chronic phase—400mg PO OD, increased if necessary to maximum dose 400mg PO BD.

Dermatofibrosarcoma protuberans
- 400mg PO BD.

GISTs
- 400mg PO OD.

Myelodysplastic/myeloproliferative diseases:
- 400mg PO OD.

Dose adjustments
Elderly
- No dose adjustments are necessary.

Hepatic/renal impairment
- Imatinib is significantly metabolized by the liver. Patients with mild, moderate or severe liver impairment should be given the minimum recommended dose of 400mg PO OD. The dose can be reduced if not tolerated.
- For patients with renal impairment (CrCl < 60mL/min) or those on dialysis, the recommended maximum starting dose is 400mg PO OD.

Dose adjustments for undesirable reactions
- If severe non-haematological undesirable effects occur, imatinib should be discontinued until the event has resolved. Imatinib can be re-introduced as appropriate at a reduced dose:
  - 400mg PO OD reduce dose to 300mg PO OD
  - 600mg PO OD reduce dose to 400mg PO OD
  - 400mg PO BD reduce dose to 600mg PO OD.
- Refer to the SmPC if haematological undesirable effects occur.

Additional information
- Tablets should be taken with a meal and a large glass of water to minimize the risk of GI irritation.
- If necessary, tablets may be dispersed in water or apple juice (approximately 50mL for a 100mg tablet, and 200mL for a 400mg tablet) immediately prior to administration.

Pharmacology
Imatinib is a Bcr-Abl tyrosine kinase inhibitor which is the product of the Philadelphia chromosome in chronic myeloid leukaemia (CML). It induces apoptosis in Bcr-Abl positive cell lines as well as in fresh leukaemic cells in Philadelphia chromosome positive CML. It also inhibits other tyrosine kinases and inhibits proliferation and induces apoptosis in GIST cells. It is well absorbed after oral administration, with a bioavailability of 98%, and is highly protein bound. It is extensively metabolized, mainly by CYP3A4, to a compound with similar activity. Imatinib and its metabolites are not excreted via the kidney to a significant extent.

Insulin: biphasic insulin aspart

NovoMix™ 30 (POM)

Biphasic insulin aspart (recombinant human insulin analogue), 30% insulin aspart, 70% insulin aspart protamine, 100 units/mL
Injection: 5 × 3mL Penfill® cartridge for Novopen® device
Injection: 5 × 3mL prefilled disposable FlexPen® injection devices; range 1–60 units, allowing 1 unit dosage adjustment)

Indications

• Diabetes mellitus.
• For end-of-life care issues see 📖 Use of drugs in end-of-life care, p.53.

Contraindications and precautions

• NovoMix® 30 has a faster onset of action than biphasic human insulin and should generally be given within 10 minutes of a meal or snack containing carbohydrates.
• It must only be administered by SC injection.
• Use with caution in the following:
  • elderly patients (see 📖 Dose adjustments, p.247)
  • renal impairment (see 📖 Dose adjustments, p.247)
  • severe hepatic impairment (see 📖 Dose adjustments, p.247)
  • systemic illness (dose increase may be necessary)
• The risk of reduced warning symptoms of hypoglycaemia is increased in the following circumstances:
  • after transfer from animal to human insulin
  • autonomic neuropathy is present
  • concurrent treatment with particular drugs (see 📖 Drug interactions, p.247)
  • elderly patients
  • gradual onset of hypoglycaemia
  • long history of diabetes
  • markedly improved glycaemic control
  • psychiatric illness.

☻ Undesirable effects

Very common

• Hypoglycaemia (also depends on other factors)

Uncommon

• Injection site reactions (generally minor, e.g. redness, pain, itching, or inflammation).
• Lipodystrophy.
• Oedema (may cause sodium retention; usually transitory during initiation).
• Peripheral neuropathy.
• Retinopathy (usually temporary deterioration associated with abrupt improvement in glycaemic control).
• Urticaria.
• Visual disturbances (usually temporary due to marked glycaemic control and associated altered lens properties).

Drug interactions

Pharmacokinetic
- None recognized.

Pharmacodynamic
- *ACEIs*—increased risk of hypoglycaemia.
- *Antipsychotics*—glucose metabolism can be affected; dose adjustments may be necessary.
- *β_2-agonists*—hypoglycaemic effect may be antagonized.
- *Corticosteroids*—hypoglycaemic effect antagonized.
- *Diuretics*—hypoglycaemic effect may be antagonized.
- *Fluoxetine*—increased risk of hypoglycaemia.
- *Octreotide*—can affect glucose metabolism; dose adjustments may be necessary.

Dose

- Biphasic insulin aspart is usually given OD–BD.
- In patients with type 1 diabetes the individual insulin requirement is usually 0.5–1.0 units/kg/day. Nonetheless, dose according to requirements.
- In patients with type 2 diabetes, biphasic insulin aspart can be combined with oral antidiabetic drugs. The usual starting dose is 6 units at breakfast and 6 units with the evening meal. It can also be initiated as 12 units with the evening meal. Doses >30 units once daily should be divided into two equal doses.
- If BD dosing results in recurrent daytime hypoglycaemic episodes, the morning dose can be split into morning and lunchtime doses (i.e. TDS regime).

Dose adjustments

Elderly
- In the elderly, progressive deterioration of renal function may lead to a steady decrease in insulin requirements.

Hepatic/renal impairment
- In patients with severe hepatic impairment, insulin requirements may be diminished because of reduced capacity for gluconeogenesis and reduced insulin metabolism.
- In patients with renal impairment, insulin requirements may be diminished because of reduced insulin metabolism.

Additional information

- During the early stages of palliative care diabetes should be managed conventionally.
- As disease progresses and prognosis becomes short term, the importance of treatment shifts to preventing symptomatic hyperglycaemia and hypoglycaemia. Fasting blood glucose should be maintained between 8 and 15mmol/L.
- As the patient deteriorates and oral intake declines, consider halving the dose of insulin.
- During use, do not refrigerate and do not store above 25°C.

⊕ Pharmacology

Biphasic insulin aspart is a suspension of human insulin aspart complexed with protamine sulphate, combined with insulin aspart. The net result is a formulation with an immediate effect, followed by a more sustained action. Onset of action is within 10–20 minutes, with a maximum effect within 1–4 hours; the duration of effect is up to 24 hours.

Insulin: biphasic insulin lispro

Humalog® Mix25 (POM)

Biphasic insulin lispro (recombinant human insulin analogue), 25% insulin lispro, 75% insulin lispro protamine, 100units/mL.
Injection: 5 × 3mL cartridge for Autopen® Classic or HumaPen® devices.
Injection: 5 × 3mL prefilled disposable injection devices; range 1–60 units, allowing 1 unit dosage adjustment.
Injection: 5 x 3mL prefilled disposable KwikPen® injection devices; range 1–60 units, allowing 1 unit dosage adjustment.

Humalog® Mix50 (POM)

Biphasic insulin lispro (recombinant human insulin analogue), 50% insulin lispro, 50% insulin lispro protamine, 100 units/mL.
Injection: 5 × 3mL cartridge for Autopen® Classic or HumaPen® devices.
Injection: 5 × 3mL prefilled disposable injection devices; range 1–60 units, allowing 1 unit dosage adjustment.
Injection: 5 × 3mL prefilled disposable KwikPen® injection devices; range 1–60 units, allowing 1 unit dosage adjustment.

Indications

- Diabetes mellitus.
- For end-of-life care issues see 📖 Use of drugs in end-of-life care, p.53.

Contraindications and precautions

- Biphasic insulin lispro has a faster onset of action than biphasic human insulin and should generally be given within 15 minutes of a meal or snack containing carbohydrates.
- It must only be administered by SC injection.
- Use with caution in the following:
  - elderly patients (see 📖 *Dose adjustments*, p.250)
  - renal impairment (see 📖 *Dose adjustments*, p.250)
  - severe hepatic impairment (see 📖 *Dose adjustments*, p.250)
  - systemic illness (dose increase may be necessary).
- The risk of reduced warning symptoms of hypoglycaemia is increased in the following circumstances:
  - after transfer from animal to human insulin
  - autonomic neuropathy is present
  - concurrent treatment with particular drugs (see 📖 *Drug interactions*, p.250)
  - elderly patients
  - gradual onset of hypoglycaemia
  - long history of diabetes
  - markedly improved glycaemic control
  - psychiatric illness.

☺ Undesirable effects

The frequency is not specifically defined, but in common with other insulin products, undesirable effects include:

- Hypoglycaemia (also depends on other factors).
- Injection site reactions (generally minor, e.g. redness, pain, itching, or inflammation).
- Lipodystrophy
- Oedema (may cause sodium retention, usually transitory during initiation).
- Peripheral neuropathy.
- Retinopathy (usually temporary deterioration associated with abrupt improvement in glycaemic control).
- Urticaria.
- Visual disturbances (usually temporary, caused by marked glycaemic control and associated altered lens properties).

Drug interactions

Pharmacokinetic
- None recognized.

Pharmacodynamic
- *ACEIs*—increased risk of hypoglycaemia.
- *Antipsychotics*—glucose metabolism can be affected; dose adjustments may be necessary.
- *β_2-agonists*—hypoglycaemic effect may be antagonized.
- *Corticosteroids*—hypoglycaemic effect antagonized.
- *Diuretics*—hypoglycaemic effect may be antagonized.
- *Fluoxetine*—increased risk of hypoglycaemia.
- *Octreotide*—can affect glucose metabolism; dose adjustments may be necessary.

⚗ Dose

- Biphasic insulin lispro is usually given within 15 minutes of meals.
- The dose is individually determined.

⚗ Dose adjustments

Elderly
- In the elderly, progressive deterioration of renal function may lead to a steady decrease in insulin requirements.

Hepatic/renal impairment
- In patients with severe hepatic impairment, insulin requirements may be diminished because of reduced capacity for gluconeogenesis and reduced insulin metabolism.
- In patients with renal impairment, insulin requirements may be diminished because of reduced insulin metabolism.

Additional information
- During the early stages of palliative care diabetes should be managed conventionally.
- As disease progresses and prognosis becomes short term, the importance of treatment shifts to preventing symptomatic hyperglycaemia and hypoglycaemia. Fasting blood glucose should be maintained between 8 and 15mmol/L.
- As the patient deteriorates and oral intake declines, consider halving the dose of insulin.
- During use, do not refrigerate and do not store above 25°C.

⊕ Pharmacology

Biphasic insulin lispro is a suspension of insulin lispro complexed with protamine sulphate, combined with insulin lispro. The net effect is a formulation with an immediate effect, followed by a more sustained action. Onset of action is within 15 minutes, with a maximum effect within 1–4 hours; the duration of effect is up to 24 hours.

Insulin: biphasic isophane insulin

Mixtard® 30 (POM)
Biphasic isophane insulin (human, pyr), 30% soluble, 70% isophane, 100 units/mL
Injection: 10mL vial
Injection: 5 × 3mL Penfill® cartridge for Novopen® device

Injection: 5 × 3mL prefilled disposable InnoLet® injection devices; range 1–50 units, allowing 1 unit dosage adjustment).

Humulin M3® (POM)
Biphasic isophane insulin (human, prb), 30% soluble, 70% isophane, 100 units/mL
Injection: 10mL vial
Injection: 5 × 3mL cartridge for most Autopen® Classic or HumaPen® devices.

Insuman® Comb 15 (POM)
Biphasic isophane insulin (human, crb), 15% soluble, 85% isophane, 100 units/mL
Injection: 5 × 3mL prefilled disposable OptiSet® injection devices; range 2–40 units, allowing 2 unit dosage adjustment.

Insuman® Comb 25 (POM)
Biphasic isophane insulin (human, crb), 25% soluble, 75% isophane, 100 units/mL
Injection: 5mL vial
Injection: 5 × 3mL cartridge for OptiPen® Pro 1 device

Injection: 5 × 3mL prefilled disposable OptiSet® injection devices; range 2–40 units, allowing 2 unit dosage adjustment.

Insuman® Comb 50 (POM)
Biphasic isophane insulin (human, crb), 50% soluble, 50% isophane, 100 units/mL
Injection: 5 × 3mL cartridge for OptiPen® Pro 1 device
Injection: 5 × 3mL prefilled disposable OptiSet® injection devices; range 2–40 units, allowing 2 unit dosage adjustment.

Hypurin® Porcine 30/70 Mix (POM)
Biphasic isophane insulin (porcine, highly purified), 30% soluble, 70% isophane, 100 units/mL
Injection: 10mL vial
Injection: 5 × 3mL cartridge for Autopen® Classic device.

Indications

- Diabetes mellitus.
- For end-of-life care issues see 📖 Use of drugs in end-of-life care, p.53.

Contraindications and precautions

- An injection should be followed within 30 minutes by a meal or snack containing carbohydrates.
- Biphasic isophane insulin must only be administered by SC injection.
- Use with caution in the following:
  - elderly patients (see 📖 Dose adjustments, p.254)
  - renal impairment (see 📖 Dose adjustments, p.254)
  - severe hepatic impairment (see 📖 Dose adjustments, p.254)
  - systemic illness (dose increase may be necessary).
- The risk of reduced warning symptoms of hypoglycaemia is increased in the following circumstances:
  - after transfer from animal insulin to human insulin
  - autonomic neuropathy is present
  - concurrent treatment with particular drugs (see 📖 Drug interactions, p.253)
  - elderly patients
  - gradual onset of hypoglycaemia
  - long history of diabetes
  - markedly improved glycaemic control
  - psychiatric illness.

☺ Undesirable effects

Very common

- Hypoglycaemia (also depends on other factors).

Uncommon

- Injection site reactions (generally minor, e.g. redness, pain, itching, or inflammation)
- Lipodystrophy
- Oedema (may cause sodium retention; usually transitory during initiation)
- Peripheral neuropathy
- Retinopathy (usually temporary deterioration associated with abrupt improvement in glycaemic control).
- Urticaria.

Very rare

- Visual disturbances (usually temporary, caused by marked glycaemic control and associated altered lens properties).

Drug interactions

Pharmacokinetic

- None recognized.

Pharmacodynamic

- *ACEIs*—increased risk of hypoglycaemia.
- *Antipsychotics*—glucose metabolism can be affected; dose adjustments may be necessary.
- *β_2-agonists*—hypoglycaemic effect may be antagonized.

- *Corticosteroids*—hypoglycaemic effect antagonized.
- *Diuretics*—hypoglycaemic effect may be antagonized.
- *Fluoxetine*—increased risk of hypoglycaemia.
- *Octreotide*—can affect glucose metabolism; dose adjustments may be necessary.

Dose
- Biphasic isophane insulin is usually given OD–BD. A suitable starting dose is 10 units SC OD; titrate according to requirements.

Dose adjustments
Elderly
- Progressive deterioration of renal function may lead to a steady decrease in insulin requirements.

Hepatic/renal impairment
- In patients with severe hepatic impairment, insulin requirements may be diminished because of reduced capacity for gluconeogenesis and reduced insulin metabolism.
- In patients with renal impairment, insulin requirements may be diminished because of reduced insulin metabolism.

Additional information
- During the early stages of palliative care diabetes should be managed conventionally.
- As disease progresses and prognosis becomes short term, the importance of treatment shifts to preventing symptomatic hyperglycaemia and hypoglycaemia. Fasting blood glucose should be maintained between 8 and 15mmol/L.
- As the patient deteriorates and oral intake declines, consider halving the dose of insulin.
- During use, do not refrigerate and do not store above 25°C.

Pharmacology
Biphasic isophane insulin is a suspension of either porcine or human insulin complexed with protamine sulphate, combined with soluble insulin. The net effect is a formulation with an immediate effect, followed by a more sustained action. Onset of action is within 30 minutes, with a maximum effect within 2–8 hours; the duration of effect is up to 24 hours.

Insulin: insulin aspart

NovoRapid® 30 (POM)

Insulin aspart (recombinant human insulin analogue), 100 units/mL
Injection: 5 × 3mL Penfill® cartridge for Novopen® devices
Injection: 5 × 3mL prefilled disposable FlexPen® injection devices; range
1–60 units, allowing 1 unit dosage adjustment).

Indications

- Diabetes mellitus.
- For end-of-life care issues see 📖 Use drugs in end-of-life care, p.53.

Contraindications and precautions

- NovoRapid® has a faster onset of action than soluble human insulin
  and should generally be given within 10 minutes of a meal or snack
  containing carbohydrates.
- Use with caution in the following:
  - elderly patients (see 📖 Dose adjustments, p.256)
  - renal impairment (see 📖 Dose adjustments, p.256)
  - severe hepatic impairment (see 📖 Dose adjustments, p.256)
  - systemic illness (dose increase may be necessary).
- The risk of reduced warning symptoms of hypoglycaemia is increased in
  the following circumstances:
  - after transfer from animal insulin to human insulin
  - autonomic neuropathy is present
  - concurrent treatment with particular drugs (see 📖 Drug interactions, p.256)
  - elderly patients
  - gradual onset of hypoglycaemia
  - long history of diabetes
  - markedly improved glycaemic control
  - psychiatric illness.

☺ Undesirable effects

Very common

- Hypoglycaemia

Uncommon

- Injection site reactions (generally minor, e.g. redness, pain, itching, or
  inflammation)
- Lipodystrophy
- Oedema (may cause sodium retention; usually transitory during
  initiation)
- Peripheral neuropathy
- Retinopathy (usually temporary deterioration associated with abrupt
  improvement in glycaemic control)
- Urticaria
- Visual disturbances (usually temporary, caused by marked glycaemic
  control and associated altered lens properties).

Drug interactions

Pharmacokinetic
- None recognized.

Pharmacodynamic
- *ACEIs*—increased risk of hypoglycaemia.
- *Antipsychotics*—glucose metabolism can be affected; dose adjustments may be necessary.
- *β_2-agonists*—hypoglycaemic effect may be antagonized.
- *Corticosteroids*—hypoglycaemic effect antagonized.
- *Diuretics*—hypoglycaemic effect may be antagonized.
- *Fluoxetine*—increased risk of hypoglycaemia.
- *Octreotide*—can affect glucose metabolism; dose adjustments may be necessary.

Dose
- Dosing must be individualized. As a rule, if blood glucose >15mmol/L and patient symptomatic, give up to 5 units SC. Recheck after an hour; if it has remained above 15mmol/L treat with the same dose only if symptomatic.

Dose adjustments

Elderly
- In the elderly, progressive deterioration of renal function may lead to a steady decrease in insulin requirements.

Hepatic/renal impairment
- In patients with severe hepatic impairment, insulin requirements may be diminished because of reduced capacity for gluconeogenesis and reduced insulin metabolism.
- In patients with renal impairment, insulin requirements may be diminished because of reduced insulin metabolism.

Additional information
- During the early stages of palliative care diabetes should be managed conventionally.
- As disease progresses and prognosis becomes short term, the importance of treatment shifts to preventing symptomatic hyperglycaemia and hypoglycaemia. Fasting blood glucose should be maintained between 8 and 15mmol/L.
- As the patient deteriorates and oral intake declines, consider halving the dose of insulin.

Pharmacology

Insulin aspart is a fast-acting insulin. Onset of action is within 10–20 minutes, with a maximum effect within 1–4 hours; the duration of effect is up to 3–5 hours.

Insulin: insulin detemir

Levemir® (POM)

Insulin detemir (recombinant human insulin analogue) 100 units/mL
Injection: 5 × 3mL cartridge for NovoPen® device
Injection: 5 × 3mL prefilled disposable FlexPen® injection devices; range 1–60 units, allowing 1 unit dosage adjustment
Injection: 5 × 3mL prefilled disposable InnoLet® injection devices; range 1–50 units, allowing 1 unit dosage adjustment

Indications

- Diabetes mellitus
- For end-of-life care issues see 📖 Use of drugs in end-of-life care, p.53.

Contraindications and precautions

- Insulin detemir is not the insulin of choice for the treatment of diabetic ketoacidosis.
- Insulin detemir must only be administered by SC injection.
- Use with caution in the following:
  - elderly patients (see 📖 Dose adjustments, p.258)
  - renal impairment (see 📖 Dose adjustments, p.258)
  - severe hepatic impairment (see 📖 Dose adjustments, p.258)
  - systemic illness (dose increase may be necessary).
- The risk of reduced warning symptoms of hypoglycaemia is increased in the following circumstances:
  - after transfer from animal insulin to human insulin
  - autonomic neuropathy is present
  - concurrent treatment with particular drugs (see 📖 Drug interactions, p.258)
  - elderly patients
  - gradual onset of hypoglycaemia
  - long history of diabetes
  - markedly improved glycaemic control
  - psychiatric illness.

☺ Undesirable effects

Common

- Hypoglycaemia (also depends on other factors)
- Injection site reactions (generally minor, e.g. redness, pain, itching, or inflammation)

Uncommon

- Lipodystrophy
- Oedema (may cause sodium retention; usually transitory during initiation)
- Retinopathy (usually temporary deterioration associated with abrupt improvement in glycaemic control)
- Visual disturbances (usually temporary, caused by marked glycaemic control and associated altered lens properties)

Rare
- Peripheral neuropathy
- Urticaria

Drug interactions

Pharmacokinetic
- None recognized.

Pharmacodynamic
- *ACEIs*—increased risk of hypoglycaemia.
- *Antipsychotics*—glucose metabolism can be affected; dose adjustments may be necessary.
- *β_2-agonists*—hypoglycaemic effect may be antagonized.
- *Corticosteroids*—hypoglycaemic effect antagonized.
- *Diuretics*—hypoglycaemic effect may be antagonized.
- *Fluoxetine*—increased risk of hypoglycaemia.
- *Octreotide*—can affect glucose metabolism; dose adjustments may be necessary.

Dose

- Initial dose 10 units SC OD (or 0.1–0.2 units/kg SC OD) at any time but at the same time each day.
- The dosage and timing of dose of insulin detemir should be individually adjusted. Some patients may require BD dosing.

Dose adjustments

Elderly
- In the elderly, progressive deterioration of renal function may lead to a steady decrease in insulin requirements.

Hepatic/renal impairment
- In patients with severe hepatic impairment, insulin requirements may be diminished because of reduced capacity for gluconeogenesis and reduced insulin metabolism.
- In patients with renal impairment, insulin requirements may be diminished because of reduced insulin metabolism.

Additional information

- During the early stages of palliative care diabetes should be managed conventionally.
- As disease progresses and prognosis becomes short term, the importance of treatment shifts to preventing symptomatic hyperglycaemia and hypoglycaemia. Fasting blood glucose should be maintained between 8 and 15mmol/L.
- As the patient deteriorates and oral intake declines, consider halving the dose of insulin. A dose of insulin detemir 10 units SC ON will provide a basal insulin level and can be used if the patient is not eating.
- During use, do not refrigerate and do not store above 25°C.

✈ Pharmacology

Insulin detemir is a long-acting human insulin analogue. It has a duration of action of 24 hours which closely resembles the basal insulin secretion of the normal pancreatic β-cells. In patients with type I diabetes, a fast-acting insulin taken with food will also be needed in order to reduce post-prandial glucose elevations.

Insulin: insulin glargine

Lantus® (POM)

Insulin glargine, 100 units/mL
Injection: 10mL vial
Injection: 5 × 3mL cartridge for Autopen® 24 device
Injection: 5 × 3mL prefilled disposable OptiSet® injection devices; range 2–40 units, allowing 2 unit dosage adjustment
Injection: 5 × 3mL prefilled disposable SoloStar® injection devices (range 1–80 units, allowing 1 unit dosage adjustment)

Indications

- Diabetes mellitus.
- For end-of-life care issues see 📖 Use of drugs in end-of-life care, p.53.

Contraindications and precautions

- Insulin glargine is not the insulin of choice for the treatment of diabetic ketoacidosis.
- Insulin glargine must only be administered by SC injection.
- Use with caution in the following:
  - elderly patients (see 📖 Dose adjustments)
  - renal impairment (see 📖 Dose adjustments)
  - severe hepatic impairment (see 📖 Dose adjustments)
  - systemic illness (dose increase may be necessary).
- The risk of reduced warning symptoms of hypoglycaemia is increased in the following circumstances:
  - after transfer from animal insulin to human insulin
  - autonomic neuropathy is present
  - concurrent treatment with particular drugs (see 📖 Drug interactions, p.261)
  - elderly patients
  - gradual onset of hypoglycaemia
  - long history of diabetes
  - markedly improved glycaemic control
  - psychiatric illness.

😧 Undesirable effects

Very common

- Hypoglycaemia (also depends on other factors).

Common

- Injection site reactions (generally minor, e.g. redness, pain, itching, or inflammation).
- Lipohypertrophy.

Rare

- Oedema (may cause sodium retention).
- Retinopathy (usually temporary deterioration associated with abrupt improvement in glycaemic control).
- Visual disturbances (usually temporary, caused by marked glycaemic control and associated altered lens properties)

Drug interactions

Pharmacokinetic

• None recognized.

Pharmacodynamic

• *ACEIs*—increased risk of hypoglycaemia.
• *Antipsychotics*—glucose metabolism can be affected; dose adjustments may be necessary.
• *β2-agonists*—hypoglycaemic effect may be antagonized.
• *Corticosteroids*—hypoglycaemic effect antagonized.
• *Diuretics*—hypoglycaemic effect may be antagonized.
• *Fluoxetine*—increased risk of hypoglycaemia.
• *Octreotide*—can affect glucose metabolism; dose adjustments may be necessary.

Dose

• Glargine should be administered OD at any time, but at the same time each day.
• The dosage and timing of the dose of insulin glargine should be individually adjusted. For type 2 patients, it can be given at the same time as oral hypoglycaemics.

Dose adjustments

Elderly

• In the elderly, progressive deterioration of renal function may lead to a steady decrease in insulin requirements.

Hepatic/renal impairment

• In patients with severe hepatic impairment, insulin requirements may be diminished because of reduced capacity for gluconeogenesis and reduced insulin metabolism
• In patients with renal impairment, insulin requirements may be diminished because of reduced insulin metabolism.

Additional information

• NICE (May 2008) has recommended that if insulin is required in patients with type 2 diabetes, insulin glargine may be considered if:
  • assistance with injecting insulin is needed, or
  • recurrent symptomatic hypoglycaemia, or
  • twice daily insulin injections necessary in addition to oral antidiabetic drugs.
• During the early stages of palliative care diabetes should be managed conventionally.
• As disease progresses and prognosis becomes short term, the importance of treatment shifts to preventing symptomatic hyperglycaemia and hypoglycaemia. Fasting blood glucose should be maintained between 8 and 15mmol/L.
• As the patient deteriorates and oral intake declines, consider halving the dose of insulin. A dose of insulin glargine 10 units SC ON will provide a basal insulin level and can be used if the patient is not eating.
• During use, do not refrigerate and do not store above 25°C.

❖ Pharmacology

Insulin glargine is a long-acting human insulin analogue. It has a duration of action of 24 hours which closely resembles the basal insulin secretion of the normal pancreatic β-cells. In patients with type I diabetes, a fast-acting insulin taken with food will also be needed in order to reduce post-prandial glucose elevations.

Insulin: insulin lispro

Humalog® (POM)

Insulin lispro (recombinant human insulin analogue), 100 units/mL
Injection: 10mL vial
Injection: 5 × 3mL cartridge for Autopen® Classic or HumaPen® devices
Injection: 5 × 3mL prefilled disposable injection devices; range 1–60 units, allowing 1 unit dosage adjustment
Injection: 5 × 3mL prefilled disposable KwikPen® injection devices; range 1–60 units, allowing 1 unit dosage adjustment

Indications

- Diabetes mellitus.
- For end-of-life care issues see 📖 Use of drugs in end-of-life care, p.53.

Contraindications and precautions

- Insulin lispro has a faster onset of action than soluble human insulin and should generally be given within 15 minutes of a meal or snack containing carbohydrates.
- Use with caution in the following:
  - elderly patients (see 📖 Dose adjustments, p.264)
  - renal impairment (see 📖 Dose adjustments, p.264)
  - severe hepatic impairment (see 📖 Dose adjustments, p.264)
  - systemic illness (dose increase may be necessary).
- The risk of reduced warning symptoms of hypoglycaemia is increased in the following circumstances:
  - after transfer from animal insulin to human insulin
  - autonomic neuropathy is present
  - concurrent treatment with particular drugs (see 📖 Drug interactions, p.264)
  - elderly patients
  - gradual onset of hypoglycaemia
  - long history of diabetes
  - markedly improved glycaemic control
  - psychiatric illness.

☺ Undesirable effects

The frequency is not specifically defined, but in common with other insulin products, undesirable effects include:

- Hypoglycaemia (also depends on other factors)
- Injection site reactions (generally minor, e.g. redness, pain, itching, or inflammation)
- Lipodystrophy
- Oedema (may cause sodium retention; usually transitory during initiation)
- Peripheral neuropathy
- Retinopathy (usually temporary deterioration associated with abrupt improvement in glycaemic control)
- Urticaria
- Visual disturbances (usually temporary, caused by marked glycaemic control and associated altered lens properties)

Drug interactions

Pharmacokinetic

- None recognized.

Pharmacodynamic

- *ACEIs*—increased risk of hypoglycaemia.
- *Antipsychotics*—glucose metabolism can be affected; dose adjustments may be necessary.
- *β$_2$-agonists*—hypoglycaemic effect may be antagonized.
- *Corticosteroids*—hypoglycaemic effect antagonized.
- *Diuretics*—hypoglycaemic effect may be antagonized.
- *Fluoxetine*—increased risk of hypoglycaemia.
- *Octreotide*—can affect glucose metabolism; dose adjustments may be necessary.

Dose

- Dosing must be individualized. As a rule, if blood glucose >15mmol/L and the patient is symptomatic, give up to 5 units SC. Recheck after an hour; if it has remained above 15mmol/L treat with the same dose only if symptomatic.

Dose adjustments

Elderly

- In the elderly, progressive deterioration of renal function may lead to a steady decrease in insulin requirements.

Hepatic/renal impairment

- In patients with severe hepatic impairment, insulin requirements may be diminished because of reduced capacity for gluconeogenesis and reduced insulin metabolism.
- In patients with renal impairment, insulin requirements may be diminished because of reduced insulin metabolism.

Additional information

- During the early stages of palliative care diabetes should be managed conventionally.
- As disease progresses and prognosis becomes short term, the importance of treatment shifts to preventing symptomatic hyperglycaemia and hypoglycaemia. Fasting blood glucose should be maintained between 8 and 15mmol/L.
- As the patient deteriorates and oral intake declines, consider halving the dose of insulin.

Pharmacology

Insulin lispro is a fast-acting insulin. Onset of action is within 15 minutes, with a maximum effect within 1–2 hours; the duration of effect is up to 2–5 hours.

Insulin: isophane insulin

Humulin I® (POM)
Isophane insulin (human, prb), 100 units/mL
Injection: 5 × 3mL cartridge for Autopen® Classic or HumaPen® devices
Injection: 5 × 3mL prefilled disposable Humulin I-Pen® injection devices;
range 1–60 units, allowing 1 unit dosage adjustment

Insulatard® (POM)
Isophane insulin (human, pyr), 100 units/mL
Injection: 5 × 3mL Penfill® cartridge for Novopen® device
Injection: 5 × 3mL prefilled disposable InnoLet® injection devices; range
1–50 units, allowing 1 unit dosage adjustment

Insuman® Basal (POM)
Isophane insulin (human, crb) 100 units/mL
Injection: 5mL vial
Injection: 5 × 3mL cartridge for OptiPen® Pro 1 device
Injection: 5 × 3mL prefilled disposable OptiSet® injection devices; range
2–40 units, allowing 2 unit dosage adjustment

Hypurin® Bovine Isophane (POM)
Isophane insulin (bovine, highly purified) 100 units/mL
Injection: 10mL vial
Injection: 5 × 3mL cartridge for Autopen® Classic device

Hypurin® Porcine Isophane (POM)
Isophane insulin (porcine, highly purified) 100 units/mL
Injection: 10mL vial
Injection: 5 × 3mL cartridge for Autopen® Classic device

Indications
- Diabetes mellitus
- For end-of-life care issues see 📖 Use of drugs in end-of-life care, p.53.

Contraindications and precautions
- Isophane insulin must only be administered by SC injection.
- Use with caution in the following:
    - elderly patients (see 📖 Dose adjustments, p.267)
    - renal impairment (see 📖 Dose adjustments, p.267)
    - severe hepatic impairment (see 📖 Dose adjustments, p.267)
    - systemic illness (dose increase may be necessary).
- The risk of reduced warning symptoms of hypoglycaemia is increased in
  the following circumstances:
    - after transfer from animal insulin to human insulin
    - autonomic neuropathy is present
    - concurrent treatment with particular drugs (see 📖 Drug
      interactions, p.266)

- elderly patients
- gradual onset of hypoglycaemia
- long history of diabetes
- markedly improved glycaemic control
- psychiatric illness.

☺ Undesirable effects

Very common
- Hypoglycaemia (also depends on other factors)

Uncommon
- Injection site reactions (generally minor, e.g. redness, pain, itching, or inflammation)
- Lipodystrophy
- Oedema (may cause sodium retention; usually transitory during initiation)
- Peripheral neuropathy
- Retinopathy (usually temporary deterioration associated with abrupt improvement in glycaemic control)
- Urticaria

Very rare
- Visual disturbances (usually temporary, because of marked glycaemic control and associated altered lens properties)

Drug interactions

Pharmacokinetic
- None recognized.

Pharmacodynamic
- *ACEIs*—increased risk of hypoglycaemia.
- *Antipsychotics*—glucose metabolism can be affected; dose adjustments may be necessary.
- *β₂-agonists*—hypoglycaemic effect may be antagonized.
- *Corticosteroids*—hypoglycaemic effect antagonized.
- *Diuretics*—hypoglycaemic effect may be antagonized.
- *Fluoxetine*—increased risk of hypoglycaemia.
- *Octreotide*—can affect glucose metabolism; dose adjustments may be necessary.

,ᔥ Dose

- Suitable initial dose 10 units SC OD; titrate according to response.
- Some patients may require BD dosing.
- Can be combined with fast-acting insulin.

♣ Dose adjustments

Elderly

- In the elderly, progressive deterioration of renal function may lead to a steady decrease in insulin requirements.

Hepatic/renal impairment

- In patients with severe hepatic impairment, insulin requirements may be diminished because of reduced capacity for gluconeogenesis and reduced insulin metabolism.
- In patients with renal impairment, insulin requirements may be diminished because of reduced insulin metabolism.

Additional information

- During the early stages of palliative care diabetes should be managed conventionally.
- As disease progresses and prognosis becomes short term, the importance of treatment shifts to preventing symptomatic hyperglycaemia and hypoglycaemia. Fasting blood glucose should be maintained between 8 and 15mmol/L.
- As the patient deteriorates and oral intake declines, consider halving the dose of insulin. A dose of isophane insulin 10 units SC ON will provide a basal insulin level and can be used if the patient is not eating.
- During use, do not refrigerate and do not store above 25°C.

♦ Pharmacology

Isophane insulin is a suspension of either porcine or human insulin complexed with protamine sulphate. Onset of action is within 90 minutes, with a maximum effect within 4–12 hours; the duration of effect is up to 24 hours.

Insulin: soluble

Actrapid® (POM)
Soluble insulin (human, pyr) 100 units/mL
Injection: 10mL vial

Humulin S® (POM)
Soluble insulin (human, prb), 100 units/mL
Injection: 10mL vial
Injection: 5 × 3mL cartridge for Autopen® Classic or HumaPen® device

Insuman® Rapid (POM)
Soluble insulin (human, crb) 100 units/mL
Injection: 5 × 3mL cartridge for OptiPen® Pro 1 device
Injection: 5 × 3mL prefilled disposable OptiSet® injection devices; range 2–40 units, allowing 2 unit dosage adjustment

Hypurin® Bovine Neutral (POM)
Soluble insulin (bovine, highly purified) 100 units/mL
Injection: 10mL vial
Injection: 5 × 3mL cartridge for Autopen® Classic device

Hypurin® Porcine Neutral (POM)
Soluble insulin (porcine, highly purified) 100 units/mL
Injection: 10mL vial
Injection: 5 × 3mL cartridge for Autopen® Classic device

Indications
- Diabetes mellitus.
- For end-of-life care issues see 📖 *Use of drugs in end-of-life care*, p.53.

Contraindications and precautions
- An injection should be followed within 30 minutes by a meal or snack containing carbohydrates.
- Use with caution in the following:
  - elderly patients (see 📖 *Dose adjustments*, p.269)
  - renal impairment (see 📖 *Dose adjustments*, p.269)
  - severe hepatic impairment (see 📖 *Dose adjustments*, p.269)
  - systemic illness (dose increase may be necessary).
- The risk of reduced warning symptoms of hypoglycaemia is increased in the following circumstances:
  - after transfer from animal insulin to human insulin
  - autonomic neuropathy is present
  - concurrent treatment with particular drugs (see 📖 *Drug interactions*, p.269)
  - elderly patients
  - gradual onset of hypoglycaemia
  - long history of diabetes
  - markedly improved glycaemic control
  - psychiatric illness.

☺ Undesirable effects

Very common
- Hypoglycaemia (also depends on other factors)

Uncommon
- Injection site reactions (generally minor, e.g. redness, pain, itching, or inflammation).
- Lipodystrophy.
- Oedema (may cause sodium retention; usually transitory during initiation).
- Peripheral neuropathy.
- Retinopathy (usually temporary deterioration associated with abrupt improvement in glycaemic control).
- Urticaria.

Very rare
- Visual disturbances (usually temporary, caused by marked glycaemic control and associated altered lens properties).

Drug interactions

Pharmacokinetic
- None recognized.

Pharmacodynamic
- *ACEIs*—increased risk of hypoglycaemia.
- *Antipsychotics*—glucose metabolism can be affected; dose adjustments may be necessary.
- *β_2-agonists*—hypoglycaemic effect may be antagonized.
- *Corticosteroids*—hypoglycaemic effect antagonized.
- *Diuretics*—hypoglycaemic effect may be antagonized.
- *Fluoxetine*—increased risk of hypoglycaemia.
- *Octreotide*—can affect glucose metabolism; dose adjustments may be necessary.

⚖ Dose

- Dosing must be individualized. As a rule, if blood glucose >15mmol/L and the patient is symptomatic, give up to 5 units SC. Recheck after an hour; if it has remained above 15mmol/L treat with the same dose only if symptomatic.

⚖ Dose adjustments

Elderly
- In the elderly, progressive deterioration of renal function may lead to a steady decrease in insulin requirements.

Hepatic/renal impairment
- In patients with severe hepatic impairment, insulin requirements may be diminished because of reduced capacity for gluconeogenesis and reduced insulin metabolism.
- In patients with renal impairment, insulin requirements may be diminished because of reduced insulin metabolism.

Additional information

- During the early stages of palliative care diabetes should be managed conventionally.
- As disease progresses and prognosis becomes short term, the importance of treatment shifts to preventing symptomatic hyperglycaemia and hypoglycaemia. Fasting blood glucose should be maintained between 8 and 15mmol/L.
- As the patient deteriorates and oral intake declines, consider halving the dose of insulin.
- During use, do not refrigerate and do not store above 25°C.

✵ Pharmacology

Soluble insulin is fast-acting. Onset of action is within 30 minutes, with the maximum effect within 1–3 hours; the duration of effect is approximately 7–8 hours.

Ipratropium bromide

Atrovent® (POM)

Dry powder for inhalation (Aerocaps® capsules for use with Aerohaler®): 40mcg (100)
Aerosol inhalation: 20mcg per metered dose (200 dose unit)
Nebulizer solution: 250mcg/mL unit-dose vials (20;60); 500mcg/2mL unit-dose vials (20;60)

Ipratropium Steri-Neb® (POM)

Nebulizer solution: 250mcg/mL unit-dose vials (20); 500mcg/2mL unit-dose vials (20)

Respontin® (POM)

Nebulizer solution: 250mcg/mL unit-dose vials (20); 500mcg/2mL unit-dose vials (20)

Generic (POM)

Nebulizer solution: 250mcg/mL unit-dose vials (20); 500mcg/2mL unit-dose vials (20)

Indications

• Reversible airways obstruction.

Contraindications and precautions

• Ipratropium bromide should be used with caution in patients with:
    • angle-closure glaucoma
    • bladder outflow obstruction
    • cystic fibrosis (may cause GI motility disturbances)
    • prostatic hyperplasia.
• If eye pain, blurred vision, or visual halos develop, treatment with miotic drops should be initiated and specialist advice sought immediately

☺ Undesirable effects

Common
• Bronchoconstriction
• Constipation
• Cough
• Dizziness
• Dry mouth
• Headache

Uncommon
• Angle-closure glaucoma
• Tachycardia
• Visual disturbances

Rare
• Ocular pain
• Urinary retention

Drug interactions

Pharmacokinetic
- None of clinical significance noted

Pharmacodynamic
- *Anticholinergics*—concurrent use with ipratropium may increase risk of adverse events

💊 Dose

Dry powder inhalation
- 40mcg TDS–QDS (may be doubled in less responsive patients).
- Note 1 Aerocap® = 2 puffs of Atrovent® metered aerosol inhalation.

Aerosol inhalation
- 20–40mcg TDS–QDS (may be doubled in less responsive patients)

Nebulized solution
- 250–500mcg TDS–QDS.
- Higher doses (>2g daily) may be given if necessary under medical supervision.

💊 Dose adjustments

Elderly
- Usual adult doses can be used. Note that the elderly are more susceptible to undesirable effects.

Hepatic/renal impairment
- No specific dose reductions stated

Additional information

- The bronchodilatory effect may not occur for up to 30 minutes (unlike β_2-agonists).
- If nebulized ipratropium therapy is initiated, ensure that any ipratropium (or tiotropium) inhaler device is withdrawn.
- If dilution of the unit dose vials is necessary, use only sterile sodium chloride 0.9%.

⟳ Pharmacology

Ipratropium bromide is an anticholinergic agent. It blocks muscarinic cholinergic receptors, without specificity for subtypes. Following inhalation, up to 30% of the dose is deposited in the lungs, with the majority of the dose being swallowed. GI absorption is negligible. Ipratropium is metabolized to inactive compounds and 40% of the dose is excreted by the kidneys unchanged.

Ketamine

Ketalar® (CD Benz POM)

Injection: 10mg/mL (20mL vial); 50mg/mL (10mL vial); 100mg/mL (10mL vial)

See *Additional information* for supply issues.

Unlicensed Special (CD Benz POM)

Oral solution: 50mg/5mL (available in a variety of volumes and flavours)

See *Additional information* for supply issues.

> Independent prescribers are **NOT** authorized to prescribe ketamine (📖 Independent prescribing: palliative care issues, p.25 and Legal categories of medicines, p.23).

Indications

- ⁺ Refractory chronic pain.
- For end-of-life care issues see 📖 Use of drugs in end-of-life care, p.53.

Contraindications and precautions

- Contraindicated for use in patients with intracranial hypertension, or where a rise in blood pressure may pose a serious hazard.
- Avoid in acute porphyria.
- Use with caution in patients with hypertension, epilepsy, cardiac failure, ischaemic heart disease, or previous cerebrovascular accidents.
- Dose adjustments may be necessary in the elderly and patients with liver impairment (see 📖 Dose adjustments, p.274).
- It is advisable to reduce any concurrent opioid dose by 30–50% prior to commencing ketamine.
- Ketamine may cause drowsiness and dizziness. Patients should be advised not to drive (or operate machinery) if affected.
- Avoid grapefruit juice with oral ketamine.

😊 Undesirable effects

Given the manner in which ketamine is used in palliative care, the incidence of undesirable effects is difficult to judge. Undesirable effects from oral use tend to be less intense. The following have been reported:

- Confusion
- Dizziness
- Excessive salivation
- Euphoria
- Hallucinations
- Hypertension
- Pain and inflammation around injection site
- Sedation
- Vivid dreams

Drug interactions
Pharmacokinetic
- Ketamine is metabolized by CYP2B6, CYP2C9, and CYP3A4. The clinical significance of co-administration with inducers or inhibitors (🕮 end cover) is unknown. Note that norketamine (see pharmacology) is produced by the action of CYP3A4 and use of drugs that inhibit or induce this isoenzyme may affect analgesia.
- The effect of grapefruit juice on the first-pass metabolism of oral ketamine is unknown.
- The prescriber should be aware of the potential for interactions and that dose adjustments may be necessary.

Pharmacodynamic
- *CNS depressants*—risk of excessive sedation
- *Opioids*—dose of opioid should be reviewed when ketamine is introduced; there is likely to be an opioid sparing effect necessitating a dose reduction

¥ Dose
¥ By CSCI
- 50–100mg over 24 hours. Dose can be increased by 50mg every 24 hours until benefit achieved. Doses above 600mg over 24 hours should be under specialist guidance only.

¥ Burst ketamine
- Treatment given by short-term CSCI, usually no longer than 7 days.
- Initial dose typically 100mg over 24 hours. The dose is increased by 100mg every 24 hours as necessary to a maximum of 500mg over 24 hours. The effect may persist for up to 2 months.

¥ Oral
- 10–25mg PO TDS–QDS. Increase in steps of 10–25mg daily to a maximum of 50mg PO QDS. Higher doses have been used under specialist guidance (e.g. up to 200mg PO QDS).

¥ Dose adjustments
Elderly
- No information is available. Nonetheless, it is advisable to initiate treatment with doses at the low end of the ranges quoted above.

Hepatic/renal impairment
- Ketamine is hepatically metabolized. Although no information exists, it is advisable to initiate treatment with doses at the low end of the ranges quoted above.
- No dose adjustments should be necessary in renal impairment.

Additional information

Supply issues

Ketamine vials

- Ketamine injection is easily available in hospitals and the community. In the community, the patient should present the prescription to the pharmacist in the usual way. The community pharmacist can then place an order through Alliance Healthcare, or directly with Pfizer (Tel 01304 645262).
- Supply should be made within 3 days of the request. The patient should be advised to request a prescription from their GP at least 5 days before the supply is needed.

Ketamine oral solution 50mg/5mL

- This unlicensed product is available as a special order from various suppliers, e.g. Martindale Pharmaceuticals (Tel 01277 266600).
- A variety of flavours (e.g. aniseed, peppermint) and volumes are available.
- It can take up to 7 days for delivery. The patient should be advised to request a prescription from their GP at least 10 days before the supply is needed.

Extemporaneous preparation of ketamine oral solution

- The injection can be used directly from the vial, although flavouring will be needed to mask the taste (e.g. fruit juice, but **not** grapefruit).
- Alternatively, the injection can be transferred from the vial (e.g. 100mg/mL vial) and diluted with a suitable vehicle (e.g. Raspberry Syrup BP or purified water) to a concentration of 50mg/5mL. If purified water is used, the patient should be advised to use a flavouring to mask the taste.
- The extemporaneous product has an expiry time of 7 days and should be refrigerated.

CSCI issues

- The injection is an irritant and infusions should be maximally diluted with NaCl 0.9%. Low-dose dexamethasone (0.5–1mg) can be added to the infusion to help prevent site reactions.
- Ketamine via CSCI is compatible with alfentanil, diamorphine, haloperidol, levomepromazine, midazolam, morphine sulphate, and oxycodone.
- Ketamine is considered to be incompatible with cyclizine, dexamethasone (higher doses), and phenobarbital.

⊕ Pharmacology

Ketamine has a variety of pharmacological actions, including interaction with *N*-methyl-D-aspartate (NMDA) receptors, opioid receptors, muscarinic receptors and Na^+ ion channels. The analgesic effect of ketamine that is seen at sub-anaesthetic doses is due to non-competitive antagonism of the NMDA receptor. Ketamine interacts with a specific binding site on the NMDA receptor, blocking the influx of Na^+ and Ca^{2+}. Binding of ketamine will only occur when the ion channel has been opened though neuronal excitation. The analgesic activity is believed to be due to attenuation of the 'wind-up' phenomenon by reducing the excitability of the neuron.

Ketamine is poorly absorbed after oral administration and undergoes extensive first-pass metabolism to norketamine. CYP3A1 is the major isoenzyme responsible (both enteric and hepatic); CYP2B6 and CYP2C9 have a minor role. On repeated administration, ketamine induces its own metabolism. Although the analgesic potencies of ketamine and norketamine are thought to be similar, the peak plasma concentration of norketamine produced after oral administration is greater than that produced after parenteral administration. With chronic use, norketamine may have a more influential analgesic effect. Consequently, on chronic dosing analgesia appears to be achieved with lower oral than parenteral doses. No direct conversion exists, but the oral analgesic dose is considered to be approximately **three times** more potent than the parenteral dose.

Ketorolac

Toradol® (POM)

Tablet: 10mg (20)
Injection: 10mg/mL (5); 30mg/mL (5)

Indications

- Short-term management of moderate to severe acute post-operative pain.
- * Short-term management of cancer pain.
- For end-of-life care issues see 📖 Use of drugs in end-of-life care, p.53.

Contraindications and precautions

- Contraindicated for use in patients with:
  - a history of, or active, peptic ulceration
  - hypersensitivity reactions to ibuprofen, aspirin, or other NSAIDs
  - moderate or severe renal impairment (SECr >160μmol/L)
  - severe heart failure
  - suspected or confirmed cerebrovascular bleeding
  - haemorrhagic diatheses, including coagulation disorders
  - complete or partial syndrome of nasal polyps, angio-oedema, or bronchospasm
  - hypovolaemia from any cause, or dehydration
  - concurrent treatment with aspirin, other NSAIDs including COX-2 inhibitors, anticoagulants including low-dose heparin, pentoxifylline, probenecid, or lithium (see 📖 Drug interactions, p.278).
- Use the minimum effective dose for the shortest duration necessary in order to reduce the risk of cardiac and GI events.
- Elderly patients are more at risk of developing undesirable effects.
- Patients with uncontrolled hypertension, congestive heart failure, established ischaemic heart disease, peripheral arterial disease, and/ or cerebrovascular disease need careful consideration because of the increased risk of thrombotic events.
- Similar consideration should be made before initiating longer-term treatment of patients with risk factors for cardiovascular events (e.g. hypertension, hyperlipidaemia, diabetes mellitus, and smoking).
- Caution should be exercised in patients with a history of cardiac failure, left ventricular dysfunction, or hypertension. Deterioration may occur due to fluid retention.
- In patients with renal, cardiac, or hepatic impairment, caution is required since the use of NSAIDs may result in deterioration of renal function.
- Refer to 📖 Selection of an NSAID, p.31 for further information, including selection.
- Ketorolac may modify reactions and patients should be advised not to drive (or operate machinery) if affected.

☺ Undesirable effects

The frequency is not defined, but reported undesirable effects include:

- Abdominal pain
- Acute renal failure
- Coagulopathy
- Diarrhoea
- Dizziness
- Drowsiness
- Dyspepsia
- Flatulence
- GI haemorrhage
- Headache
- Hypertension
- Oedema
- Pain at injection site (less for CSCI)
- Rash
- Stomatitis
- Vomiting

Drug interactions

Pharmacokinetic

- *Lithium*—increased risk of lithium toxicity due to reduced renal clearance.
- *Methotrexate*—reduced excretion of methotrexate.

Pharmacodynamic

- Anticoagulants—increased risk of bleeding (concurrent use contraindicated).
- Antihypertensives—reduced hypotensive effect.
- Antiplatelet drugs—increased risk of bleeding (concurrent use contraindicated).
- Corticosteroids—increased risk of GI toxicity.
- Ciclosporin—increased risk of nephrotoxicity.
- Diuretics—reduced diuretic effect; nephrotoxicity of ketorolac may be increased.
- Rosiglitazone—increased risk of oedema.
- SSRIs—increased risk of GI bleeding.

♨ Dose

Gastroprotective treatment must be prescribed concurrently if appropriate. Consider misoprostol or a proton pump inhibitor. Alternatively, ranitidine via CSCI can be considered.

¥ Cancer pain

- Initial dose 10–30mg SC TDS PRN. Alternatively, 60mg OD via CSCI, increasing to 90mg if necessary.

.ⁱ Dose adjustments

Elderly
- The elderly are at an increased risk of undesirable effects due to an increased plasma half-life and reduced plasma clearance of ketorolac. Doses >60mg/day are not recommended.

Hepatic/renal impairment
- In liver impairment, no specific dose recommendations are available. However, the lowest dose possible should be used for the shortest duration possible.
- Ketorolac must not be used in patients with moderate to severe renal impairment. In patients with mild renal impairment, the dose used should not exceed 60mg/day.

Additional information

- Ensure concurrent opioid requirements are reviewed; since ketorolac is such a potent analgesic, it may have opioid-sparing effects.
- The risk of clinically serious GI bleeding is dose dependent. This is particularly true in elderly patients who receive an average daily ketorolac dose >60mg.
- Ketorolac via CSCI should be diluted with NaCl 0.9% and administered in a separate infusion, unless compatibility data are available. There is a risk of incompatibility with many drugs given via CSCI since ketorolac has an alkaline pH. However, it is compatible with diamorphine and oxycodone.
- Ketorolac may precipitate in solutions with a low pH and is reportedly incompatible with cyclizine, haloperidol, morphine, and promethazine. There are mixed reports of incompatibility with hydromorphone. Glycopyrronium is likely to be incompatible because of the alkaline pH of ketorolac.

⊕ Pharmacology

Ketorolac exhibits anti-inflammatory, analgesic, and antipyretic activity, although the analgesic effect appears to be the predominant action. The mechanism of action of ketorolac, like that of other NSAIDs, is not completely understood but may be related to inhibition of COX-1 and COX-2. The major metabolic pathway is glucuronic acid conjugation, and about 90% of a dose is excreted in urine as unchanged drug metabolites.

Lactulose

Generic (P)
Solution: 3.1–3.7g/5mL (300mL; 500mL)

Indications
- Treatment of constipation.
- Treatment of hepatic encephalopathy.

Contraindications and precautions
- Contraindicated for use in:
  - galactosaemia
  - intestinal obstruction.
- Use with caution in patients with lactose intolerance.

☻ Undesirable effects
The frequency is not defined, but reported undesirable effects include:
- Abdominal pain
- Diarrhoea
- Flatulence (should improve after a few days treatment)
- Nausea
- Vomiting

Drug interactions
Pharmacokinetic
- None known

Pharmacodynamic
- *Anticholinergics*—antagonizes the laxative effect.
- *Cyclizine*—antagonizes the laxative effect.
- *Opioids*—antagonizes the laxative effect.
- *5-HT$_3$ antagonists*—antagonizes the laxative effect.
- *Tricyclic antidepressants*—antagonizes the laxative effect.

♣ Dose
Constipation
- Initial dose 15mL PO BD, adjusted to the patient's needs.

Hepatic encephalopathy
- Initial dose 30–50mL PO TDS, adjusted to produce 2–3 soft stools daily.

♣ Dose adjustments
Elderly
- No dose adjustment necessary.

Hepatic/renal impairment
- No dose adjustment necessary.

Additional information
• Can take up to 48 hours for the laxative effect to work.

✈ Pharmacology

Lactulose is a synthetic sugar consisting of fructose and galactose. In the colon, it is broken down primarily to lactic acid by the action of colonic bacteria. This results in an increase in osmotic pressure and a slight reduction of colonic pH, which cause an increase in stool water content and softens the stool. In the treatment of hepatic encephalopathy, it is thought that the low pH reduces the absorption of ammonium ions and other toxic nitrogenous compounds.

Lansoprazole

Zoton Fastabs® (POM)
Orodispersible tablet: 15mg (28); 30mg (7; 14; 28)

Generic (POM)
Capsule (enclosing enteric-coated granules): 15mg (28); 30mg (28)

Indications
- Treatment of benign gastric and duodenal ulcer.
- Treatment and prophylaxis of gastro-oesophageal reflux disease.
- Treatment and prophylaxis of NSAID-associated benign gastric and duodenal ulcers requiring continual therapy.

Contraindications and precautions
- Do not administer with atazanavir or erlotinib.
- Treatment with lansoprazole may lead to a slightly increased risk of developing GI infections (e.g. *Clostridium difficile*). Therefore avoid unnecessary use or high doses.
- Zoton Fastabs® contain aspartame—avoid in phenylketonuria.
- Lansoprazole may modify reactions and patients should be advised not to drive (or operate machinery) if affected.
- Rebound acid hypersecretion may occur on discontinuation of the patient has received more than 8 weeks treatment.

☺ Undesirable effects
Common
- Abnormal LFTs
- Diarrhoea
- Dry mouth
- Fatigue
- Flatulence
- Headache
- Nausea and vomiting
- Rash

Uncommon
- Arthralgia
- Blood dyscrasias
- Myalgia
- Oedema

Rare
- Confusion
- Gynaecomastia
- Hepatitis
- Insomnia
- Pancreatitis
- Taste disturbances

Very rare
- Stevens–Johnson syndrome

Drug interactions

Pharmacokinetic
- Lansoprazole is metabolized mainly by CYP2C19 with a minor role involving CYP3A4.
- Lansoprazole also has a moderate inhibitory effect on CYP2C19 and can induce CYP1A2.
- P-gp is inhibited by lansoprazole, but the clinical significance is presently unknown.
- Drugs with pH-dependent absorption can be affected:
  - *atazanavir*—avoid combination because of substantially reduced absorption
  - *digoxin*—increased plasma concentrations possible
  - *erlotinib*—avoid combination as bioavailability of erlotinib can be significantly reduced
  - *ketoconazole/itraconazole*—risk of sub-therapeutic plasma concentrations
  - *metronidazole suspension*—lansoprazole may reduce/prevent the absorption of metronidazole.
- *Antacids*—should be given at least 1 hour before lansoprazole (reduced bioavailability).
- *Clopidogrel*—antiplatelet action may be reduced (avoid combination).
- *Theophylline*—lansoprazole can reduce the plasma concentration (CYP1A2 induction).
- The clinical significance of co-administration with CYP2C19 inducers or inhibitors (see 📖 end cover) is unknown. The prescriber should be aware of the potential for interactions and that dose adjustments may be necessary.
- Although the clinical significance is unknown, co-administration of lansoprazole may increase the levels/effects of CYP2C19 substrates (📖 end cover). The prescriber should be aware of the potential for interactions and that dose adjustments may be necessary.
- Although the clinical significance is unknown, co-administration with CYP3A4 inducers (📖 end cover) may decrease the levels/effects of lansoprazole. The prescriber should be aware of the potential for interactions and that dose adjustments may be necessary.

Pharmacodynamic
- No clinically significant interactions noted.

⚖ Dose

Treatment of peptic ulcer disease
- 30mg PO OD for 2–4 weeks
- Gastric ulcer treatment may need to continue for 4–8 weeks.

Reflux oesophagitis
- Treatment: 30mg PO OD for 4–8 weeks.
- Prophylaxis: 15–30mg PO OD as necessary.

NSAID-associated benign gastric and duodenal ulcers
- Treatment: 30mg PO OD for 4 weeks, continuing to 8 weeks if not fully healed. 30mg PO BD can be considered.
- Prophylaxis: 15–30mg PO OD.

NB: There is little evidence to recommend routine prescribing of lansoprazole 30mg PO OD for dyspeptic symptoms. If 30mg PO OD fails to control such symptoms, treatment should be combined with antacids such as Gaviscon® (given at least 1 hour before lansoprazole).

Dose adjustments
Elderly
- 30mg PO OD should not usually be exceeded unless there are compelling clinical reasons.

Hepatic/renal impairment
- A 50% dose reduction is recommended in moderate to severe hepatic impairment.
- No dose adjustment is necessary in renal impairment.

Additional information
- Lansoprazole capsules may be opened and emptied into a glass of orange juice or apple juice, mixed, and swallowed immediately. The glass should be rinsed with additional juice to ensure complete delivery of the dose.
- The intact enteric-coated granules should not be chewed or crushed.
- Zoton Fastabs® may block NG tubes. Lansoprazole capsules cannot be used to form a suspension suitable to put through an NG tube. Use Losec MUPS® (📖 Omeprazole, p.367) if PPI therapy is required.
- Symptoms can be relieved following the first dose.

Pharmacology
Lansoprazole is a gastric proton pump inhibitor, reducing the release of H^+ from parietal cells by inhibiting H^+/K^+-ATPase. It is rapidly inactivated by gastric acid; hence oral formulations are enteric coated. Oral bioavailability is high (~90%) but administration with food can reduce this. It is extensively metabolized, mainly by CYP2C19, although an alternative pathway involves CYP3A4. Note that CYP2C19 poor metabolizers (or patients taking CYP2C19 inhibitors) can have significantly higher plasma concentrations, leading to unexpected results. Metabolites are virtually inactive and are eliminated by both renal and biliary excretion.

Letrozole

Femara® (POM)
Tablet: 2.5mg (14; 28)

Indications
- Treatment (primary or adjuvant) of postmenopausal women with hormone-receptor-positive invasive early breast cancer.

Contraindications and precautions
- Letrozole is contraindicated for use in patients with:
  - severe hepatic impairment
  - unknown or negative receptor status.
- It should be used with caution in patients with severe renal impairment (CrCl <10mL/min).
- May cause reduction in bone mineral density; treatment for osteoporosis may be required.
- Fatigue and dizziness have been reported with letrozole. Caution should be observed when driving (or operating machinery) while such symptoms persist.

☺ Undesirable effects

Very common
- Arthralgia
- Hot flushes

Common
- Alopecia
- Anorexia
- Bone fractures
- Bone pain
- Constipation
- Depression
- Diarrhoea
- Dizziness
- Dyspepsia
- Fatigue
- Headache
- Myalgia
- Osteoporosis
- Nausea
- Peripheral oedema
- Raised serum cholesterol
- Sweating
- Vomiting

Uncommon
- Anxiety
- Drowsiness
- Dyspnoea
- Hypertension
- Ischaemic cardiac events
- Leucopenia
- Tumour pain
- Urinary tract infection
- Vaginal bleeding/discharge
- Visual disturbances

Drug interactions
Pharmacokinetic
- Letrozole is metabolized by CYP2A6 and CYP3A4. The contribution of each isoenzyme is unknown. It inhibits CYP2A6 and also moderately affects CYP2C19.
- Letrozole is unlikely to be a cause of many drug interactions since CYP2A6 does not have a major role in drug metabolism. At usual doses, letrozole is unlikely to affect CYP2C19 substrates, although the prescriber should be aware of potential additive interactions, particularly with substrates with a narrow therapeutic index.
- The clinical significance of co-administration with CYP3A4 inducers or (📖 end cover) is unknown. The prescriber should be aware that dose adjustments may be necessary.

Pharmacodynamic
- None known.

♪ Dose
- 2.5mg PO OD.

♪ Dose adjustments
Elderly
- No dose adjustments are necessary for elderly patients.

Hepatic/renal impairment
- No dose adjustments are necessary for patients with mild to moderate hepatic impairment or mild to moderate renal impairment (CrCl ≥10mL/min)
- Letrozole is contraindicated for use in severe hepatic impairment and should be used with caution in severe renal impairment (because of lack of data).

♦ Pharmacology
Letrozole is a non-steroidal aromatase inhibitor. It is believed to work by significantly lowering serum oestradiol concentrations through inhibition of aromatase (converts adrenal androstenedione to oestrone, which is a precursor of oestradiol). Many breast cancers have oestrogen receptors and growth of these tumours can be stimulated by oestrogens.

Levomepromazine

Nozinan® (POM)
Tablet (*scored*): 25mg (84)
Injection: 25mg/mL (10)

Levinan® (POM) (*unlicensed product—see* 📖 *Additional Information*, p.289)
Tablet (*scored*): 6mg (30)

Indications
- ⚸ Psychosis (injection unlicensed)
- Terminal agitation
- ⚸ Nausea and vomiting (tablets unlicensed)
- For end-of-life care issues see 📖 Use of Drugs in End-of-Life Care, p.53.

Contraindications and precautions
- There are no absolute contraindications to the use of levomepromazine in terminal care.
- Avoid using in patients with dementia unless patient is at immediate risk of harm or severely distressed (increased mortality reported).
- Levomepromazine should be used with caution in patients with:
  - concurrent anti-hypertensive medication (see 📖 *Drug interactions*, p.288)
  - diabetes (risk of hyperglycaemia in elderly)
  - epilepsy
  - liver dysfunction
  - Parkinson's disease
  - postural hypotension.
- Electrolyte disturbances (e.g. hypokalaemia) must be corrected because of the risk of QT prolongation.
- Levomepromazine should be used with caution in ambulant patients over 50 years of age because of the risk of a hypotensive reaction.
- Levomepromazine may modify reactions and patients should be advised not to drive (or operate machinery) if affected.

☺ Undesirable effects
The frequency is not defined, but commonly reported undesirable effects include:
- Asthenia
- Drowsiness
- Dry mouth and other anticholinergic symptoms
- Postural hypotension (especially the elderly)

Drug interactions
Pharmacokinetic
- Levomepromazine is an inhibitor of CYP2D6. Although metabolized by the liver, involvement of specific pathways is unclear.
- The clinical significance of co-administration with substrates of CYP2D6 (📖 end cover) is unknown. Caution is advised if

levomepromazine is co-administered with drugs that are predominantly metabolized by CYP2D6 (e.g. haloperidol, risperidone, tricyclic antidepressants). The prescriber should be aware of the potential for interactions and that dose adjustments may be necessary, particularly for drugs with a narrow therapeutic index.

- The clinical significance of co-administration with prodrug substrates of CYP2D6 (e.g. codeine, tramadol) is unknown. The prescriber should be aware of the potential for interactions and that dose adjustments may be necessary.

Pharmacodynamic

- Levomepromazine can cause dose-related prolongation of the QT interval. There is a potential risk that co-administration with other drugs that also prolong the QT interval (e.g. amiodarone, erythromycin, haloperidol, quinine) may result in ventricular arrhythmias.
- *Anticholinergics*—increased risk of undesirable effects.
- *Antiepileptics*—dose may need to be increased to take account of the lowered seizure threshold.
- *Antihypertensives*—increased risk of hypotension.
- *CNS depressants*—additive sedative effect.
- *Haloperidol*—may be an additive hypotensive effect; increased risk of extrapyramidal symptoms.
- *Levodopa and dopamine agonists*—effect antagonized by levomepromazine.
- *Metoclopramide*—increased risk of extrapyramidal symptoms.
- *Opioids*—may be an additive hypotensive effect.
- *Trazodone*—may be an additive hypotensive effect.

♣ Dose

When prescribing levomepromazine, the subcutaneous dose should be lower than the corresponding oral dose (which undergoes significant first-pass metabolism). There should be a separate prescription for each route, ensuring that the same dose cannot be given PO or by SC/CSCI.

Psychosis

- Initial dose 25–50mg PO daily in 2–3 divided doses. Larger doses can be given at bedtime. Doses can be increased as necessary to the most effective level compatible with sedation and other undesirable effects.
- ¥ Alternatively, by 12.5–25mg SC OD or via CSCI. Can increase as necessary up to a maximum of 200mg daily via CSCI.

Terminal agitation

- Initial dose 12.5–25mg SC(¥) OD or via CSCI. The dose can be increased as necessary up to a maximum of 200mg daily via CSCI, although higher doses may be necessary.

Nausea and vomiting

- ¥ 6–12mg PO PRN or OD to a max of 50mg daily. Regular daily doses are generally administered at bedtime.
- ¥ Alternatively, 6.25–12.5mg SC PRN or via CSCI to a maximum of 25mg daily.

⚖ Dose adjustments

Elderly

- No specific adjustments required. However, patients over the age of 50 years may be more susceptible to undesirable effects, such as postural hypotension and anticholinergic effects (with an increased risk for cognitive decline and dementia). Wherever possible, the lowest effective dose should be used

Hepatic/renal impairment

- Wherever possible, lower doses should be used. Patients may be more susceptible to undesirable effects.

Additional information

- Tablets can be dispersed in water immediately prior to administration if necessary.
- The injection may change colour if placed in direct sunlight (e.g. deep purple) and is incompatible with alkaline solutions (e.g. dexamethasone).
- In order to reduce the risk of site reactions, levomepromazine via CSCI should be diluted with NaCl 0.9%.
- Levomepromazine via CSCI has been shown to be compatible with alfentanil, clonazepam, cyclizine, diamorphine, dihydrocodeine, fentanyl, glycopyrronium, haloperidol, hyoscine butylbromide, hyoscine hydro-bromide, ketamine, methadone, metoclopramide, midazolam, octre-otide, ondansetron, oxycodone, and tramadol.
- Levinan® tablets are presently an unlicensed product and are available on a named-patient basis only. Contact Archimedes Pharma UK Ltd on (0118) 931 5060 for further information.

⟳ Pharmacology

Levomepromazine is an antipsychotic drug that shares similar properties with chlorpromazine. It is an antagonist at dopamine D_2 receptors, serotonin 5-HT_2 receptors, α_1-adrenergic receptors, histamine H_1 receptors, and acetylcholine muscarinic receptors. Consequently it has a wide spectrum of undesirable effects.

Lidocaine

Versatis® (POM)

Medicated plaster: 5% w/w lidocaine (700mg); 10 cm × 14 cm (30)

Indications

- Symptomatic relief of neuropathic pain associated with post-herpetic neuralgia.
- ¥ Post-thoracotomy pain.
- ¥ Post-mastectomy pain.
- ¥ There is developing experience suggesting that topical lidocaine may be useful in other localized neuropathies and musculoskeletal pain.

Contraindications and precautions

- Contraindicated in patients with known hypersensitivity to lidocaine or other local anaesthetics of the amide type (e.g. bupivacaine).
- Do not apply to inflamed or broken skin.
- Although only 3±2% of the total applied dose is systemically available, lidocaine plasters should be used with caution in patients with severe cardiac impairment, severe renal impairment, or severe hepatic impairment.

☺ Undesirable effects

Very common

- Administration site reactions (e.g. erythema, rash, pruritus)

Uncommon

- Site injury (e.g. skin lesion)

Very rare

- Anaphylaxis

Drug interactions

Pharmacokinetic

- None have been reported. Given the low systemic absorption, it is unlikely that lidocaine plasters will be involved in pharmacokinetic interactions.

Pharmacodynamic

- Although none have been reported, lidocaine plasters may have an opioid-sparing effect, so regular review of analgesia requirements should be performed.

⚖ Dose

- Apply up to three plasters over the affected area(s) for 12 hours, followed by a 12-hour plaster-free period.
- The plasters can be cut to size before removal of the backing material.
- Response to treatment can occur with application of the first plaster, but it may take up to 4 weeks for a response to occur. Treatment outcome should be reassessed after 2–4 weeks.
- ¥ Patches may be kept *in situ* for up to 18 hours if necessary.

♪ Dose adjustments

Elderly
- No adjustments are necessary.

Hepatic/renal impairment
- No adjustments are necessary, but the manufacturer recommends that the plasters should be used with caution.

Additional information

- Do not refrigerate or freeze the plasters.
- Hair in the area to which the plaster is to be applied should be cut with scissors prior to application. The area must not be shaved.
- After 12 hours, 650mg lidocaine remains in the plaster, so it must be disposed of carefully by folding the adhesive sides in half.

♦ Pharmacology

Lidocaine prevents the generation and conduction of nerve impulses by blocking Na^+ channels. As a general rule, small nerve fibres are more susceptible to the action of lidocaine than large fibres. C and Aδ fibres, which mediate pain and temperature, are blocked before larger fibres which mediate, for example, touch and pressure (Aβ). Lidocaine binds more tightly and rapidly to open channels and appears to preferentially inhibit abnormal excessive activity at ectopic foci with increased Na^+-channel density. These conditions are present after peripheral nerve injury and in nociceptors sensitized by inflammatory modulators. The release characteristics of the lidocaine plaster are such that only very low concentrations penetrate the skin. Spontaneous ectopic discharges are suppressed by lidocaine applied topically and normal function is unaffected, i.e. the lidocaine plaster produces analgesia rather than anaesthesia.

Loperamide

Imodium® (POM)
Capsule: 2mg (30)
Syrup: 1mg/5mL (100mL)

Generic (POM)
Capsule: 2mg (30)
Tablet: 2mg (30)

Note: Loperamide can be sold over the counter provided that it is licensed and labelled for the treatment of acute diarrhoea and the maximum daily dose does not exceed 16mg (**P**) or 12mg (**GSL**).

Imodium® Instants (GSL)
Orodispersible tablet: 2mg (6)
Note: This product is licensed for the acute treatment of diarrhoea, with a maximum daily dose of 12mg.

Indications
- Acute diarrhoea
- Chronic diarrhoea (**POM** only)
- ⁺ Bowel colic
- ⁺ Reduction of stoma output

Contraindications and precautions
- Contraindicated for use in:
    - abdominal distension
    - acute ulcerative colitis
    - antibiotic-associated colitis
    - ileus
    - toxic megacolon.
- Use with caution in patients with hepatic impairment (risk of CNS toxicity).
- Avoid use of Imodium® Instants in patients with phenylketonuria—orodispersible tablets contain aspartame, a source of phenylalanine.
- Patients with diarrhoea treated with loperamide may experience dizziness or drowsiness and should not drive (or operate machinery) if affected.

☻ Undesirable effects
The frequency is not defined, but reported undesirable effects include:
- Abdominal bloating
- Abdominal cramps
- Dizziness
- Drowsiness
- Paralytic ileus
- Urticaria

Drug interactions

Pharmacokinetic

- Loperamide is metabolized by CYP2C8 and CYP3A4. It is also a substrate of P-gp.
- The clinical significance of co-administration with inducers and inhibitors of CYP2C8 and CYP3A4 (📖 end cover) is unknown. The prescriber should be aware of the potential for interactions and that dosage adjustments may be necessary.
- The effect of grapefruit juice on the bioavailability of loperamide is unknown.
- Co-administration with P-gp inhibitors (e.g. lansoprazole, quinidine) may result in raised plasma levels. The clinical significance of this interaction remains unclear, but the prescriber should be aware of the potential for interactions and that dose adjustments may be necessary.

Pharmacodynamic

- *Anticholinergic drugs*—additive constipating effects.
- *Erythromycin*—antagonism of antidiarrhoeal effect.
- *Domperidone*—antagonism of antidiarrhoeal effect.
- *Metoclopramide*—antagonism of antidiarrhoeal effect.
- *Octreotide*—enhanced constipating effect.

⚖ Dose

Acute diarrhoea

- Initial dose 4mg PO, followed by 2mg PO after each loose stool. Maximum 16mg PO daily (**POM** and **P**) or 12mg PO daily (**GSL**)

Chronic diarrhoea

- Initial dose 4–8mg PO daily in divided doses, adjusted to response. Maximum dose 16mg PO daily in two or more divided doses.

¥ Bowel colic

- 2–4mg PO QDS.

Reduction of stoma output

- Initial dose 8mg PO QDS, adjusted to response. Maximum dose may be as high as 64mg PO daily in divided doses.

⚖ Dose adjustments

Elderly

- No dose adjustment is necessary.

Hepatic/renal impairment

- No specific guidance is available for patients with hepatic impairment. However, the manufacturer advises caution, given the extensive hepatic metabolism.
- No dose adjustment is necessary in renal impairment.

⟳ Pharmacology

Loperamide is an opioid receptor agonist and acts on μ-opioid receptors in the bowel. It works specifically by reducing peristalsis and increasing intestinal transit time. Loperamide is well absorbed orally and is extensively metabolized by CYP2C8 and CYP3A4.

Lorazepam

Generic (CD Benz POM)

Tablet: 1mg (28); 2.5mg (28). Note that not all generic formulations are scored, so the prescriber should specify if a scored tablet is required.
Injection: 4mg/mL (midazolam generally preferred).

Note: Independent prescribers are authorized to prescribe lorazepam
See 📖 Independent prescribing—palliative care issues, p.25 Note that
sublingual lorazepam is an unlicensed route of administration. See 📖
Unlicensed use of medicines, p.22.

Indications

- Anxiety
- Insomnia
- Status epilepticus (injection)
- ¥ Dyspnoea

Contraindications and precautions

- Contraindicated for use in patients with
  - acute pulmonary insufficiency
  - myasthenia gravis
  - severe hepatic insufficiency
  - sleep apnoea syndrome.
- Use with caution if there is a history of drug or alcohol abuse.
- Lorazepam should be used with caution in patients with chronic respiratory disease, renal impairment, or moderate hepatic impairment.
- Dose reductions may be necessary in the elderly (see 📖 *Dose adjustments*).
- Avoid abrupt withdrawal, even if short-duration treatment. Prolonged use of benzodiazepines may result in the development of dependence with subsequent withdrawal symptoms on cessation of use, e.g. agitation, anxiety, confusion, headaches, restlessness, sleep disturbances, sweating, and tremor. The risk of dependence increases with dose and duration of treatment. Gradual withdrawal is advised.
- Lorazepam may modify reactions and patients should be advised not to drive (or operate machinery) if affected.

☺ Undesirable effects

The frequency is not defined, but reported undesirable effects include:

- Anterograde amnesia
- Ataxia
- Confusion
- Depression
- Dizziness
- Drowsiness
- Fatigue
- Hallucinations
- Headache

- Muscle weakness
- Nightmares
- Paradoxical events such as agitation, irritability and restlessness
- Sexual dysfunction
- Sleep disturbance
- Visual disturbances

Drug interactions

Pharmacokinetic

- Given the fact that the metabolism of lorazepam does not involve the cytochrome P450 system, pharmacokinetic interactions are likely to be minimal compared with the other benzodiazepines.

Pharmacodynamic

- *Alcohol*—may precipitate seizures.
- *Antidepressants*—reduced seizure threshold.
- *Antipsychotics*—reduced seizure threshold.
- *CNS depressants*—additive sedative effect.

♣ Dose

Anxiety

- Initial dose 0.5–1mg SL stat (¥) or 0.5mg PO BD. Dose can be increased as necessary to 4mg daily.
- ¥ Alternatively, 0.5mg SL PRN, to a maximum of 4mg daily.

Insomnia

- 1–2mg PO before bedtime.

Status epilepticus

- 4mg IV stat.
- The injection may be diluted 1:1 with NaCl 0.9% or WFI immediately before administration.

¥ Dyspnoea

- 0.5mg SL PRN, to a maximum of 4mg daily.

♣ Dose adjustments

Elderly

- No specific guidance is available. Use the lowest effective dose.

Hepatic/renal impairment

- No specific guidance is available. The dose must be carefully adjusted to individual requirements.

Additional information

- Although the injection has been administered via CSCI, this is generally not recommended and midazolam or clonazepam are the preferred choices.
- Tablets can be crushed and dispersed in water if necessary. A low volume of water can be used (e.g. ≤2mL).

Pharmacology

Potentiates action of GABA, resulting in increased neuronal inhibition and CNS depression, especially in the limbic system and reticular formation. Metabolism of lorazepam is through direct glucuronide conjugation, avoiding the cytochrome P450 system.

Macrogol '3350'

Laxido® (P)
Oral powder: macrogol '3350' 13.125g, sodium bicarbonate 178.5mg, sodium chloride 350.7mg, potassium chloride 46.6mg/sachet (20; 30)

Movicol® (P)
Oral powder: macrogol '3350' 13.125g, sodium bicarbonate 178.5mg, sodium chloride 350.7mg, potassium chloride 46.6mg/sachet (20; 30; 50)

Movicol Half®
Oral powder: macrogol '3350' 6.563g, sodium bicarbonate 89.3mg, sodium chloride 175.4mg, potassium chloride 23.3mg/sachet (20; 30)

Indications
- Constipation
- Faecal impaction

Contraindications and precautions
- Contraindicated for use in the following conditions:
  - Crohn's disease
  - ileus
  - intestinal perforation or obstruction
  - toxic megacolon
  - ulcerative colitis.
- Patients with cardiovascular disease should not take more than two sachets in any one hour.

☺ Undesirable effects
The frequency is not defined, but reported undesirable effects include:
- Abdominal distension
- Abdominal pain
- Anal discomfort
- Borborygmi
- Diarrhoea
- Flatulence
- Nausea
- Vomiting

Drug interactions
Pharmacokinetic
- No known pharmacokinetic interactions.

Pharmacodynamic
- *Anticholinergics*—antagonizes the laxative effect.
- *Cyclizine*—antagonizes the laxative effect.
- *Opioids*—antagonizes the laxative effect.
- *5-HT₃ antagonists*—antagonizes the laxative effect.
- *Tricyclic antidepressants*—antagonizes the laxative effect.

Dose

The contents of each sachet should be dissolved in 125mL of water.

Constipation
- Usual dose 1 sachet OD-TDS
- * The dose can be increased to 2 sachets TDS if necessary.

Faecal impaction
- 8 sachets, to be taken within a 6-hour period.
- Patients with cardiovascular disease should not take more than 2 sachets in one hour.
- The dose can be repeated on days 2 and 3 if necessary.

Dose adjustments

Elderly
- No dose adjustment is necessary.

Hepatic/renal impairment
- No dose adjustment is necessary

Additional information

- After reconstitution the solution should be kept in a refrigerator and discarded if unused after 6 hours.
- An effect should be seen within 1–3 days.

Pharmacology

Macrogol '3350' is a polymer that produces an osmotic laxative effect.

Magnesium hydroxide

Generic (GSL)
Oral suspension: magnesium hydroxide BP (100mL; 200mL)

Indications
- Constipation

Contraindications and precautions
- Contraindicated in acute GI conditions (e.g. acute inflammatory bowel diseases, abdominal pain of unknown origin, intestinal obstruction).
- Use with caution in patients with:
  - renal impairment—risk of hypermagnesaemia
  - severe dehydration
  - severe hepatic impairment (see ☐ *Dose adjustments*, p.300).

☻ Undesirable effects
The frequency is not stated, but undesirable effects include:
- Diarrhoea
- Symptoms of hypermagnesaemia (e.g. nausea, vomiting, confusion, drowsiness)

Drug interactions
Pharmacokinetic
- Magnesium hydroxide should not be given within 1 hour of the following drugs/formulations:
  - *bisacodyl*—may remove the enteric coat and increase the risk of dyspepsia
  - *demeclocycline*—reduced absorption
  - *enteric coated formulations*
  - *gabapentin*—reduced absorption
  - *lansoprazole*—reduced absorption
  - *paroxetine*—reduced absorption of suspension
  - *rabeprazole*—reduced absorption.

Pharmacodynamic
- *Anticholinergics*—antagonizes the laxative effect.
- *Cyclizine*—antagonizes the laxative effect.
- *Opioids*—antagonizes the laxative effect; risk of respiratory depression (associated with hypermagnesaemia).
- *5-HT₃ antagonists*—antagonizes the laxative effect,
- *Tricyclic antidepressants*—antagonizes the laxative effect.

♂ Dose
Antacid
- 5–10mL PO as necessary, to a maximum of 60mL daily.

Laxative
- 30–45mL PO at bedtime. May be taken with water if necessary.

⚖ Dose adjustments

Elderly
- No specific dose adjustments recommended by the manufacturer.

Hepatic/renal impairment
- No specific dose adjustments recommended by the manufacturer.
- Magnesium hydroxide should be used with caution in patients with severe hepatic impairment because of the possible risk of subsequent renal impairment.
- Magnesium can accumulate in patients with renal impairment. Use lower doses or choose an alternative.

Additional information

- The laxative effect can work within 1–6 hours, so administration times may need to be adjusted. The dose may need to be adjusted if co-administered with a stimulant laxative.

⊷ Pharmacology

Magnesium hydroxide has an indirect laxative effect caused by water retention in the intestinal lumen.

Magnesium-L-aspartate

Magnaspartate® (GSL)
Oral powder: 6.5g (10mmol Mg^{2+}) per sachet (10)

Indications
• Hypomagnesaemia

Contraindications and precautions
• Contraindicated in severe renal impairment.
• Use with caution in patients with:
  • diabetes (sucrose content of product)
  • mild to moderate renal impairment—risk of hypermagnesaemia
  • severe dehydration
  • severe hepatic impairment (see 📖 *Dose adjustments,* p.301).

☺ Undesirable effects
The frequency is not stated, but undesirable effects include:
• Diarrhoea
• Symptoms of hypermagnesaemia (e.g. nausea, vomiting, confusion, drowsiness)

Drug interactions
Pharmacokinetic
• None known.

Pharmacodynamic
• *Opioids*—risk of respiratory depression (associated with hypermagnesaemia).

⚗ Dose
• Initial dose 10mmol (1 sachet) PO OD in 200mL water, increasing to 10mmol PO BD and above as necessary dependent on serum magnesium. High doses will lead to the development of diarrhoea.

⚗ Dose adjustments
Elderly
• No specific dose adjustments recommended by the manufacturer.

Hepatic/renal impairment
• No specific dose adjustments recommended by the manufacturer.
• Magnesium-L-aspartate should be used with caution in patients with severe hepatic impairment because of the possible risk of subsequent renal impairment.
• Magnesium can accumulate in patients with renal impairment. Use lower doses or choose an alternative.

Additional information
- Low serum Mg^{2+} can cause secondary low serum Ca^{2+}, Na^+, and K^+.
- Compared with oral magnesium supplements, Magnaspartate® has excellent bioavailability.
- Magnaspartate® is available from KoRa Healthcare (Tel: 0114 299 4979).

✈ Pharmacology

Magnaspartate® is a food supplement used in the management of magnesium deficiency. Magnesium is an essential electrolyte and is involved in many enzyme systems. The largest body stores are found in bone. Magnesium salts, with the exception of Magnaspartate®, are generally poorly absorbed orally, necessitating replacement therapy for symptomatic hypomagnesaemia by the IV route. Magnesium is excreted renally and can accumulate in renal impairment.

Magnesium sulphate

Generic (POM)
Magnesium sulphate 50%
Injection (ampoule): 1g/2mL; 2g/4mL; 2.5g/5mL; 5g /10mL
NB: 50% − 500mg/mL−2mmol/mL

Indications
- Symptomatic hypomagnesaemia.

Contraindications and precautions
- Contraindicated in severe renal impairment.
- Use with caution in patients with:
  - mild to moderate renal impairment—risk of hypermagnesaemia
  - severe dehydration
  - severe hepatic impairment (see 📖 *Dose adjustments*, p.304).

☺ Undesirable effects
The frequency is not stated, but undesirable effects include:
- Diarrhoea
- Symptoms of hypermagnesaemia (e.g. nausea, vomiting, confusion, drowsiness)

Drug interactions
Pharmacokinetic
- None known.

Pharmacodynamic
- *Opioids*—risk of respiratory depression (associated with hypermagnesaemia).

🜪 Dose
- Up to 160mmol Mg^{2+} via IV infusion over up to 5 days may be required to replace the deficiency.
- Serum Mg^{2+} should be measured throughout treatment.
- There are several suggested methods of replacement therapy:
  - 35–50mmol (8.75–12.5g magnesium sulphate, or 17.5–25mL of 50% solution) diluted in 1L of NaCl 0.9% or glucose 5% via an infusion pump over 12–24 hours. Subsequent daily doses can be reviewed as per serum Mg^{2+}.
  - 20mmol (5g magnesium sulphate, or 10mL of 50% solution) diluted in 1L of NaCl 0.9% or glucose 5% via an infusion pump over 3 hours. Subsequent daily doses can be reviewed as per serum Mg^{2+}.

Dose adjustments

Elderly
- No specific dose adjustments recommended by the manufacturer.

Hepatic/renal impairment
- No specific dose adjustments recommended by the manufacturer.
- Magnesium sulphate should be used with caution in patients with severe hepatic impairment because of the possible risk of subsequent renal impairment.
- Magnesium can accumulate in patients with renal impairment. Use lower doses or choose an alternative.

Additional information

- To reduce venous irritation, IV infusion dilution to a concentration up to 200mg/mL (or 0.8mmol/mL) is recommended.
- The administration rate should not exceed 150mg/min (0.6mmol/min) in order to avoid excessive renal losses.
- Low serum Mg^{2+} can cause secondary low serum Ca^{2+}, Na^+, and K^+.

Pharmacology

Magnesium is an essential electrolyte and is involved in many enzyme systems. The largest body stores are found in bone. Magnesium salts are generally poorly absorbed orally, with the exception of Magnaspartate®, necessitating replacement therapy by the IV route. Magnesium is excreted renally and can accumulate in renal impairment.

Medroxyprogesterone

Provera® (POM)
Tablet (*scored*): 100mg (60; 100); 200mg (30); 400mg (30)

Indications
- Endometrial carcinoma.
- Renal cell carcinoma.
- Carcinoma of breast in postmenopausal women.
- ⌁ Anorexia and cachexia.

Contraindications and precautions
- Medroxyprogesterone is contraindicated in patients with:
  - acute porphyria
  - angina
  - atrial fibrillation
  - cerebral infarction
  - deep vein thrombosis
  - endocarditis
  - heart failure
  - hypercalcaemia associated with bone metastases
  - impaired liver function or active liver disease
  - pulmonary embolism
  - thromboembolic ischaemic attack
  - thrombophlebitis
  - undiagnosed vaginal bleeding.
- May cause hypercalcaemia in patients with breast cancer and bone metastases.
- Unexpected vaginal bleeding during treatment should be investigated.
- Treatment with medroxyprogesterone can cause Cushingoid symptoms.
- Discontinue treatment if the following develop:
  - jaundice or deterioration in liver function
  - significant increase in blood pressure
  - new onset of migraine-type headache
  - sudden change in vision.
- Use with caution in patients with:
  - continuous treatment with relatively large doses (monitor for signs of hypertension, sodium retention, oedema)
  - depression
  - diabetes
  - epilepsy
  - hyperlipidaemia
  - hypertension
  - migraine
  - renal impairment.

☻ Undesirable effects

The frequency is not defined, but reported undesirable effects include:

- Congestive heart failure
- Depression
- Dizziness
- Headache
- Hypercalcaemia
- Hypertension
- Increased appetite
- Insomnia
- Malaise
- Menstrual irregularities
- Nervousness
- Oedema
- Reduced libido
- Somnolence
- Thromboembolic disorders (e.g. pulmonary embolism, retinal thrombosis)
- Weight gain

Drug interactions

Pharmacokinetic

- Medroxyprogesterone is metabolized by CYP3A4. Despite this, the clearance of medroxyprogesterone is believed to be approximately equal to hepatic blood flow. Therefore medroxyprogesterone would not be expected to be affected by drugs that alter hepatic enzyme activity.
- Nonetheless, the clinical significance of co-administration with inducers or inhibitors of CYP3A4 (🕮 end cover) is unknown. The prescriber should be aware of the potential for interactions and that dose adjustments may be necessary.
- Avoid excessive amounts of grapefruit juice as it may increase the bioavailability of medroxyprogesterone through inhibition of intestinal CYP3A4.

Pharmacodynamic

- *NSAIDs*—increased risk of fluid retention.
- *Warfarin*—possible effect on bleeding times; INR should be monitored.

♃ Dose

Endometrial and renal cell carcinoma

- 200–600mg PO daily.

Breast carcinoma

- 400–1500mg PO daily.

¥ Anorexia and cachexia

- Initial dose 400mg PO OM. Increase as necessary to 400mg BD.

♣ Dose adjustments

Elderly
- No dose adjustments are necessary.

Hepatic/renal impairment
- Although specific guidance is unavailable, the lowest effective dose should be used. Medroxyprogesterone is contraindicated in severe impaired liver function.
- Although specific guidance is unavailable, the lowest effective dose should be used. Medroxyprogesterone should be used with caution in patients with renal impairment.

Additional information

- As with corticosteroids and megestrol, the increase in body mass is likely to be due to retention of fluid or increase in body fat.
- Medroxyprogesterone has a catabolic effect on skeletal muscle which could further weaken the patient.

♦ Pharmacology

Medroxyprogesterone is a synthetic progestin and has the same physiological effects as natural progesterone. It has a similar effect to megestrol.

Megestrol

Megace® (POM)
Tablet: 160mg (30)

Indications
- Breast cancer.
- Endometrial cancer.
- ¥ Anorexia and cachexia.

Contraindications and precautions
- Use with caution in patients with:
  - history of thrombophlebitis
  - severe impaired liver function.
- Glucose intolerance and Cushing's syndrome have been reported with the use of megestrol. The possibility of adrenal suppression should be considered in all patients taking or withdrawing from chronic megestrol treatment. Glucocorticoid replacement treatment may be necessary.

☺ Undesirable effects
The frequency is not defined, but commonly reported undesirable effects include:
- Weight gain
- Increased appetite and food intake
- Nausea
- Vomiting
- Oedema
- Breakthrough uterine bleeding
- Headache

Other reported undesirable effects include:
- Dyspnoea
- Heart failure
- Hypertension
- Hot flushes
- Mood changes
- Cushingoid facies
- Tumour flare (with or without hypercalcaemia)
- Hyperglycaemia
- Alopecia
- Carpal tunnel syndrome
- Thrombophlebitis
- Pulmonary embolism

Drug interactions
Pharmacokinetic
- None stated.

Pharmacodynamic
- None stated.

♪ Dose

Breast cancer
- 160mg PO OD.

Endometrial cancer
- 40–320mg PO daily, in two or more divided doses

¥ *Anorexia and cachexia*
- Initial dose 160mg PO OD, increased as necessary up to 800mg daily in two or more divided doses.

♪ Dose adjustments

Elderly
- No dose adjustment is necessary.

Hepatic/renal impairment
- Undergoes complete hepatic metabolism. Although specific guidance is unavailable, the lowest effective dose should be used. Megestrol is contraindicated in severely impaired liver function.
- Dose adjustments are not necessary in renal impairment.

Additional information

- Although oral suspensions can be imported (unlicensed, named-patient supply), these are expensive. The tablet can be dispersed in water immediately prior to administration.
- As with corticosteroids and medroxyprogesterone, the increase in body mass is likely to be due to retention of fluid or increase in body fat.
- Megestrol has a catabolic effect on skeletal muscle which could further weaken the patient.

⊙ Pharmacology

Megestrol is a synthetic progestin and has the same physiological effects as natural progesterone. It interferes with the oestrogen cycle and suppresses luteinizing hormone release from the pituitary. It has a slight but significant glucocorticoid effect and a very slight mineralocorticoid effect. The precise mechanism of the effect on anorexia and cachexia is unknown. Megestrol has direct cytotoxic effects on breast cancer cells in tissue culture and may also have a direct effect on the endometrium.

Metformin

Standard release

Glucophage® (POM)
Tablet: 500mg (84); 850mg (56)
Powder for oral solution: 500mg (30); 1000mg (30)

Generic (POM)
Tablet: 500mg (28; 84); 850mg (56)
Oral solution: 500mg/5mL (100mL—*sugar-free*)

Modified release

Glucophage SR® (POM)
Generic (POM)
Tablet: 500mg (28; 56)

Indications

- Type II diabetes (particularly in overweight patients) not controlled by diet or exercise.

Contraindications and precautions

- Do not use metformin in conditions that may increase the risk of developing lactic acidosis:
  - Liver impairment
  - Renal impairment where CrCl <60mL/min
  - Severe congestive heart failure
  - Severe COPD.
- *Glucophage®* powder for oral solution contains aspartame. Avoid in patients with phenylketonuria.
- Metformin must be discontinued prior to and not restarted until 48 hours post administration of iodinated contrast agent.
- Discontinue metformin 48 hours prior to elective surgery requiring a general anaesthetic. Restart not less than 48 hours afterwards

☻ Undesirable effects

Very common
These tend to be gastrointestinal in nature and can be reduced with slow titration; they usually resolve spontaneously.
- Diarrhoea
- Loss of appetite
- Nausea/vomiting

Common
- Metallic taste

Very rare
- Lactic acidosis

NB—Hypoglycaemia should not occur with metformin at normal doses

Drug interactions

Pharmacokinetic

- Drugs excreted by renal tubular secretion (e.g. amiloride, cefalexin, digoxin, morphine, quinine) have the potential to interact with metformin, increasing plasma concentrations. The clinical significance is unknown and until further information is available, the following is suggested:
  - if metformin is co-administered with these drugs, a slow and cautious titration is advisable.
  - if these drugs are prescribed for a patient already using metformin, it is advisable to review the metformin dose (lower doses may be required).
- Drugs which affect renal function have the potential to interact with metformin. If such drugs are co-administered, regular monitoring of renal function is advisable. Such drugs include:
  - ACE inhibitors
  - NSAIDs
  - iodinated contrast agent (see *Contraindications and precautions*)

Pharmacodynamic

- Drugs that may precipitate hyperglycaemia may interfere with blood glucose control, e.g.
  - corticosteroids
  - diuretics
  - nifedipine
- ACE inhibitors can cause hypoglycaemia by an unknown mechanism. Severe symptomatic cases have been reported when used in combination with antidiabetic drugs.
- Alcohol (increased risk of lactic acidosis with acute intoxication).

,ḏ Dose

Standard release

- Initial dose 500mg PO BD with or after meals; allow 1–2 weeks before increasing the dose. A slower titration improves GI tolerance.
- Dose increases of 500mg PO OD can be made at 1–2 weekly intervals to a maximum dose of 3g daily, in 2–3 divided doses, with or after meals.

Modified release

- Initial dose 500mg PO OD with evening meal.
- Dose can be increased every 1–2 weeks by 500mg OD to a maximum of 2g OD with evening meal (or 1g BD with meals to improve blood glucose control).
- If blood glucose control is not achieved, change to standard-release formulations or review treatment.

,⅃ Dose adjustments

Elderly
- Renal function must be assessed. Must not be used if CrCl <60mL/min.

Hepatic/renal impairment
- Avoid in hepatic impairment because of increased risk of lactic acidosis.
- Must not be used if CrCl <60mL/min.

Additional information

- Metformin is occasionally combined with insulin to improve blood glucose control. Metformin dosage as described above.
- In the absence of the oral solution, metformin tablets can be crushed and dispersed in water immediately prior to administration. The suspension can be flushed through an NG tube.

↬ Pharmacology

Metformin is a biguanide which delays the intestinal absorption of glucose, reduces hepatic glucose production (inhibits glycogenolysis and gluconeogenesis), and increases peripheral glucose uptake and utilization in muscle. It lowers basal and postprandial plasma glucose concentrations, but does not stimulate insulin secretion (minimal risk of hypoglycaemia). The pharmacodynamics of metformin may rely upon a type of transport protein (▥ Pharmacogenetics, p.11), the organic cation transporter (OCT). OCT1 is involved in the uptake of metformin by hepatocytes, while OCT2 is involved in renal excretion. Unexpected responses to metformin may be due to genetic polymorphisms (▥ Pharmacogenetics, p.11) in OCT1 and OCT2 genes, or by drug interactions (mainly with OCT2—see ▥ Drug interactions, p.15). Metformin is excreted unchanged in the urine.

Methadone

Generic (CD POM)
Tablet: 5mg (50)
Injection: 10mg/mL; 20mg/2mL; 35mg/3.5mL; 50mg/5mL; 50mg/2mL; 50mg/mL
Oral solution: 1mg/mL (various volumes); 5mg/mL (various volumes)
Note: *some generic formulations are sugar free.*
Oral concentrate: 10mg/mL (blue, 150mL); 20mg/mL (brown, 150mL)
Note: *prescriptions should only be dispensed after appropriate dilution with Methadose® Diluent*
Linctus: 2mg/5mL

Methadone is a Schedule 2 controlled drug (see 📖 Legal categories, p.23). Independent prescribers are NOT authorized to prescribe methadone (📖 Independent prescribing: palliative care issues, p.25).

Indications
- Moderate to severe pain.
- Treatment of opioid dependence.
- Cough (linctus).

Contraindications and precautions
- If the dose of an opioid is titrated correctly, it is generally accepted that there are no absolute contraindications to the use of such drugs in palliative care, although there may be circumstances where one opioid is favoured over another (e.g. renal impairment, constipation). Nonetheless, manufacturers state that methadone is contraindicated for use in patients with:
  - concurrent administration of MAOIs or within 2 weeks of discontinuation of their use
  - head injury
  - obstructive airways disease (may cause histamine release)
  - paralytic ileus
  - respiratory depression.
- Use with caution in the following instances:
  - Addison's disease (adrenocortical insufficiency)
  - asthma (may cause histamine release)
  - cardiac disease (methadone may increase QT interval)
  - concurrent administration of drugs that:
    - have a potential for QT prolongation
    - are CYP3A4 and CYP2B6 inhibitors (see 📖 *Drug interactions*, p.314)
  - diseases of the biliary tract
  - epilepsy (morphine may lower seizure threshold)
  - hepatic impairment
  - hypotension
  - hypothyroidism
  - inflammatory bowel disorders
  - myasthenia gravis

- prostatic hypertrophy
- raised intracranial pressure
- renal impairment (if sodium bicarbonate is co-prescribed—see 📖 *Drug interactions*, p.314)
- Electrolyte disturbances must be corrected (e.g. hypokalaemia) because of the risk of QT prolongation. ECG monitoring is recommended for doses >100mg daily (unlikely in palliative care).

☹ Undesirable effects

Strong opioids tend to cause similar undesirable effects, albeit to varying degrees. The frequency is not defined, but reported undesirable effects include:

- Anorexia
- Asthenia
- Biliary pain
- Confusion
- Constipation
- Drowsiness
- Dry mouth
- Dyspepsia
- Exacerbation of pancreatitis
- Euphoria
- Insomnia
- Headache
- Hyperhidrosis
- Myoclonus
- Nausea
- Pruritus
- Sexual dysfunction (e.g. amenorrhea, decreased libido, erectile dysfunction)
- Urinary retention
- Vertigo
- Visual disturbance
- Vomiting

The following can occur with excessive dose:
- Agitation
- Exacerbation of pain
- Hallucinations
- Miosis
- Paraesthesia
- Respiratory depression
- Restlessness

Drug interactions

Pharmacokinetic
- Methadone is metabolized by CYP3A4 and CYP2B6. To a lesser extent, CYP1A2 and CYP2D6 are involved. Methadone weakly inhibits CYP2D6.
- *Amiodarone*—may increase plasma concentration of methadone.
- *Carbamazepine*—reduces effect of methadone.
- *Ciprofloxacin*—may increase plasma concentration of methadone.
- *Clopidogrel*—may increase plasma concentration of methadone.
- *Erythromycin*—may increase plasma concentrations of methadone.
- *Fluconazole*—may increase plasma concentration of methadone.
- *Fluoxetine*—may increase plasma concentration of methadone.
- *Paroxetine*—may increase plasma concentration of methadone.
- *Phenobarbital*—reduces effect of methadone.
- *Sertraline*—may increase plasma concentration of methadone.
- *Sodium bicarbonate*—increases plasma concentration of methadone because of reduced renal excretion.

- The clinical significance of co-administration with other CYP3A4 and CYP2B6 inhibitors or inducers (📖 end cover) is unknown. The prescriber should be aware of the potential for interactions and that dose adjustments may be necessary.
- The clinical significance of co-administration with substrates of CYP2D6 (📖 end cover) is unknown. Caution is advised if methadone is co-administered with drugs that are predominantly metabolized by CYP2D6. The prescriber should be aware of the potential for interactions and that dose adjustments may be necessary, particularly for drugs with a narrow therapeutic index.
- Avoid grapefruit juice as it may increase the bioavailability of methadone through inhibition of intestinal CYP3A4.

Pharmacodynamic

- Methadone can cause dose-related prolongation of the QT interval. There is a potential risk that co-administration with other drugs that also prolong the QT interval (e.g. amiodarone, erythromycin, quinine) may result in ventricular arrhythmias.
- *Antihypertensives*—increased risk of hypotension.
- *CNS depressants*—risk of excessive sedation.
- *Haloperidol*—may be an additive hypotensive effect and additive QT effect.
- *Ketamine*—there is a potential opioid-sparing effect with ketamine and the dose of morphine may need reducing.
- *Levomepromazine*—may be an additive hypotensive effect and additive QT effect.

♃ Dose

Oral

- Initial dose depends upon the patient's previous opioid requirements.
- Methadone is rarely initiated in opioid-naive patients and such use is not mentioned here.
- If converting from oral hydromorphone or oxycodone, convert the total daily dose to morphine (see 📖 Opioid substitution, p.33 for information regarding opioid dose equivalences).
- The following method is suggested when switching from oral morphine. It involves a 5 day titration phase using an initial *loading dose*, followed by administration of a *fixed dose* of methadone 3 hourly PO PRN.
- The loading dose is calculated as 1/10th of the previous total daily morphine dose, to a **maximum of 30mg**.
- The fixed dose is calculated as 1/30th of the previous total daily morphine dose.
- For example:
  - 120mg PO BD morphine—*loading dose* of PO methadone = 24mg
  - 120mg PO BD morphine—*fixed dose* of PO methadone = 8mg.

Procedure
- Stop morphine abruptly (or hydromorphone/oxycodone).
- If switching from 12-hourly modified-release morphine (or other oral opioid):
  - in pain—give the *loading dose* of methadone 6 hours after the last dose
  - pain free—give the *loading dose* of methadone 12 hours after last dose.
- If switching from 24-hourly modified-release morphine:
  - in pain—give the *loading dose* of methadone 12 hours after last dose
  - pain free—give the *loading dose* of methadone 24 hours after the last dose.
- If switching from transdermal fentanyl:
  - in pain—give the *loading dose* of methadone 12 hours after the patch removal.
  - pain free—give the *loading dose* of methadone 24 hours after patch removal.
- Administer the *fixed dose* 3 hourly PRN for 5 days.
- On day 6, review the amount of methadone used in the preceding 48 hours (i.e. days 4 and 5). Divide this by **four** to arrive at a 12 hourly maintenance dose. Rescue doses are 1/6th of the total daily maintenance dose. For example, 64mg methadone in 48 hours:
  - maintenance dose = 16mg BD
  - suggested rescue dose = 5mg PRN.
- If more than **two** PRN doses are given in a 24-hour period, the maintenance dose should be increased weekly.
- If the patient experiences pain within 3 hours of the last PRN methadone dose, give a rescue dose as per the previously taken opioid (dose between 50% and 100%).

Subcutaneous
- Methadone can be administered via SC injection or CSCI (¥), but it is never initiated this way. To convert from oral to subcutaneous methadone, halve the oral dose, although some patients may require a fairly rapid dose escalation as their ratio approaches 1:1.
- SC injection can be painful and CSCI is preferred.

♣ Dose adjustments
Elderly
- No specific guidance is available; dose requirements should be individually titrated.

Hepatic/renal impairment
- No specific guidance is available, although the plasma concentration is expected to be increased in patients with hepatic impairment. In view of its hepatic metabolism, caution is advised when giving methadone to patients with hepatic impairment. Dose requirements should be individually titrated.

- No specific guidance is available for patients with renal impairment. The manufacturers suggest that dose reductions may be necessary in moderate or severe renal impairment. Dose requirements should be individually titrated.

Additional information

- It is probably safer to manage conversions in an inpatient unit where the patient can be observed closely for toxic effect.
- Concentrated methadone oral solution is intended for dilution for the treatment of addiction but can be a useful preparation if high oral doses are required for pain. If being used in this way, it may be more convenient to dilute each dose individually.
- To reduce the incidence of CSCI site reactions, ensure the infusion is diluted maximally with NaCl 0.9%. The addition of 1mg dexamethasone may improve tolerability, although check for compatibility. Changing to a 12-hourly infusion with site rotation may also help.
- Methadone by CSCI is stated to be compatible with dexamethasone, haloperidol, hyoscine butylbromide, ketorolac, levomepromazine, metoclopramide, and midazolam.

⟿ Pharmacology

Methadone is less sedating than morphine and, as it exerts opioid and NMDA activity, it may be more useful than other opioids for the management of neuropathic pain. Its metabolism is not linear and it has a long half-life so accumulation can occur. The half-life of a single injected dose is 6–8 hours but for a single oral dose it is 12–18 hours. However, as the drug is lipid soluble, it accumulates and its half-life on repeated doses can extend to 12–48 hours. For this reason and because of great inter-individual variations in metabolism it must be introduced carefully and gradually, starting with low doses and gradually increasing the dosing interval to the usual 12-hourly regime.

Methylnaltrexone

Relistor® (POM)

Injection: 12mg (0.6mL ampoule); 20mg/mL prefilled syringe (7 × 1mL)

Indications

- Treatment of opioid-induced constipation in advanced illness patients who are receiving palliative care when response to usual laxative therapy has not been sufficient.

Contraindications and precautions

- Must not be used in patients with known or suspected mechanical bowel obstruction, or acute surgical abdomen.
- Should not be used for treatment of patients with constipation not related to opioid use.
- Administer with caution to patients with:
  - colostomy
  - peritoneal catheter
  - active diverticular disease
  - faecal impaction.
- A bowel movement can occur within 30–60 minutes of administration. Patients should be made aware and be in close proximity to toilet facilities.
- Treatment should not be continued beyond 4 months.
- Methylnaltrexone should be added to usual laxative treatment, not replace it.
- Not recommended in patients with severe hepatic impairment or with endstage renal impairment requiring dialysis (see 📖 *Dose adjustments*, p.319).

☹ Undesirable effects

Very common
- Abdominal pain
- Nausea
- Flatulence
- Diarrhoea

Common
- Dizziness
- Injection site reactions (e.g. stinging, burning, pain, redness, oedema)

Drug interactions

Pharmacokinetic
- Methylnaltrexone is a weak inhibitor of CYP2D6. It is unlikely to cause clinically significant interactions.
- Drugs excreted by renal tubular secretion (e.g. amiloride, digoxin, morphine, quinine) have the potential to interact with methylnaltrexone, increasing plasma concentrations. The clinical significance is unknown.

Pharmacodynamic
- While none have currently been observed, there is the theoretical risk that peripheral opioid analgesia will be antagonized.

♪ Dose
- Given by subcutaneous injection:
  - 38–61 kg, 8mg (0.4mL)
  - 62–114kg, 12mg (0.6mL).
- Patients whose weight falls outside the ranges quoted should be dosed at 0.15mg/kg.
- The recommended administration schedule is a single dose every other day. Doses may also be given at longer intervals, as per clinical need. Patients may receive two consecutive doses 24 hours apart only when there has been no response (bowel movement) to the dose on the preceding day.

Dose adjustments
Elderly
- No dose adjustments are necessary based on age alone.

Hepatic/renal impairment
- No dose adjustments are necessary for patients with mild to moderate hepatic impairment. No data exist for use in patients with severe hepatic impairment, and caution is advised.
- If creatinine clearance <30mL/min, the dose should be reduced to:
  - 8mg (0.4 mL) for weight 62–114 kg
  - 0.075mg/kg for weight outside the 62–114 kg range.
- No information is currently available for patients with endstage renal failure undergoing dialysis.

Additional information
- Initial response to treatment can produce abdominal pain, cramping, or colic. If severe, it can be managed by administration of an opioid or anticholinergic agent (e.g. morphine, glycopyrronium).
- Areas for injection include upper legs, abdomen, and upper arms.
- Rotate injection site.
- Avoid areas where skin is tender, bruised, red, or hard. Scars or stretch marks should also be avoided.

♦ Pharmacology
Methylnaltrexone is a peripherally acting selective μ-opioid receptor antagonist. It does not penetrate the blood–brain barrier to any significant extent because of its chemical structure. Opioid-derived analgesia is not affected by treatment with methylnaltrexone.

Following SC administration, methylnaltrexone is rapidly absorbed, with peak concentrations achieved within 30 minutes. It does not affect the cytochrome P450 system to any significant degree, although it is a weak inhibitor of CYP2D6. Methylnaltrexone is primarily eliminated as the unchanged drug; approximately half the dose is excreted in the urine.

Methylphenidate

Ritalin® (CD POM)
Tablet (*scored*): 10mg (30)

Generic® (CD POM)
Tablet: 5mg (30); 10mg (30); 20mg (30)

Methylphenidate is a Schedule 2 controlled drug (see 📖 Legal categories for medicines, p.23 for further information). Independent prescribers are **NOT** authorized to prescribe methylphenidate (📖 Independent prescribing: palliative care issues, p.25).

Indications
- ⌇ Cancer-related fatigue.
- ⌇ Depression.

Contraindications and precautions
- Methylphenidate is contraindicated for use in patients with:
    - agitation
    - arrhythmia
    - glaucoma
    - hyperthyroidism
    - marked anxiety,
    - motor tics, tics in siblings, or a family history or diagnosis of Tourette's syndrome
    - severe angina pectoris
    - thyrotoxicosis.
- It should be avoided in patients with severe hypertension.
- Use with caution in patients with:
    - epilepsy (withdraw treatment if seizures occur)
    - hepatic impairment
    - pre-existing hypertension, heart failure, recent myocardial infarction.
- Avoid concurrent use with an irreversible MAOI, or within 14 days of stopping one. In exceptional cases, concurrent use of the reversible MAOI linezolid is allowed but the patient must be closely monitored (see 📖 Drug interactions, p.321).
- If affected by drowsiness and dizziness, patients should be warned about driving.

☺ Undesirable effects
Very common
- Insomnia (give last dose no later than 2p.m.)
- Nervousness

Common
- Abdominal pain
- Arrhythmias
- Arthralgia
- Dizziness

- Drowsiness
- Dyskinesia
- Fever
- Headache
- Hypertension
- Nausea and vomiting (usually occurs during initiation; may improve if administered with food)
- Palpitations
- Pruritus
- Rash
- Scalp hair loss
- Tachycardia
- Urticaria

Rare
- Blurred vision

Very rare
- Seizures

Unknown
- Serotonin syndrome (see 📖 *Drug interactions*, p.321)

Drug interactions

Pharmacokinetic

- Methylphenidate undergoes fairly significant first-pass metabolism and the carboxylesterase CES1A1 is involved. The cytochrome system may also be involved, as methylphenidate appears to be a major substrate of CYP2D6 and a weak inhibitor of CYP2D6.
- The clinical significance of co-administration with inhibitors of CYP2D6 (📖 end cover) is unknown. The prescriber should be aware of the potential for interactions and that dose adjustments may be necessary.
- *Carbamazepine*—may reduce plasma concentration of methylphenidate
- May inhibit the metabolism of tricyclic antidepressants, SSRIs, and warfarin. Caution is advised if methylphenidate is co-administered with other drugs that are predominantly metabolized by CYP2D6 as a degree of competitive inhibition may develop. The prescriber should be aware of the potential for interactions and that dose adjustments may be necessary.

Pharmacodynamic

- *Antiepileptics*—methylphenidate may antagonize the effects of antiepileptics.
- *Antihypertensives*—effect may be reduced by methylphenidate.
- *Antidepressants*—may increase the risk of serotonin syndrome; note that SSRIs have been combined successfully with methylphenidate to augment antidepressant action (see 📖 *Dose*, p.322).
- *Haloperidol*—reverses the wakefulness effect of methylphenidate (other dopamine antagonists may do the same).

- *Linezolid*—risk of hypertension; in exceptional circumstances linezolid may be given with methylphenidate, but the patient must be closely monitored.
- *MAOI*—avoid concurrent use; risk of serotonin syndrome and may lead to increase in blood pressure.

⚡ Dose
Blood pressure should be monitored at appropriate intervals in all patients taking methylphenidate.

¥ *Depression and fatigue*
- Initial dose 2.5mg PO OM. Increase dose by 2.5mg every 2–3 days as tolerated. Doses above 2.5mg are usually divided, with the final dose being no later than 2p.m.. Usual maximum dose is 20mg PO daily.

⚡ Dose adjustments
Elderly
- No specific information available. Use the lowest effective dose.

Hepatic/renal impairment
- There are no specific instructions for dose reduction in hepatic impairment. However, given the fact that methylphenidate is extensively metabolized, if the drug has to be used, the patient should be closely monitored and the lowest effective dose should be prescribed.
- There are no specific instructions for dose adjustment in renal impairment. However, since methylphenidate undergoes significant first-pass metabolism (to relatively inactive compounds) renal impairment is unlikely to have a great effect. Nonetheless, caution is advised and the lowest effective dose should be prescribed.

Additional information
- Methylphenidate can be cautiously combined with SSRIs in the treatment of resistant depression. It should be introduced slowly and the patient should be closely monitored.

⊕ Pharmacology
Methylphenidate is a mild CNS stimulant with more prominent effects on mental than on motor activities. Its mode of action in humans is not completely understood, but it appears to blocks the reuptake mechanism of dopaminergic neurons and has a similar action to amphetamines.

Metoclopramide

Standard release

Maxolon® (POM)
Tablet (*scored*): 10mg (84)
Syrup (*sugar-free*): 5mg/5mL (200mL)
Paediatric liquid (*sugar-free*): 1mg/mL (15mL)
Injection: 10mg/2mL (12)

Generic (POM)
Tablet (*scored*): 10mg (84)
Syrup (*sugar-free*): 5mg/5mL (200mL)
Injection: 10mg/2mL (12)

Modified release

Maxolon SR® (POM)
Capsule: 15mg (56)

Indications

- Nausea and vomiting
- Dyspepsia
- Reflux
- For end-of-life care issues see 📖 *Use of drugs in end-of-life care*, p.53.

Contraindications and precautions

- Contraindicated in patients with:
  - phaeochromocytoma
  - GI obstruction, perforation, or haemorrhage.
- Avoid within 3 days of GI surgery.
- Use with caution in patients with:
  - severe renal and hepatic insufficiency (see 📖 *Dose adjustments*, p.324)
  - acute porphyria
  - concurrent use of serotonergic drugs (e.g. SSRIs) and antipsychotics (see 📖 *Drug interactions*, p.324)
  - Parkinson's disease.
- The elderly and young adults <20 years of age (especially female) are more susceptible to undesirable effects.
- Metoclopramide may modify reactions and patients should be advised not to drive (or operate machinery) if affected.

☉ Undesirable effects

The frequency is not defined, but reported undesirable effects include:

- Breast tenderness
- Confusion
- Depression
- Diarrhoea
- Drowsiness
- Extrapyramidal symptoms
- Galactorrhoea
- Gynaecomastia
- Headache
- Insomnia
- Neuroleptic malignant syndrome (rare)
- Restlessness

Drug interactions

Pharmacokinetic

- *Carbamazepine* — possible risk of neurotoxicity due to increased speed of absorption.
- *Paracetamol*—potential increase in onset of analgesia.

Pharmacodynamic

- *Anticholinergics*—may antagonize the prokinetic effect
- *Antipsychotics*—increased risk of extrapyramidal effects.
- *Cyclizine*—may antagonize the prokinetic effect.
- *Levodopa and dopamine agonists*—effect antagonized by metoclopramide.
- *Opioids*—antagonize the prokinetic effect.
- *Serotonergic drugs*—caution is advisable if metoclopramide is co-administered with serotonergic drugs (e.g. methadone, methylphenidate, mirtazapine, oxycodone, SSRIs, tricyclic antidepressants, trazodone, venlafaxine) because of the risk of serotonin syndrome (📖 Box 1.10, p.19).
- *5-HT$_3$ antagonists*—antagonize the prokinetic effect.
- *Tricyclic antidepressants*—may antagonize the prokinetic effect.

💊 Dose

- Initial dose, 10mg PO TDS PRN. This can be increased to 20mg PO TDS (¥).
- Maxolon SR® is given 15mg PO BD.
- Alternatively, 30mg OD via CSCI (¥). The dose can be increased to a maximum of 120mg daily (¥).

💊 Dose adjustments

Elderly

- The elderly are more susceptible to undesirable effects. Therapy should be initiated at a reduced dose and maintained at the lowest effective dose.

Hepatic/renal impairment

- The manufacturer recommends that in patients with hepatic or renal impairment, therapy should be initiated at a reduced dose and maintained at the lowest effective dose. Metoclopramide is metabolized in the liver and the predominant route of elimination of metoclopramide and its metabolites is via the kidney.

Additional information

- Metoclopramide via CSCI is reportedly compatible with alfentanil, dexamethasone, diamorphine, dimenhydrinate (not in UK), fentanyl, glycopyrronium, granisetron, hydromorphone, levomepromazine, methadone, midazolam, morphine, octreotide, ondansetron, and tramadol.

✑ Pharmacology

Metoclopramide is primarily a D_2 antagonist. It also has serotonergic properties, as it is a 5-HT$_3$ antagonist and a 5-HT$_4$ agonist. The anti-emetic action of metoclopramide results from its antagonist activity at D_2 receptors in the chemoreceptor trigger zone (CTZ), making it a suitable choice for drug-induced causes of nausea and vomiting. At higher doses, the 5-HT$_3$ antagonist activity may also contribute to the anti-emetic effect. D_2 antagonism in the GI tract enhances the response to acetylcholine, thereby indirectly increasing GI motility and accelerating gastric emptying. The 5-HT$_4$ agonist effect also has a direct stimulatory effect on the bowel, and both properties contribute to the prokinetic effect (which will in turn contribute to the anti-emetic effect). The D_2 antagonism can lead to increases in prolactin secretion, with consequences such as galactorrhoea, gynaecomastia and irregular periods.

Metoclopramide is rapidly and almost completely absorbed from the GI tract after oral doses, although conditions such as vomiting or impaired gastric motility may reduce absorption. It is a minor substrate of CYP2D6 and CYP1A2. About 20% of the dose is excreted unchanged and plasma concentrations can increase in renal impairment.

Metronidazole

Anabact® (POM) Gel: 0.75% (15g, 30g)
Flagyl® (POM)
Tablet: 200mg (21); 400mg (14)
Suppository: 500mg (10); 1g (10)
Injection: 500mg/100mL

Flagyl S® (POM)
Oral suspension: 200mg/5mL (100mL)

Metrogel® (POM)
Gel: metronidazole 0.75% (40g)

Generic (POM)
Tablet: 200mg (21); 400mg (21); 500mg (21)
Oral suspension: 200mg/5mL (100mL)
Injection: 100mg/20mL; 500mg/100mL

Indications
- Refer to local guidelines.
- Anaerobic infections.
- *Helicobacter pylori* eradication.
- Malodorous fungating tumours (topical).
- ¥ Pseudomembranous colitis.

Contraindications and precautions
- Avoid in acute porphyria.
- Use with caution in hepatic impairment (see 📖 *Dose adjustments*, p.327).
- If treatment exceeds 10 days, the manufacturer recommends laboratory monitoring.
- Use the infusion with caution in patients on a low-sodium diet.

☺ Undesirable effects
The frequency is not defined, but reported undesirable effects include:
- Abnormal LFTs
- Anorexia
- Arthralgia
- Ataxia
- Blood dyscrasias (e.g. agranulocytosis, neutropenia, thrombocytopenia)
- Cholestatic hepatitis
- Dark urine (due to metronidazole metabolite)
- Dizziness
- Drowsiness
- Furred tongue
- Headache
- Myalgia
- Nausea
- Pancreatitis
- Skin rashes
- Transient visual disorders
- Unpleasant taste
- Vomiting

Drug interactions

Pharmacokinetic

- Metronidazole is metabolized by CYP3A4 and CYP2C9. It inhibits CYP2C9.
- *Warfarin*—risk of raised INR.
- *Alcohol*—concurrent use can give rise to the disulfiram reaction (includes that present in medication).
- The clinical significance of co-administration with CYP3A4 and/or CYP2C9 inducers or inhibitors (📖 end cover) is unknown. The prescriber should be aware of the potential for interactions and that dose adjustments may be necessary.
- The clinical significance of co-administration with CYP2C9 substrates (📖 end cover) is unknown. The prescriber should be aware of the potential for interactions and that dose adjustments may be necessary.

Pharmacodynamic

- None known.

Dose

Standard doses are described here. Refer to local guidelines for specific advice.

Anaerobic infections

- Initial dose 400mg PO TDS, or 1g PR TDS for 3 days, then 1g PR BD.
- Alternatively, if rectal administration is inappropriate, 500mg by IV infusion TDS.
- In most cases, a course of 7–10 days should be sufficient.

Malodorous fungating tumour

- Apply gel to clean wound OD–BD and cover with non-adherent dressing.

¥ Pseudomembranous colitis

- 400mg PO TDS for 7–10 days
- IV therapy may be appropriate for the first 48 hours, after which effectiveness is reduced because of reduced penetration into the bowel lumen.

Dose adjustments

Elderly

- No dose adjustments are necessary.

Hepatic/renal impairment

- In patients with severe hepatic impairment, the manufacturer advises that the daily dose should be reduced to one-third and be administered once daily.
- No dose adjustments are necessary in patients with renal impairment.

Additional information

• Metronidazole suspension should not be used in patients with an in situ feeding tube, or in those receiving a PPI. The suspension contains the metronidazole benzoate salt and the absorption of this is significantly reduced in the presence of food. In addition, it requires the action of stomach acids to convert it to the active metronidazole base.
• Administer the IV infusion over 20 minutes (i.e. 5mL/min).

⟩ Pharmacology

Metronidazole is a nitroimidazole antibiotic with specific activity against anaerobic bacteria and some protozoa. Metronidazole diffuses into the organism where it is converted to its active form which then disrupts the helical structure of DNA, inhibiting bacterial nucleic acid synthesis and resulting in bacterial cell death. Metronidazole is well absorbed and penetrates well into body tissues. It is extensively metabolized by CYP3A4 and CYP2C9 and any unchanged drug along with metabolites are excreted renally.

Midazolam

Hypnovel® (CD No Register POM)
Injection: 10mg/5mL (10); 10mg/2mL (10)

Generic (CD No Register POM)
Injection: 2mg/2mL; 5mg/5mL; 50mg/50mL; 10mg/5mL; 10mg/2mL; 50mg/10mL

Unlicensed Special (CD No Register POM)
Oral liquid: 2.5mg/mL (100mL)
Buccal liquid: 50mg/5mL; 250mg/25mL

Midazolam is a Schedule 3 controlled drug (see 📖 Legal categories for medicines, p.23 for further information). It can be prescribed for parental or buccal administration by Nurse Independent Prescribers. (📖 Independent prescribing: palliative care issues, p.25).

Indications
- ¥ Dyspnoea
- ¥ Epilepsy
- ¥ Hiccup
- ¥ Major haemorrhage
- ¥ Myoclonus
- ¥ Status epilepticus
- ¥ Terminal agitation or anxiety
- For end-of-life care issues see 📖 Use of drugs in end-of-life care, p.53.

Contraindications and precautions
- Must not be used in patients with severe respiratory failure or acute respiratory depression.
- Use with caution in patients with:
  - myasthenia gravis
  - chronic renal failure
  - impaired hepatic function
  - impaired cardiac function
  - chronic respiratory insufficiency.
- Prolonged treatment with midazolam can lead to the development of physical dependence. Abrupt cessation of treatment may precipitate withdrawal symptoms, such as anxiety, confusion, convulsions, hallucinations, headaches, insomnia, and restlessness. Note such changes can occur after the introduction of a CYP3A4 inducer (see 📖 Drug interactions, p.330).
- Midazolam may modify reactions and patients should be advised not to drive (or operate machinery) if affected.

☻ Undesirable effects

The frequency is not defined, but reported undesirable effects include

- Amnesia
- Anterograde amnesia
- Confusion
- Drowsiness
- Hiccups
- Nausea
- Vomiting

Drug interactions

Pharmacokinetic

- Midazolam is metabolized by CYP3A4. It does not affect the pharma-cokinetics of other drugs.
- Interactions with CYP3A4 inhibitors or inducers will be more pro-nounced for oral administration (compared with parenteral, buccal, or intranasal) because midazolam undergoes significant first-pass metabolism.
- *Carbamazepine*—reduces the plasma concentrations of midazolam (CYP3A4 induction); the dose of midazolam may need to be titrated accordingly if carbamazepine is added or discontinued.
- *Clarithromycin*—increased risk of midazolam toxicity; use lower initial doses. Dose adjustments may be necessary if clarithromycin is added or discontinued.
- *Diltiazem*—increased risk of midazolam toxicity; use lower initial doses. Dose adjustments may be necessary if diltiazem is added or discontinued.
- *Erythromycin*—increased risk of midazolam toxicity; use lower initial doses. Dose adjustments may be necessary if erythromycin is added or discontinued.
- *Fluconazole*—may inhibit the metabolism of midazolam (although more likely to occur when fluconazole dose >200mg daily).
- *Grapefruit juice*—significantly increases the effect of midazolam administered orally. Avoid concurrent use.
- The clinical significance of co-administration with other CYP3A4 inhibitors or inducers (📖 end cover) is unknown. The prescriber should be aware of the potential for interactions and that dose adjustments may be necessary.

Pharmacodynamic

- *Alcohol*—may precipitate seizures and significantly increases sedative effect of midazolam.
- *Antidepressants*—reduced seizure threshold.
- *Antipsychotics*—reduced seizure threshold.
- *CNS depressants*—additive sedative effect.

♪ Dose

¥ Dyspnoea
- Dose should be titrated and adjusted to individual requirements.
- Typical initial dose is 2.5–5mg SC PRN, or 10mg via CSCI.
- Dose can be increased as necessary to 5–10mg SC PRN, or 60mg via CSCI.
- Midazolam can be used as an adjunct to morphine for breathlessness

¥ Epilepsy/myoclonus
- Dose should be titrated and adjusted to individual requirements.
- Typical initial dose is 10mg SC PRN, or 10–20mg via CSCI increasing to 30–60mg via CSCI.
- If the patient has not settled with 60mg midazolam via CSCI, an alternative treatment such as phenobarbital should be considered.

¥ Hiccup
- Typical dose 10–60mg via CSCI
- Note that midazolam is also implicated as a cause of hiccup.

¥ Major haemorrhage
- 5–10mg IV/IM/intranasal titrated to the patient's requirements to a maximum dose of 30mg per episode.
- Avoid the SC route because of poor and erratic absorption.

¥ Status epilepticus
- The intranasal route can be appropriate for the treatment of seizures and the dose is determined by weight:
  - <50kg–5mg intranasal midazolam
  - >50kg–10mg intranasal midazolam.
- The buccal route can be used as an alternative to the intranasal route if there is excessive head movement due to seizures:
  - 10mg buccal midazolam.
- Doses of intranasal or buccal midazolam may be repeated after 10 minutes if necessary. Further doses should not be given without further medical assessment.

¥ Terminal agitation or anxiety
- Typical dose 2.5–10mg SC PRN, or 10–60mg via CSCI. The dose should be titrated and adjusted to individual requirements.
- If the patient has not settled at 60mg via CSCI, addition of an antipsychotic such as levomepromazine should be considered.

♪ Dose adjustments

Elderly
- No specific guidance is available, but the dose should be carefully adjusted to individual requirements

Hepatic/renal impairment
- No specific guidance is available but in liver impairment empirical dose reductions may be necessary.
- In patients with CrCl < 10mL/min, a dose reduction should be considered because of an increased risk of sedation as accumulation of an active metabolite can occur.

Additional information

- A buccal liquid is available from Special Products Ltd (Tel: 01932 690325)
- Although the injection can be administered buccally, the volume may be too much for some patients.
- The injection can also be administered intranasally (*) (see 📖 *Dose*, p.331) using a mucosal atomization device (MAD). This is available from Wolfe-Tory Medical (see *http://www.wolfetory.com/nasal.php* for further information regarding supply).
- Midazolam precipitates in solutions containing bicarbonate and it is likely to be unstable in solutions with alkaline pH (e.g. dexamethasone, dimenhydrinate, ranitidine).
- Midazolam via CSCI is reportedly compatible with alfentanil, cyclizine, diamorphine, fentanyl, glycopyrronium, haloperidol, hydromorphone, hyoscine butylbromide, hyoscine hydrobromide, levomepromazine, metoclopramide, morphine (hydrochloride, sulphate, tartrate), midazolam, promethazine, octreotide, and oxycodone.

➔ Pharmacology

The exact mechanism of action is unknown, but it is believed to act via enhancement of GABA-ergic transmission in the CNS. It is extensively metabolized by CYP3A4 and has an active metabolite (α-hydroxymidazolam glucuronide).

Mirtazapine

Zispin SolTab® (POM)
- **Orodispersible tablet**: 15mg (30), 30mg (30), 45mg (30)

Generic (POM)
- **Tablet**: 15mg (28), 30mg (28), 45mg (28)
- **Orodispersible tablet**: 15mg (30); 30mg (30); 45mg (30)
- **Oral solution**: 15mg/mL (66mL bottle)

Indications
- Depression
- ¥ Appetite
- ¥ Nausea and vomiting
- ¥ Pruritus

Contraindications and precautions
- Do not use with an MAOI, or within 14 days of stopping one; avoid concomitant use with linezolid or moclobemide.
- Use with caution in epilepsy (lowers seizure threshold).
- Depression is associated with an increased risk of suicidal thoughts, self-harm, and suicide which persists until remission. Note that that the risk of suicide may increase during initial treatment.
- Hyponatraemia should be considered in all patients who develop drowsiness, confusion, or convulsions while taking an antidepressant. Hyponatraemia has been associated with all types of antidepressants, although it is reportedly more common with SSRIs.
- May precipitate psychomotor restlessness, which usually appears during early treatment.
- Avoid abrupt withdrawal as symptoms such as dizziness, agitation, anxiety, headache, and nausea and vomiting can occur. Mirtazapine should be withdrawn gradually over several weeks whenever possible. Refer to 📖 Discontinuing and/or switching antidepressants, p.45 for information about switching or stopping antidepressants.
- Avoid in patients with phenylketonuria—orodispersible tablets contain aspartame, a source of phenylalanine.
- Mirtazapine may modify reactions and patients should be advised not to drive (or operate machinery) if affected.

☺ Undesirable effects
Very common
- Constipation
- Drowsiness (improves as dose increases)
- Increased appetite
- Weight gain (≥7% bodyweight)
- Xerostomia

Common
- Abnormal dreams
- Asthenia

- Dizziness
- Flu-like symptoms
- Peripheral oedema

Uncommon
- Headache

Rare
- Agranulocytosis (usually appears after 4–6 weeks' treatment)
- Convulsions
- Myoclonus
- Nightmares
- Psychomotor restlessness
- Restless legs

Drug interactions

Pharmacokinetic

- Mirtazapine is metabolized by CYP1A2, CYP2D6, and CYP3A4.
- Carbamazepine and phenytoin can reduce mirtazapine levels by at least 50%.
- The clinical significance of co-administration with other CYP3A4 inducers or inhibitors (📖 end cover) is unknown. The prescriber should be aware of the potential for interactions and that dose adjustments may be necessary.
- The clinical significance of co-administration with inhibitors of CYP2D6 (📖 end cover) is unknown, but plasma concentrations of mirtazapine may increase. The prescriber should be aware of the potential for interactions and that dose adjustments may be necessary.
- Dose adjustments may be necessary upon smoking cessation. The clinical significance of co-administration with CYP1A2 inducers or inhibitors (📖 end cover) is unknown. The prescriber should be aware of the potential for interactions and that dose adjustments may be necessary.
- MAOIs, including linezolid, should be avoided
- The effect of grapefruit juice on the absorption of mirtazapine is unknown.

Pharmacodynamic

- *CNS depressants*—risk of excessive sedation.
- *MAOIs*—risk of serotonin syndrome (see *Contraindications and precautions*).
- *Serotonergic drugs*, e.g. duloxetine, methadone, SSRIs, tricyclic antidepressants, tramadol and trazodone—risk of serotonin syndrome (📖 Box 1.10, p.19).
- *SSRIs*—increased risk of seizures and serotonin syndrome.
- *Tramadol*—increased risk of seizures and serotonin syndrome; may reduce effect of tramadol by blocking 5-HT$_3$ receptor mediated analgesia.

♪ Dose

Depression
- Initial dose 15mg PO ON.
- Adjust dose as clinically appropriate; review within 2–4 weeks and increase dose to a maximum of 45mg/day.

¥ *Nausea and vomiting/appetite*
- Initial dose 7.5–15mg PO ON. Review dose within 1 week and increase as necessary to a maximum of 45mg/day.
- Patient may show improved response to a BD dosing schedule.

¥ *Pruritus*
- Initial dose 7.5–15mg PO ON. Higher doses may be of no further benefit.

♪ Dose adjustments

Elderly
- Initial dose as above.
- 7.5mg dose may actually be more sedative.
- Adjust dose as clinically appropriate.

Hepatic/renal impairment
- Clearance is reduced in moderate to severe renal or hepatic impairment
- Specific dose recommendations not warranted; adjust as clinically appropriate
- Prescriber must be aware that plasma levels may be raised in these patients

Additional information

- Relief of insomnia and anxiety can start shortly after initiation of dosing, but in general it begins to exert an antidepressant effect after 1–2 weeks of treatment.
- Weight gain more likely in women and unlikely to see benefit after 6 weeks treatment.
- Orodispersible tablets may block feeding tubes; in such instances, the oral solution should be used.
- Warn the patient about the importance of reporting signs of infection such as sore throat and fever during initial treatment (risk of agranulocytosis).

♦ Pharmacology

Mirtazapine is an antidepressant that is believed to produce its effect through a presynaptic α_2-adrenoreceptor antagonism, increasing central noradrenergic and serotonergic neurotransmission. It is also an antagonist at 5-HT_2, 5-HT_3, and H_1 receptors which explains its anti-emetic activity. Mirtazapine actually has similar binding affinity for the 5-HT_3 receptor as the 5-HT_3 antagonists. At low doses, the H_1 antagonistic effect predominates and causes sedation during initial treatment, which improves as the dose escalates.

Misoprostol

Cytotec® (POM)
Tablet (*scored*): 200mcg (60)

With diclofenac (📖 Diclofenac, p.143)

Arthrotec® 50 (POM)
Tablet: diclofenac sodium 50mg, misoprostol 200mcg (60)

Arthrotec® 75 (POM)
Tablet: diclofenac sodium 75mg, misoprostol 200mcg (60)

With naproxen (📖 Naproxen, p.351)

Napratec OP® Combination Pack (POM)
Tablets: naproxen 500mg + misoprostol 200mcg (56)

Indications
- Healing of duodenal and gastric ulcers including those induced by NSAIDs.
- Prophylaxis of NSAID-induced ulcers.

Contraindications and precautions
- Contraindicated for use in pregnancy (causes uterine contractions). Additionally, women of child-bearing potential must use effective contraception.
- Misoprostol should be used with caution in conditions where hypotension may precipitate severe complications, e.g. cerebrovascular disease, coronary artery disease.

☺ Undesirable effects
- The frequency is not defined, but reported undesirable effects include:
- Abdominal pain
- Diarrhoea (occasionally severe, necessitating discontinuation)
- Dizziness
- Flatulence
- Intermenstrual bleeding
- Nausea and vomiting
- Uterine contractions
- Vaginal bleeding (both pre- and postmenstrual women)

Drug interactions
Pharmacokinetic
- No clinically significant interactions noted

Pharmacodynamic
- No clinically significant interactions noted

♪ Dose

Healing of duodenal and gastric ulcers
- Initial dose 200mcg PO QDS or 400mcg PO BD with food.
- ¥ Patients may not tolerate this dose initially and a more gradual dose titration may be warranted.

Prophylaxis of NSAID-induced ulcers
- 200mcg PO BD-QDS.
- ¥ Patients may not tolerate this dose initially and a more gradual dose titration may be warranted.

♪ Dose adjustments

Elderly
- No dose adjustments are necessary based on age alone.

Hepatic/renal impairment
- No dose adjustments are necessary in patients with liver or renal impairment.

Additional information

- Diarrhoea is often a dose-limiting undesirable effect. It can be minimized by using single doses ≤200mcg with food and by avoiding the use of magnesium-containing antacids.
- Misoprostol has been used to treat intractable constipation.
- Although the tablets can be crushed and dispersed in water prior to administration, this should not be performed by pregnant women, or women of child-bearing potential, due to risk of inducing uterine contractions.

♪ Pharmacology

Misoprostol is a prostaglandin E_1 (PGE_1) analogue which acts by binding to the prostaglandin receptor on parietal cells. The resulting cytoprotective actions include:
- Enhanced mucosal blood flow as a result of direct vasodilatation.
- Inhibiting gastric acid secretion.
- Reducing the volume and proteolytic activity of gastric secretions.
- Increasing bicarbonate and mucus secretion.

Modafinil

Provigil® (POM)
Tablet: 100mg (30 per pack), 200mg (30 per pack)

Indications
- ¥ Cancer-related fatigue

Contraindications and precautions
- Modafinil is contraindicated for use in patients with uncontrolled moderate to severe hypertension or arrhythmia.
- Avoid in patients with left ventricular hypertrophy or cor pulmonale.
- Use with caution in patients with a history of psychosis, mania, major anxiety, depression, or substance/alcohol abuse.
- Withdraw treatment if patient develops a rash or psychiatric symptoms.
- Modafinil may modify reactions and patients should be advised not to drive (or operate machinery) if affected.

☺ Undesirable effects
Very common
- Headache (up to 21% of patients may be affected)

Common
- Abnormal LFTs
- Anxiety
- Blurred vision
- Confusion
- Dizziness
- Dry mouth
- Insomnia
- Nausea
- Tachycardia

Uncommon
- Amnesia
- Arrhythmia
- Cough
- Diabetes mellitus
- Hypertension
- Migraine
- Peripheral oedema
- Rhinitis

Unknown
- Serious skin reactions, e.g. Stevens–Johnson syndrome (usually within first 5 weeks of treatment).
- Psychosis, mania, and hallucinations have been reported.

Drug interactions

Pharmacokinetic

- Modafinil is metabolized by CYP3A4 and is also a strong inhibitor of CYP2C19. It is a weak inhibitor of CYP2C9 and weak inducer of CYP3A4 and CYP2B6.
- The clinical significance of co-administration of modafinil with CYP2C19 and CYP2C9 substrates (📖 end cover) is unknown but dose adjustments may be necessary.
- In patients who are CYP2D6 deficient (or taking inhibiting drugs) the metabolism of SSRIs and TCAs via CYP2C19 becomes more important. Consequently, lower doses of the antidepressants may be necessary in patients co-administered modafinil.
- The clinical significance of co-administration with CYP3A4 inducers or inhibitors (📖 end cover) is unknown. The prescriber should be aware of the potential for interactions and that dose adjustments may be necessary.

Pharmacodynamic

- None of significance noted.

⚗ Dose

- 200mg PO OM

⚗ Dose adjustments

Elderly

- 100mg PO OM initially.

Hepatic/renal impairment

- 100mg PO OM initially in severe liver disease.
- 100mg PO OM initially if CrCl <10mL/min.

Additional information

- An effect should be seen within a few hours of the first dose. If no effect is seen, discontinue.
- Monitor blood pressure and heart rate in hypertensive patients.
- Patients who complain of headaches may find that taking tablets with or after food may ameliorate the symptom.
- Effect can be seen within 2 hours of dosing although it may take several days to achieve optimal clinical response.
- Tablets are dispersible in water. If necessary, they can be crushed and dispersed in water prior to use. The resulting solution can be flushed down a feeding tube.

⟳ Pharmacology

The mechanism of action is unknown but its therapeutic effects are similar to methylphenidate. Unlike the amphetamine, the effect of modafinil does not appear to be related to dopamine and drugs such as haloperidol do not reduce its effect.

Morphine

It is not possible to ensure the interchangeability of different makes of modified-release oral morphine preparations in individual patients. Therefore it is recommended that patients should remain on the same product once treatment has been stabilized. Inclusion of the brand name on the prescription is suggested.

Standard oral release

Oramorph® oral solution (POM)
Solution: 10mg/5mL (100mL; 300mL; 500mL)
Note: Discard 90 days after opening

Oramorph® concentrated oral solution (CD POM)
Solution (*sugar-free*): 10mg/mL (30mL; 120mL)
Note: Discard 120 days after opening

Sevredol® (CD POM)
Tablet (*scored*): 10mg (*blue*, 56); 20mg (*pink*, 56); 50mg (*pale green*, 56)

Generic (POM)
Solution: 10mg/5mL (100mL)

Standard-release rectal products

Generic (CD POM)
Suppository: 10mg (12); 15mg (12); 20mg (12); 30mg (12)
Note: Products contain morphine sulphate or hydrochloride. Prescription must state the morphine salt to be dispensed.

Parenteral products

Generic (CD POM)
Injection: 10mg/mL; 15mg/mL; 20mg/mL; 30mg/mL. All in 1mL and 2mL ampoules

12 hourly modified release

Morphgesic® (CD POM)
Tablet: 10mg (*buff*, 60); 30mg (*violet*, 60); 60mg (*orange*, 60); 100mg (*grey*, 60)

MST Continus® (CD POM)
Tablet: 5mg (*white*, 60); 10mg (*brown*, 60); 15mg (*green*, 60); 30mg (*purple*, 60); 60mg (*orange*, 60); 100mg (*grey*, 60); 200mg (*green*, 60)
Suspension (*granules*): 20mg (30); 30mg (30); 60mg (30); 100mg (30); 200mg (30)

Zomorph® (CD POM)
Capsule: 10mg (*yellow/clear*, 60); 30mg (*pink/clear*, 60); 60mg (*orange/clear*, 60); 100mg (*white/clear*, 60); 200mg (*clear*, 60)

24 hourly modified release

MXL® (CD POM)

Capsule: 30mg (*light blue*, 28); 60mg (*brown*, 28); 90mg (*pink*, 28); 120mg (*green*, 28); 150mg (*blue*, 28); 200mg (*red-brown*, 28)

> Morphine is a Schedule 2 controlled drug (see 📖 Legal categories of medicines, p.23 for further information). Oral, parenteral, and rectal products **can** be prescribed by nurse independent prescribers (📖 Independent prescribing: palliative care issues, p.25).

Indications

- Relief of severe pain.
- ⁛ Relief of moderate pain.
- ⁛ Painful skin lesions (topical).
- ⁛ Mucositis (topical).
- ⁛ Cough.
- ⁛ Dyspnoea.
- For end-of-life care issues see 📖 Use of drugs in end-of-life care, p.53.

Contraindications and precautions

- If the dose of an opioid is titrated correctly, it is generally accepted that there are no absolute contraindications to the use of such drugs in palliative care, although there may be circumstances where one opioid is favoured over another (e.g. renal impairment, constipation). Nonetheless, manufacturers state that morphine is contraindicated for use in patients with:
  - acute abdomen
  - acute diarrhoeal conditions associated with antibiotic-induced pseudomembranous colitis
  - acute hepatic disease
  - concurrent administration of MAOIs or within 2 weeks of discontinuation of their use (NB: *initial low doses, careful titration, and close monitoring may permit safe combination.*)
  - delayed gastric emptying
  - head injury
  - obstructive airways disease (diamorphine may release histamine)
  - paralytic ileus
  - phaeochromocytoma (due to the risk of pressor response to histamine release)
  - respiratory depression.
- Use with caution in the following instances:
  - Addison's disease (adrenocortical insufficiency)
  - asthma (morphine may release histamine)
  - constipation
  - delirium tremens
  - diseases of the biliary tract
  - elderly patients
  - epilepsy (morphine may lower seizure threshold)
  - hepatic impairment (see above)
  - history of alcohol and drug abuse

- hypotension associated with hypovolaemia (morphine may result in ⟨ severe hypotension ⟩)
- hypothyroidism
- inflammatory bowel disorders
- pancreatitis
- prostatic hypertrophy
- raised intracranial pressure
- significantly impaired hepatic and renal function.
- Morphine may modify reactions and patients should be advised not to drive (or operate machinery) if affected.

☻ Undesirable effects

Strong opioids tend to cause similar undesirable effects, albeit to varying degrees. The frequency is not defined, but reported undesirable effects include:

- Anorexia
- Asthenia
- Biliary pain
- Confusion
- Constipation
- Drowsiness
- Dry mouth
- Dyspepsia
- Exacerbation of pancreatitis
- Euphoria
- Insomnia
- Headache

- Hyperhidrosis
- Myoclonus
- Nausea
- Pruritus
- Sexual dysfunction (e.g. amenor-rhea, decreased libido, erectile dysfunction)
- Urinary retention
- Vertigo
- Visual disturbance
- Vomiting

The following can occur with excessive dose:

- Agitation
- Exacerbation of pain
- Hallucinations
- Miosis
- Paraesthesia
- Respiratory depression
- Restlessness

Drug interactions

Pharmacokinetic
- A minor pathway involves CYP2D6.
- No clinically significant pharmacokinetic interactions reported

Pharmacodynamic
- *Antihypertensives*—increased risk of hypotension.
- *CNS depressants*—risk of excessive sedation.
- *Haloperidol*—may be an additive hypotensive effect.
- *Ketamine*—there is a potential opioid-sparing effect with ketamine and the dose of morphine may need reducing.
- *Levomepromazine*—may be an additive hypotensive effect.

♣ Dose

Pain

The initial dose of morphine depends upon the patient's previous opioid requirements. Refer to ◻ Opioid substitution, p.33 for information regarding opioid dose equivalences and ◻ Breakthrough cancer pain, p.35 for guidance relating to BTcP.

Oral

- Standard release
  - For opioid-naive patients, initial dose is 10mg PO every 4–6 hours and PRN. The dose is then increased as necessary until a stable dose is attained. The patient should then be converted to a modified-release formulation.
  - ¥ Lower initial doses (e.g. 2.5mg PO every 4–6 hours and PRN) can be used for opioid-naive patients to treat moderate pain (i.e. instead of using codeine).
- Modified release
  - For opioid-naive patients, initial dose is 5–10mg PO BD. The dose can then be titrated as necessary.
  - MXL® can be introduced once a total daily dose of 30mg is reached.

Subcutaneous

- Initial dose in opioid-naive patients is 5mg SC 4-hourly PRN. Alternatively, 10mg via CSCI over 24 hours and increase as necessary.
- The maximum dose per injection site that should be given by SC bolus injection is 60mg (= 2mL).

Rectal

- Initial dose 15–30mg PR every 4 hours, adjusted according to response.

¥ Painful skin lesions

- Often use 0.1% or 0.125% w/w gels initially. These can be prepared immediately prior to administration by adding 10mg morphine injection to 8g Intrasite® gel (making a 0.125% w/w gel). Higher-strength gels, typically up to 0.5%, can be made if necessary.
- Initial dose: 5–10mg morphine in Intrasite® gel to affected area at dressing changes (up to twice daily).
- Use within 1 hour of preparation and discard any remaining product.

¥ Mucositis

- Often use 0.1% w/v initially. Preparations should be prepared immediately prior to administration by adding 10mg morphine injection to 10mL of a suitable carrier (e.g. Gelclair®, Oralbalance Gel®).
- Higher-strength preparations (up to 0.5% w/v) can be used if required.
- Initial dose: 10mg to the affected area BD–TDS.
- Use within 1 hour of preparation and discard any remaining product.

¥ Dyspnoea

Oral
- Standard release
  - For opioid-naive patients, initial dose is 2.5–5mg PO PRN. A regular prescription every 4 hours plus PRN may be necessary.
  - For patients established on opioids, a dose equivalent to 25% of the current PRN rescue analgesic dose may be effective. This can be increased up to 100% of the rescue dose in a graduated fashion.

Subcutaneous
- For opioid-naive patients, initial dose is 1.25–2.5mg SC PRN. If patients require more than 2 doses daily, a CSCI should be considered.
- For patients established on opioids, a dose equivalent to 25% of the current PRN rescue analgesic dose may be effective. This can be increased up to 100% of the rescue dose in a graduated fashion.

¥ Cough
- Standard release:
  - Initial dose 5mg PO every 4 hours, and increase as necessary.

⚖ Dose adjustments

Elderly
- No specific guidance is available, although lower starting doses in opioid-naive patients may be preferable (e.g. for severe pain, 2.5–5mg PO 4 hourly and PRN). Dose requirements should be individually titrated.

Hepatic/renal impairment
- No specific guidance is available, although the plasma concentration is expected to be increased in patients with hepatic impairment. In view of its hepatic metabolism, caution is advised when giving morphine to patients with hepatic impairment. Lower starting doses in opioid-naive patients may be preferable, and dose requirements should be individually titrated.
- No specific guidance is available for patients with renal impairment. However, in view of the fact that the active metabolite morphine-6-glucuronide is renally excreted, lower starting doses in opioid-naive patients may be preferable and dose requirements should be individually titrated. Alternatively, a different opioid may be more appropriate (e.g. oxycodone or fentanyl).

Additional information
- Oramorph® oral solution 10mg/5mL contains alcohol. It may cause stinging in patients with mucositis.
- MXL® and Zomorph® capsules should be swallowed whole, or the capsules can be opened and the contents sprinkled on soft food.
- MST® tablets provide an initial immediate release of morphine, coupled with the modified release. There is no need to administer a dose of a standard-release preparation at the same time.

- Morphine sulphate via CSCI is stated to be compatible with clonazepam, cyclizine, dexamethasone, glycopyrronium, haloperidol, hyoscine butylbromide, hyoscine hydrobromide, ketamine, ketorolac, levomepromazine, metoclopramide, midazolam, octreotide, ondansetron, and ranitidine. Refer to Dickman A *et al.*, *The Syringe Driver* (2nd edn), Oxford University Press, 2005, for further information.

⌖ Pharmacology

Morphine is a strong opioid that interacts predominantly with the μ-opioid receptor. Following oral administration, morphine undergoes extensive first-pass metabolism; bioavailability is approximately 30%, but can range from 10% to 65%. The major pathway for morphine metabolism is glucuronidation, catalysed by UDP glucuronyltransferase, in the liver and GI tract to produce morphine-3-glucuronide (M3G) and morphine-6-glucuronide (M6G). The latter metabolite is considered to make a significant contribution to the analgesic effect of morphine, while M3G is devoid of analgesic action and may even antagonize the action of morphine. Enterohepatic circulation of metabolites probably occurs. Approximately 90% of the dose is excreted renally within 24 hours.

Nabumetone

Relifex[®] (POM)
Tablet: 500mg (56)
Suspension (*sugar-free*): 500mg/5mL (300mL)

Generic (POM)
Tablet: 500mg (56)

Indications
- Pain and inflammation associated with osteoarthritis and rheumatoid arthritis.
- [¥] Pain associated with cancer.

Contraindications and precautions
- Contraindicated for use in patients with:
  - a history of, or active, peptic ulceration
  - hypersensitivity reactions to ibuprofen, aspirin, or other NSAID
  - severe heart, hepatic, or renal failure.
- Certain NSAIDs are associated with an increased risk of thrombotic events. There are insufficient data at present to exclude such a risk for nabumetone.
- Use the minimum effective dose for the shortest duration necessary in order to reduce the risk of cardiac and GI events.
- Elderly patients are more at risk of developing undesirable effects.
- Use with caution in the following circumstances:
  - concurrent use of diuretics, corticosteroids, and NSAIDs (see 📖 *Drug interactions*, p.347)
  - congestive heart failure and/or left ventricular dysfunction
  - diabetes mellitus
  - established ischaemic heart disease, peripheral arterial disease, and/or cerebrovascular disease need careful consideration because of the increased risk of thrombotic events
  - hepatic impairment
  - hyperlipidaemia
  - hypertension (particularly uncontrolled)
  - recovery from surgery
  - renal impairment
  - smoking.
- Patients on long-term therapy need regular monitoring of renal and liver function.
- Abnormal LFTs can occur; discontinue NSAID if this persists.
- Nabumetone may prevent the development of signs and symptoms of inflammation/infection (e.g. fever).
- Nabumetone is believed to have an improved GI tolerability compared with other NSAIDs. Nonetheless, consider co-prescription of misoprostol or a proton pump inhibitor if:
  - long-term NSAID therapy
  - concurrent use of drugs that increase the risk of GI toxicity (see 📖 *Drug interactions*, p.347).

- Refer to 📖 Selection of an NSAID, p.31 for further information, including selection.
- Nabumetone may modify reactions and patients should be advised not to drive (or operate machinery) if affected.

☺ Undesirable effects

The frequency is not defined, but reported undesirable effects include:

- Abdominal pain
- Diarrhoea
- Dizziness
- Dyspepsia
- Flatulence
- Haematemesis
- Melaena
- Nausea
- Oedema
- Rash
- Ulcerative stomatitis
- Vomiting

Drug interactions

Pharmacokinetic

- *Methotrexate*—reduced excretion of methotrexate

Pharmacodynamic

- *Anticoagulants*—increased risk of bleeding.
- *Antihypertensives*—reduced hypotensive effect.
- *Antiplatelet drugs*—increased risk of bleeding.
- *Corticosteroids*—increased risk of GI toxicity.
- *Ciclosporin*—increased risk of nephrotoxicity.
- *Diuretics*—reduced diuretic effect; nephrotoxicity of nabumetone may be increased.
- *Rosiglitazone*—increased risk of oedema.
- *SSRIs*—increased risk of GI bleeding.

⚖ Dose

The dose should preferably be taken with or after food.

¥ Cancer pain

- Initial dose 1g PO ON. The dose can be increased if necessary to 500mg PO OM and 1g PO ON, followed by a further increase to 1g PO BD. Use the lowest effective dose for the shortest duration possible.

⚖ Dose adjustments

Elderly

- Initial dose 500mg PO ON, increased to a maximum of 1g PO ON. Use the lowest effective dose for the shortest duration possible.

Hepatic/renal impairment

- Since the formation of the active metabolite depends on biotransformation in the liver, plasma concentrations could be decreased in patients with severe hepatic impairment; therefore the manufacturer states that the drug should be used cautiously in such patients.
- Modification of nabumetone dose is generally not necessary in patients with mild renal impairment (creatinine clearance of 50mL/min or greater).

- In patients with severe renal impairment (CrCl <30mL/min), the initial dose should not exceed 500mg PO OD. After careful monitoring of renal function, dose may be increased, if needed, to a maximum of 1g PO daily.

✧ Pharmacology

Nabumetone is a prodrug and has little pharmacological activity until it undergoes oxidation in the liver to form an active metabolite, 6-methoxy-2-naphthylacetic acid (6-MNA), that is structurally similar to naproxen. 6-MNA is a relatively selective COX-2 inhibitor.

Naloxone

Generic (POM)
Injection (*ampoule*): 400mcg/mL
Injection (*pre-filled syringe*): 2mg/2mL

Indications
- Treatment of opioid overdose (use only if respiratory rate is <8 breaths/min, or <10–12 breaths/min and patient is difficult to rouse and cyanosed).

Contraindications and precautions
- No absolute contraindication when used for life-threatening respiratory depression.
- Do not use to treat opioid-induced drowsiness.

☻ Undesirable effects
The frequency is not defined, but reported undesirable effects include:
- Cardiac arrest
- Hypertension
- Nausea
- Reversal of opioid analgesia
- Seizures
- Sweating
- Tachycardia
- Vomiting

Drug interactions
Pharmacokinetic
- None known

Pharmacodynamic
- *Opioids*—antagonism of effects

⚕ Dose
- Initial dose 0.4–2mg IV injection, repeated every 2–3 minutes if necessary to a maximum of 10mg.
- SC or IM route can be used (same dose) if IV access is unavailable
- The duration of action of some opioids or modified-release formulations may exceed that of naloxone. In such situations, an IV infusion of naloxone will provide sustained antagonism of the opioid and avert the need for repeated injections.

⚕ Dose adjustments
Elderly
- No specific guidance is available. The dose should be titrated to effect.

Hepatic/renal impairment
- No specific guidance is available. The dose should be titrated to effect. The manufacturer advises caution and close monitoring of the patient.

Additional information
- To prepare an IV infusion for the reversal of opioid overdose, add 2mg naloxone to 500mL NaCl 0.9% or dextrose 5%. The rate of administration should be titrated in accordance with the patient's response.
- Naloxone has an onset of action of 1–2 minutes by IV injection and 2–5 minutes by SC/IM injection

❧ Pharmacology
Naloxone is an opioid antagonist, with strong affinity for the μ-opioid receptor. It competes with and displaces opioids at receptor sites.

Naproxen

Naprosyn® (POM)
Tablet (*scored*): 250mg (56); 500mg (56)

Naprosyn EC® (POM)
Tablet (*enteric-coated*): 250mg (56); 375mg (56); 500mg (56)

Synflex® (POM)
Tablet: 275mg (60) (NB: Synflex® is naproxen sodium; 275mg naproxen sodium = 250mg naproxen)

Generic (POM)
Tablet: 250mg (28); 500mg (28)
Tablet (*enteric-coated*): 250mg (56); 375mg (56); 500mg (56)

With misoprostol (📖 Misoprostol, p.336)
Napratec OP® (POM)
Tablet: naproxen 500mg, misoprostol 200mcg (56)

Indications
- Pain and inflammation in musculoskeletal disorders

Contraindications and precautions
- Contraindicated for use in patients with:
  - a history of, or active, peptic ulceration
  - hypersensitivity reactions to ibuprofen, aspirin, or other NSAIDs
  - severe heart, hepatic, or renal failure.
- To date, naproxen has not shown an increased risk of thrombotic events, as have many other NSAIDs. It has been suggested that naproxen possesses significant antiplatelet activity when administered regularly, twice daily.
- Use the minimum effective dose for the shortest duration necessary in order to reduce the risk of cardiac and GI events.
- Elderly patients are more at risk of developing undesirable effects.
- Use with caution in the following circumstances:
  - concurrent use of diuretics, corticosteroids, and NSAIDs (see 📖 *Drug interactions*, p.352)
  - congestive heart failure and/or left ventricular dysfunction
  - diabetes mellitus
  - established ischaemic heart disease, peripheral arterial disease, and/or cerebrovascular disease need careful consideration because of the increased risk of thrombotic events
  - hepatic impairment
  - hyperlipidaemia
  - hypertension (particularly uncontrolled)
  - recovery from surgery
  - renal impairment
  - smoking.

- Patients taking long-term therapy need regular monitoring of renal and liver function.
- Abnormal LFTs can occur; discontinue NSAID if this persists.
- Naproxen may prevent the development of signs and symptoms of inflammation/infection (e.g. fever).
- Consider co-prescription of misoprostol or a proton pump inhibitor if:
  - long-term NSAID therapy
  - concurrent use of drugs that increase the risk of GI toxicity (see 📖 *Drug interactions*, p.352)
- Refer to 📖 *Selection of an NSAID*, p.31 for further information, including selection.
- Naproxen may modify reactions and patients should be advised not to drive (or operate machinery) if affected.

☺ Undesirable effects

The frequency is not defined, but reported undesirable effects include:

- Abdominal pain
- Congestive heart failure
- Constipation
- Diarrhoea
- Dyspepsia
- Dyspnoea
- Fatigue
- Flatulence
- GI haemorrhage
- Headache
- Hypersensitivity reactions (e.g. anaphylaxis, asthma, dyspnoea, pruritus, rash, severe skin reactions)
- Hypertension
- Jaundice
- Melaena
- Nausea
- Oedema
- Peptic ulcer
- Renal failure
- Stomatitis
- Tinnitus
- Vomiting

Drug interactions

Pharmacokinetic

- Naproxen is a minor substrate of CYP1A2 and CYP2C8/9 and is unlikely to be affected by enzyme inhibitors.
- *Methotrexate*—reduced excretion of methotrexate
- *Warfarin*—possible increased risk of bleeding through inhibition of warfarin metabolism (5–11% of Caucasians have a variant of CYP2C9, requiring lower maintenance doses of warfarin. Combination with naproxen may further reduce warfarin metabolism).

Pharmacodynamic

- *Anticoagulants*—increased risk of bleeding.
- *Antihypertensives*—reduced hypotensive effect.
- *Antiplatelet drugs*—increased risk of bleeding.
- *Corticosteroids*—increased risk of GI toxicity.
- *Ciclosporin*—increased risk of nephrotoxicity.
- *Diuretics*—reduced diuretic effect; nephrotoxicity of naproxen may be increased.
- *Rosiglitazone*—increased risk of oedema.
- *SSRIs*—increased risk of GI bleeding.

₰ Dose

Naprosyn EC® should be swallowed whole, while the other products should be taken with or after food.

- Initial dose: 500–1000mg PO daily in 1–2 divided doses.
- Maximum daily dose is 1250mg PO daily, which can be taken in 2–3 divided doses.
- For Naprotec® the usual dose is one tablet PO BD.

₰ Dose adjustments

Elderly

- Use the lowest effective dose for the shortest duration possible

Hepatic/renal impairment

- In liver impairment, no specific dose recommendations are available. However, the lowest dose possible should be used for the shortest duration possible.
- Naproxen should be used with extreme caution in renal impairment. Close monitoring of renal function is recommended. Naproxen is contraindicated for use in patients with CrCl <30mL/min.

Additional information

- If Naprotec® is used, ensure that a PPI is not co-prescribed.

✥ Pharmacology

Naproxen is an NSAID with analgesic, anti-inflammatory, and antipyretic properties. The sodium salt of naproxen is more rapidly absorbed. The mechanism of action of naproxen, like that of other NSAIDs, is not completely understood but may be related to inhibition of COX-1 and COX-2. Naproxen and naproxen sodium are rapidly and completely absorbed after oral administration. It is highly protein bound and extensively metabolized in the liver (involving CYP1A2 and CYP2C8/9); the metabolites are excreted renally.

Nifedipine

Standard release
Adalat® (POM)
Capsule: 5mg (90); 10mg (90)

Generic (POM)
Capsule: 5mg (84); 10mg (84)

Modified release
Different versions of modified-release preparations may not have the same clinical effect; prescribers should specify the brand to be dispensed.

Adalat LA® (POM)
Tablet: 20mg (28); 30mg (28); 60mg (28)

Adalat Retard® (POM)
Tablet: 10mg (56); 20mg (56)

A variety of other products are available, including Adipine® MR, Adipine® XL, Coracten SR®, Coracten XL®, Fortipine LA, Hypolar® Retard 20, Nifedipress® MR, Tensipine MR® and Valni XL®. Consult the *BNF* for more information.

Indications
- Prophylaxis of chronic stable angina.
- Hypertension *(modified release only)*.
- Raynaud's phenomenon *(standard release only)*.
- ⁑ Smooth muscle spasm pain.
- ⁑ Intractable hiccup.

Contraindications and precautions
- Contraindicated for use in:
  - clinically significant aortic stenosis
  - during or within 4 weeks of a myocardial infarction
  - unstable angina.
- Standard-release formulations cause a dose-dependent increase in the risk of cardiovascular complications (e.g. myocardial infarction); only use if no other treatment suitable.
- Once-daily modified-release formulations are contraindicated for use in inflammatory bowel disease or Crohn's disease.
- Use with caution in patients with:
  - concurrent administration of CYP3A4 inducers or inhibitors (see 📖 *Drug interactions*, p.355)
  - concurrent administration of other anti-hypertensive drugs (see 📖 *Drug interactions*, p.355)
  - diabetes (can impair glucose tolerance)
  - hepatic impairment
  - low systolic blood pressure (<90mmHg).

☺ Undesirable effects

Common
- Constipation
- Headache
- Oedema
- Vasodilatation

Uncommon
- Anxiety
- Dizziness
- Dry mouth
- Dyspepsia
- Migraine
- Nausea
- Sexual dysfunction
- Sleep disorder
- Tremor
- Vertigo
- Visual disturbances

Drug interactions

Pharmacokinetic
- Nifedipine is metabolized mainly by CYP3A4; it is an inhibitor of CYP1A2.
- *Erythromycin*—increased effect of nifedipine.
- *Rifampicin*—significant reduction in effect of nifedipine.
- The clinical significance of co-administration with other CYP3A4 inhibitors or inducers (☐ end cover) is unknown. The prescriber should be aware of the potential for interactions and that dosage adjustments may be necessary.
- The clinical significance of co-administration with CYP1A2 substrates, (☐ end cover) is unknown. The prescriber should be aware of the potential for interactions and that dosage adjustments may be necessary.
- Avoid grapefruit juice as it may increase the bioavailability of nifedipine through inhibition of intestinal CYP3A4.

Pharmacodynamic
- *Alcohol*—potentiates the hypotensive effect of nifedipine.
- The risk of hypotension is increased if nifedipine is taken concurrently with the following drugs:
  - β-blockers
  - diuretics
  - haloperidol
  - levomepromazine
  - opioids
  - phosphodiesterase inhibitors (e.g. sildenafil, tadalafil, or vardenafil)
  - Tricyclic antidepressants

♊ Dose

Smooth muscle spasm, intractable hiccup

Standard release
- Initial dose 5mg PO TDS with food (or 30 minutes before food in oesophageal spasm); increase dose as necessary to a maximum of 20mg PO TDS.

Modified release
- Initial dose 20mg PO OD, or 10mg PO BD; increase dose as necessary to a maximum of 60mg PO daily.

♊ Dose adjustments

Elderly
- No specific guidance is available; use the lowest effective dose.

Hepatic/renal impairment
- No specific guidance is available for patients with hepatic impairment. Manufacturers advise caution, given the hepatic metabolism. Use the lowest effective dose.
- Patients with renal impairment are unlikely to need dose adjustments.

✣ Pharmacology

Nifedipine is a dihydropyridine calcium-channel antagonist. It inhibits the entry of calcium through cell membranes by blocking channels. The decrease in intracellular calcium inhibits the contractile processes of smooth muscle cells, thereby attenuating spasm.

Nitrofurantoin

Standard release
Macrodantin® (POM)
- **Capsule**: 50mg (30); 100mg (30)

Furadantin® (POM)
- **Tablet** *(scored)*: 50mg; 100mg

Generic (POM)
- **Tablet**: 50mg; 100mg
- **Oral suspension**: 25mg/5mL (300mL)

Modified release

Macrobid® (POM)
- **Capsule**: 100mg (14)

Indications
- Refer to local guidelines.
- Prophylaxis against and treatment of acute or recurrent uncomplicated lower urinary tract infections.

Contraindications and precautions
- Avoid in patients with:
  - CrCl <60mL/min (ineffective as inadequate urine concentrations achieved)
  - glucose-6-phosphate dehydrogenase (G6PD) deficiency.
- Because of the risk of peripheral neuropathy, use with caution in patients with:
  - anaemia
  - diabetes mellitus (may also obtain false-positive result for glucose in urinary tests)
  - electrolyte imbalance
  - folate deficiency
  - vitamin B deficiency.
- Use with caution in the following conditions as undesirable pulmonary and hepatic effects can be masked:
  - allergic diathesis
  - hepatic impairment
  - neurological disorders
  - pulmonary disease.
- Monitor lung and hepatic function in long-term therapy, especially in the elderly.

☺ Undesirable effects
The frequency is not defined, but reported undesirable effects include:
- Acute pulmonary reactions (can occur within the first week)
- Allergic skin reactions
- Anorexia
- Asthenia

- Blood dyscrasias (e.g. agranulocytosis, leucopenia, haemolytic anaemia, thrombocytonenia)
- Cholestatic jaundice
- Chronic pulmonary reactions
- Diarrhoea
- Dizziness
- Drowsiness
- Erythema multiforme
- Headache
- Hepatitis
- Nausea (reduce dose)
- Peripheral neuropathy
- Vomiting

Drug interactions

Pharmacokinetic

- *Magnesium trisilicate*—reduced absorption of nitrofurantoin.
- *Probenecid*—reduced renal excretion (reduced effect) and increased plasma concetration.

Pharmacodynamic

- *Quinolones*——increased risk of undesirable effects.

Dose

Standard doses are described here. Refer to local guidelines for specific advice.

Standard release

Prophylaxis
- 50–100mg PO ON.

Treatment
- 50–100mg PO QDS for 7days.

Modified release
- 100mg PO BD for 7 days (treatment)

Dose adjustments

Elderly
- No dose adjustment necessary.

Hepatic/renal impairment
- No specific guidance is available for use in hepatic impairment, but refer to *Contraindications and precautions*
- Nitrofurantoin should not be used in patients with CrCl <60mL/min

Additional information

- Patients should be warned that urine may be coloured yellow, orange, or brown.

➔ Pharmacology

Nitrofurantoin is a broad-spectrum bactericidal antibacterial agent active against many Gram-negative and some Gram-positive bacteria. It inhibits bacterial acetyl-coenzyme A, interfering with the carbohydrate metabolism. Nitrofurantoin may also disrupt bacterial cell wall formation. Approximately 20–25% of the total single dose of nitrofurantoin is excreted unchanged.

Nystatin

Nystan® (POM)
Oral suspension: 100,000units/mL (30mL)

Indications
• Candidal infections of the oral cavity, oesophagus.

Contraindications and precautions
• None stated.

☺ Undesirable effects
Frequency is not stated, but reported undesirable effects include:
• Diarrhoea (more likely with high doses)
• Nausea
• Oral irritation
• Vomiting

Drug interactions
Pharmacokinetic
• None known

Pharmacodynamic
• *Chlorhexidine*—nystatin inactivated by chlorhexidine; separate administration by at least 1 hour

⚗ Dose
• Initial dose 1mL PO QDS, rinsed around the mouth for 1 minute before swallowing.
• If necessary, dose can be increased to 5mL PO QDS.
• Patients with dentures should remove them before using nystatin and clean them before re-insertion. Overnight, dentures should be soaked in an appropriate antiseptic solution (and rinsed before reinsertion).

⚗ Dose adjustments
Elderly
• Dose adjustments are unnecessary.

Hepatic/renal impairment
• Dose adjustments are unnecessary.

⟐ Pharmacology
Nystatin is a polyene antifungal drug active against a wide range of yeasts and yeast-like fungi, including *Candida albicans*. It acts by binding to the cell membrane, causing a change in membrane permeability and the subsequent leakage of intracellular components. *C.albicans* (the organism responsible for the majority of oral candidiasis) does not develop resistance to nystatin. Other *Candida* species can become quite resistant during treatment, resulting in cross-resistance to amphotericin. This resistance is lost once nystatin is discontinued. Absorption of nystatin from the GI tract is negligible; excessive doses tend only to produce undesirable GI effects such as diarrhoea, nausea, and vomiting.

Octreotide

Sandostatin® (POM)

Injection: 50mcg/mL (5); 100mcg/mL (5); 1mg/5mL (multidose vial); 500mcg/mL (5)

Generic (POM)

Injection: 50mcg/mL (5); 100mcg/mL (5); 1mg/5mL (multidose vial); 500mcg/mL (5)

Indications

- Relief of symptoms associated with functional gastroenteropancreatic (GEP) endocrine tumours (e.g. carcinoid, VIPomas, glucagonomas).
- Anti-secretory effect:
  - ¥ large-volume vomiting associated with bowel obstruction
  - ¥ excessive diarrhoea
  - ¥ bronchorrhoea
  - ¥ ascites
  - ¥ rectal discharge.
- For end-of-life care issues see 📖 Use of drugs in end-of-life care, p.53.

Contraindications and precautions

- Abrupt withdrawal of subcutaneous octreotide is associated with biliary colic and pancreatitis.
- Octreotide reduces gall-bladder motility and there is a risk of gallstone development.
- Use with caution in patients with:
  - type 1 diabetes (insulin and oral hypoglycaemic doses may need reducing)
  - type 2 diabetes (dose adjustment may be needed)
  - hepatic impairment (e.g. cirrhosis)—dose reduction may be needed.
- Monitor thyroid function if on long-term treatment

☺ Undesirable effects

Common
- Abdominal pain
- Constipation
- Diarrhoea
- Flatulence
- Local injection site pain, swelling, and irritation

Uncommon
- Hair loss
- Cholecystitis

Rare
- Abdominal bloating
- Gallstones
- Nausea
- Steatorrhoea
- Vomiting

Drug interactions

Pharmacokinetic

- Through suppression of growth hormone, octreotide may reduce the metabolic clearance of drugs metabolized by the cytochrome P450 system. The prescriber should be aware that drugs mainly metabolized by CYP3A4 and with a narrow therapeutic index may need dose adjustments.
- Octreotide can reduce the absorption of ciclosporin, potentially resulting in reduced plasma levels and possible treatment failure.

Pharmacodynamic

- *Anticholinergics*—additive antisecretory effect

♪ Dose

GEP tumours

- Initial dose 50mcg SC OD–BD. Increase according to response to a maximum of 200mcg TDS. To reduce pain on administration, ensure that the ampoule is warmed to room temperature beforehand.
- ¥ Alternatively, 100mcg daily via CSCI. Increase as necessary to 600mcg daily.
- Discontinue after a week if no improvement.

¥ Anti-secretory effect

- Initial dose 200–500mcg daily via CSCI. Dose can be increased to a usual maximum of 600mcg daily. Higher doses (e.g. 1mg) have been used successfully.
- Alternatively, 50–100mcg SC TDS, increased as necessary to 200mcg SC TDS. To reduce pain on administration, ensure that the ampoule is warmed to room temperature beforehand.

♪ Dose adjustments

Elderly

- Normal doses can be used.

Hepatic/renal impairment

- Manufacturer advises that a dose reduction may be necessary in patients with hepatic impairment.
- No dose adjustments are necessary for patients with renal impairment.

Additional information

- Octreotide via CSCI is reportedly compatible with alfentanil, clonazepam, cyclizine, diamorphine, glycopyrronium, haloperidol, hydromorphone, hyoscine butylbromide, hyoscine hydrobromide, levomepromazine, metoclopramide, midazolam, morphine, ondansetron, oxycodone, and ranitidine.
- Combination with an anticholinergic drug such as glycopyrronium may have an additive anti-secretory effect.

⟿ Pharmacology

Octreotide is a somatostatin analogue that has multitude of inhibitory actions (e.g. reduction of insulin and glucagon secretion; reduction of pancreatic and intestinal secretions of water and sodium), in addition to stimulating absorption of water and electrolytes.

Olanzapine

Zyprexa® (POM)
Tablet: 2.5mg (28); 5mg (28); 7.5mg (56); 10mg (28); 15mg (28); 20mg (28)
Injection: 10mg (see 📖 *Additional information*)

Zyprexa Velotab® (POM)
Orodispersible tablet: 5mg (28); 10mg (28); 15mg (28); 20mg (28)

Indications
- Psychosis
- ¥ Nausea and vomiting
- ¥ Delirium
- ¥ Terminal agitation refractory to conventional treatment

Contraindications and precautions

> *Warning*
> - Olanzapine should not be used to treat behavioural symptoms of dementia. Elderly patients with dementia-related psychosis treated with olanzapine are at an increased risk of CVA.
> - The risks associated with CVA (e.g. diabetes, hypertension, smoking) should be assessed before commencing treatment with olanzapine.

- Use with caution in:
  - diabetes (risk of hyperglycaemia in elderly)
  - epilepsy (seizure threshold may be lowered)
  - hepatic/renal impairment (see below)
  - Parkinson's disease (olanzapine may worsen Parkinsonian symptomatology and cause hallucinations).
- Must not be used in patients with known risk for narrow-angle glaucoma.
- Phenylketonuria—Zyprexa Velotab® contains aspartame, a source of phenylalanine.
- Avoid sudden discontinuation as this may lead to the development of acute withdrawal symptoms (e.g. sweating, insomnia, tremor, anxiety, nausea, and vomiting).
- Olanzapine may modify reactions and patients should be advised not to drive (or operate machinery) if affected.

☺ Undesirable effects

Very common
- Drowsiness
- Weight gain (≥7% of baseline body weight with short-term treatment; with long term exposure, defined as >48 weeks, weight gain may be ≥25% of baseline body weight)

Common

■ Akathisia

- Dizziness
- Fatigue
- Increased appetite
- Increased cholesterol and triglyceride plasma concentrations
- Orthostatic hypotension
- Weight gain (≥15% of baseline body weight with short-term treatment)

Uncommon

- Bradycardia
- Neutropenia
- QT prolongation

Unknown

- Diabetes (development or exacerbation)
- Neuroleptic malignant syndrome
- Pancreatitis
- Seizures
- Thrombocytopenia
- Withdrawal symptoms upon sudden discontinuation

Drug interactions

Pharmacokinetic

- Metabolized mainly by glucuronidation, but CYP1A2 is involved to a lesser degree. CYP2D6 has a minor role.
- Co-administration of CYP1A2 inducers may lead to reduced olanzapine concentrations. The clinical significance is likely to be limited, but clinical monitoring is recommended and an increase of olanzapine dose may be considered if necessary.
- Smoking may lead to faster metabolism of olanzapine. Dose adjustments may be necessary upon smoking cessation (📖 Box 1.9, p.17).
- CYP1A2 inhibitors can significantly inhibit the metabolism of olanzapine. Lower initial doses of olanzapine should be considered in patients receiving a CYP1A2 inhibitor. A dose reduction of olanzapine should be considered if treatment with a CYP1A2 inhibitor is initiated.
- Co-administration of CYP2D6 inhibitors is unlikely to be of any clinical significance.

Pharmacodynamic

- Olanzapine can cause dose-related prolongation of the QT interval. There is a potential risk that co-administration with other drugs that also prolong the QT interval (e.g. amiodarone, erythromycin, haloperidol, quinine) may result in ventricular arrhythmias.
- *Antihypertensives*—increased risk of hypotension.
- *CNS depressants*—additive sedative effect.
- *Haloperidol*—increased risk of extrapyramidal reactions.
- *Levodopa and dopamine agonists*—effect antagonized by olanzapine.
- *Levomepromazine*—increased risk of extrapyramidal reactions.
- *Metoclopramide*—increased risk of extrapyramidal reactions.

♪ Dose

The dose is usually administered in the early evening.

Psychosis
- Initial dose 10mg PO OD, adjusted on the basis of individual clinical response within the range 5–20mg/day.

¥ *Nausea and vomiting*
- Initial dose 2.5mg PO ON, increased as necessary to a maximum of 10mg PO ON.

¥ *Delirium*
- Initial dose 2.5mg PO ON, increased as necessary to a maximum of 10mg PO ON.

¥ *Terminal agitation*
- Initial dose 5–10mg via CSCI increased as necessary to a maximum of 20mg/day.

♪ Dose adjustments

Elderly
- Note that the elderly are more susceptible to the undesirable anti-cholinergic effects which may increase the risk for cognitive decline and dementia.
- For psychosis, initial dose 5mg daily.
- For delirium, nausea, and vomiting increase dose gradually to improve tolerance.
- For terminal agitation, initial dose 5mg via CSCI.

Hepatic/renal impairment
- For psychosis, initial dose 5mg daily (in both cases)
- For delirium, nausea, and vomiting increase dose gradually to improve tolerance.
- For terminal agitation, initial dose 5mg via CSCI.

Additional information

- The Velotab® may be placed on the tongue and allowed to dissolve or disperse in water, orange juice, apple juice, milk, or coffee.
- Therapeutic doses of olanzapine can precipitate an acute confusional state in vulnerable individuals. This may be related to the anticholinergic effects of olanzapine.
- Risk factors for a poor response to olanzapine in cancer patients with delirium include:
  - age >70 years
  - history of dementia
  - CNS metastases.
- Olanzapine injection should be reconstituted as follows:
  - withdraw 2.1mL of WFI into a sterile syringe; inject into the vial and completely dissolve the contents
  - the vial contains olanzapine 5mg/mL
  - there is a deliberate overage; withdrawal of 10mg/2mL will leave 1mg olanzapine in the vial.

• Compatibility information for olanzapine injection is presently limited and it is recommended to be given via separate CSCI. Saline 0.9% or WFI can be used as a diluent.

❖ Pharmacology

Olanzapine interacts with a wide range of receptors in producing its therapeutic effects, including $5HT_{2A/2C}$, D_1, D_2, D_3, and D_4. It also interacts with additional receptors which explain the range of effects that are produced; these include $5HT_3$, muscarinic, α_1-adrenergic, and H_1 receptors. Olanzapine is well absorbed after oral administration, reaching peak plasma concentrations within 5–8 hours. It is mainly metabolized in the liver by glucuronidation, although some oxidation via CYP1A2 occurs. CYP2D6 also has a minor role in the metabolism of olanzapine. The main metabolite of olanzapine is inactive.

Omeprazole

Losec® (POM)
Capsule: 10mg (28); 20mg (28); 40mg (7)
IV infusion: 40mg
IV injection: 40mg

Losec® MUPS® (POM)
Dispersible tablet: 10mg (28); 20mg (28); 40mg (7)

Generic (POM)
Capsule: 10mg (28); 20mg (28); 40 mg (28)
Tablet: 10mg (28); 20mg (28); 40mg (7;28)
IV infusion: 40mg

Indications
- Treatment of duodenal and benign gastric ulcers.
- Treatment of oesophageal reflux disease.
- Treatment and prophylaxis of NSAID-associated peptic ulcer disease.
- Dyspepsia.

Contraindications and precautions
- Do not administer with atazanavir or erlotinib.
- Treatment with omeprazole may lead to a slightly increased risk of developing GI infections (e.g. *Clostridium difficile*). Therefore avoid unnecessary use or high doses.
- Omeprazole may modify reactions and patients should be advised not to drive (or operate machinery) if affected.
- Rebound acid hypersecretion may occur on discontinuation if the patient has received treatment for more than 8 weeks.

☺ Undesirable effects
Common
- Abdominal pain
- Constipation
- Diarrhoea
- Flatulence
- Headache
- Nausea and vomiting

Uncommon
- Dermatitis
- Dizziness
- Drowsiness
- Insomnia
- Light-headedness
- Paraesthesia
- Pruritus
- Raised liver enzymes
- Rash
- Urticaria
- Vertigo

Rare

- Agranulocytosis
- Agitation
- Confusion
- Depression
- Dry mouth
- Gynaecomastia
- Hallucinations
- Hepatitis
- Muscular weakness
- Stomatitis

Drug interactions

Pharmacokinetic

- Omeprazole is metabolized mainly by CYP2C19, but minor pathways involve CYP2C8/9, CYP2D6, and CYP3A4. It is a strong inhibitor of CYP2C19, a moderate inhibitor of CYP2C8/9, and a weak inhibitor of CYP2D6 and CYP3A4.
- Drugs with pH-dependent absorption can be affected:
  - *atazanavir*—avoid combination because of substantially reduced absorption.
  - *digoxin*—increased plasma concentrations possible.
  - *erlotinib*—avoid combination as bioavailability of erlotinib can be significantly reduced.
  - *ketoconazole/itraconazole*—risk of sub-therapeutic plasma concentrations.
  - *metronidazole suspension*—omeprazole may reduce/prevent the absorption of metronidazole.
- *Citalopram*—omeprazole can increase the plasma concentration of citalopram through inhibition of CYP2C19.
- *Clopidogrel*—antiplatelet action may be reduced (avoid combination).
- *Diazepam*—plasma concentrations of diazepam can be increased through inhibition of CYP2C19.
- *Warfarin*—possible increase in INR.
- The clinical significance of co-administration with CYP2C19 inducers or inhibitors (🕮 end cover) is unknown. The prescriber should be aware of the potential for interactions and that dose adjustments may be necessary.
- The clinical significance of co-administration of CYP2C19 or CYP2C8/9 substrates (🕮 end cover) is unknown. Caution is advised if omeprazole is co-administered with drugs that are predominantly metabolized by CYP2C19 or CYP2C8/9. The prescriber should be aware of the potential for interactions and that dose adjustments may be necessary, particularly for drugs with a narrow therapeutic index.

Pharmacodynamic

- No clinically significant interactions noted.

⚕ Dose

Duodenal and benign gastric ulcers

- Initial dose 20mg PO OD for 4 weeks in duodenal ulceration or 8 weeks in gastric ulceration.
- In severe or recurrent cases the dose may be increased to 40mg PO OD.
- Maintenance treatment for recurrent duodenal ulcer is recommended at a dose of 20mg PO OD.
- Alternatively, in patients unable to tolerate oral therapy, 40mg IV or IV infusion OD for up to 5 days.

Oesophageal reflux disease

- Initial dose 20mg PO OD for 4–12 weeks. For refractory disease, 40mg PO OD has been given for 8 weeks.
- Maintenance 10mg PO OD, increasing to 20mg PO OD if necessary.
- Alternatively, in patients unable to tolerate oral therapy, 40mg IV or IV infusion OD for up to 5 days.

Treatment of NSAID-associated peptic ulcer disease

- Initial dose 20mg PO OD, continued for 4–8 weeks.
- Alternatively, in patients unable to tolerate oral therapy, 40mg IV injection or IV infusion OD for up to 5 days.

Prophylaxis of NSAID-associated peptic ulcer disease

- 20mg PO OD.

Dyspepsia

- 10–20mg PO OD for 2–4 weeks depending on the severity and persistence of symptoms.

⚕ Dose adjustments

Elderly

- Dose adjustments are not necessary in the elderly.

Hepatic/renal impairment

- In liver impairment, the dose should not exceed 20mg PO OD.
- Dose adjustments are not required for patients with renal impairment.

Additional information

- Losec® MUPS® tablets can be dispersed in 10mL of water prior to administration. Alternatively, fruit juice (e.g. apple, orange) can be used. The mixture should be stirred before drinking and it is recommended that half a glass of water is taken afterwards.
- The content of Losec® capsules can be swallowed directly with half a glass of water, or may be suspended in 10mL of water prior to administration. Alternatively, fruit juice can be used. The mixture should be stirred before drinking and it is recommended that half a glass of water is taken afterwards.
- Omeprazole IV injection is to be given slowly over a period of 5 minutes.
- Omeprazole IV infusion should be administered in either 100mL NaCl 0.9% or 100mL 5% dextrose over 20–30 minutes.

♦ Pharmacology

Omeprazole is a proton pump inhibitor that suppresses gastric acid secretion in a dose-related manner by specific inhibition of the H+/K+ ATPase in the gastric parietal cell. Oral bioavailability is low (~40%). It is extensively metabolized, mainly by CYP2C19 although several alternative pathways are involved (e.g. CYP2C8/9, CYP2D6, and CYP3A4). Note that poor CYP2C19 metabolizers (or patients taking CYP2C19 inhibitors) can have significantly higher plasma concentrations, leading to unexpected results.

Ondansetron

Zofran® (POM)
Tablet: 4mg (30); 8mg (10)
Syrup (*sugar-free*): 4mg/5mL (50mL)
Injection: 4mg/2mL (5); 8mg/2mL (5)
Suppository: 16mg (1)

Zofran Melt® (POM)
Oral lyophilisate: 4mg (10); 8mg (10)

Generic (POM)
Tablet: 4mg; 8mg
Injection: 4mg/2mL; 8mg/4mL

Indications
- Nausea and vomiting (postoperative, induced by chemotherapy or radiotherapy).
- ¥ Nausea and vomiting (e.g. drug-induced, cancer-related, refractory)
- ¥ Pruritus (e.g. cholestatic, uraemic, opioid-induced).
- For end-of-life care issues see 📖 Use of drugs in end-of-life care, p.53.

Contraindications and precautions
- Since ondansetron increases large bowel transit time, use with caution in patients with signs of sub-acute bowel obstruction.
- Use with caution in patients with:
  - cardiac rhythm or conduction disturbances
  - concurrent use of anti-arrhythmic agents or β-adrenergic blocking agents (see 📖 Drug interactions, p.372)
  - significant electrolyte disturbances
  - hepatic impairment (see 📖 Dose adjustments, p.372).

☺ Undesirable effects
Very common
- Headache

Common
- Constipation
- Flushing

Uncommon
- Abnormal LFTs
- Arrhythmias
- Extrapyramidal symptoms
- Hiccups
- Seizures

Rare
- Anaphylaxis

Drug interactions

Pharmacokinetic
- Metabolized by a variety of cytochromes (e.g. CYP1A2, CYP2D6), but is a major substrate of CYP3A4.
- Carbamazepine and phenytoin can reduce ondansetron levels and reduce the effect.
- The clinical significance of co-administration with other CYP3A4 inducers or inhibitors (☐ end cover) is unknown. The prescriber should be aware of the potential for interactions and that dose adjustments may be necessary.
- *Paracetamol*—possible reduced analgesic benefit.
- *Tramadol*—reduced analgesic benefit.
- The effect of grapefruit juice on the absorption of ondansetron is unknown.

Pharmacodynamic
- Ondansetron can cause prolongation of the QT interval. There is a potential risk that co-administration with other drugs that also prolong the QT interval (e.g. amiodarone, erythromycin, haloperidol, quinine) may result in ventricular arrhythmias.
- Ondansetron increases bowel transit time. This effect can be enhanced by drugs such as opioids, TCAs, and anticholinergics.
- *Domperidone/metoclopramide*—ondansetron reduces the prokinetic effect.
- *SSRIs*—risk of serotonin syndrome.

⚖ Dose

¥ *Nausea and vomiting (e.g. drug-induced, cancer-related, refractory)*
- Initial dose 4–8mg PO/SC BD–TDS.
- Alternatively, 8–16mg via CSCI daily. The dose can be increased if necessary to a maximum of 32mg daily.
- Alternatively, 16mg PR OD.

¥ *Pruritus*
- Initial dose 4mg PO/SC BD, increasing if necessary to 8mg PO/SC TDS. Treatment may be continued via CSCI if necessary.

⚖ Dose adjustments

Elderly
- Adult doses can be used.

Hepatic/renal impairment
- In moderate or severe impairment hepatic impairment, the manufacturer advises that a total daily dose of 8mg should not be exceeded (no dose adjustment necessary for granisetron)
- No dose adjustments are necessary for patients with renal impairment.

Additional information

- 5-HT$_3$ antagonists differ in chemical structure, pharmacokinetics, and pharmacodynamics. There may be individual variation in response and it may be worth considering an alternative 5-HT$_3$ antagonist if response to ondansetron is not as expected.
- Treatment with ondansetron should be used regularly for 3 days and then response assessed. Avoid using on a PRN basis.
- Response in pruritus is highly variable.
- Ondansetron via CSCI is compatible with alfentanil, dexamethasone, diamorphine, fentanyl, glycopyrronium, metoclopramide, midazolam, morphine, octreotide, and oxycodone.

⟿ Pharmacology

Ondansetron is a selective 5-HT$_3$ receptor antagonist, blocking serotonin peripherally on vagal nerve terminals and centrally in the chemoreceptor trigger zone. It is a particularly useful in the treatment of nausea and vomiting associated with serotonin release (e.g. damage to enterochromaffin cells due to bowel injury, chemotherapy, or radiotherapy).

Oxybutynin

Standard release

Cystrin® *(POM)*
Tablet: 3mg (56); 5mg (*scored*-84)

Ditropan® *(POM)*
Tablet (*scored*): 2.5mg (84); 5mg (84)
Elixir: 2.5mg/5mL (150mL)

Modified release

Lyrinel® *XL* *(POM)*
Tablet: 5mg (30); 10mg (30)

Kentera® *(POM)*
Transdermal patch: 3.9mg/24 hours (applied for 72–96 hours)

Indications
- Urinary incontinence.
- Urinary frequency.

Contraindications and precautions
- Oxybutynin is contraindicated for use in patients with:
  - myasthenia gravis
  - narrow-angle glaucoma
  - porphyria
  - severe ulcerative colitis
  - toxic megacolon
  - urinary retention.
- It should be used with caution in patients with the following:
  - cardiac arrhythmia
  - congestive heart failure
  - dementia
  - elderly (see 📖 *Dose adjustments*)
  - GI reflux disease
  - hepatic impairment
  - hypertension
  - hyperthyroidism
  - prostatic hypertrophy
  - pyrexia (reduces sweating)
  - renal impairment.
- Oxybutynin may modify reactions and patients should be advised not to drive (or operate machinery) if affected.

☻ Undesirable effects

Very common
- Application site reaction (patch)
- Dry mouth

Common
- Asthenia
- Confusion
- Constipation
- Depression
- Diarrhoea (overflow)
- Dizziness
- Drowsiness
- Dyspepsia
- Fatigue
- Headache
- Hypertension
- Insomnia
- Urinary retention
- Visual disturbances

Uncommon
- Anorexia
- Anxiety
- Dehydration
- Dysphagia
- Hyperglycaemia
- Mouth ulceration

Drug interactions

Pharmacokinetic
- Metabolized by CYP3A4.
- The clinical significance of co-administration with inducers or inhibitors of CYP3A4 (📖 end cover) is unknown. The prescriber should be aware of the potential for interactions and the need for dose adjustments.
- The effect of grapefruit juice on the bioavailability of oxybutynin is unknown.

Pharmacodynamic
- *Donepezil*—effect may be antagonized.
- *β_2-agonists*—increased risk of tachycardia.
- *Cyclizine*—increased risk of undesirable anticholinergic effects.
- *Domperidone*—may inhibit prokinetic effect.
- *Galantamine*—effect may be antagonized.
- *Metoclopramide*—may inhibit prokinetic effect.
- *Nefopam*—increased risk of undesirable anticholinergic effects.
- *Rivastigmine*—effect may be antagonized.
- *Tricyclic antidepressants*—increased risk of undesirable anticholinergic effects.

.§ Dose

Standard release

- Initial dose 5mg PO BD. Can be increased as necessary up to a maximum of 5mg PO QDS.

Modified release

- Patients may be transferred from the standard-release product.
- Initial dose 5mg PO OD. The dose can be increased after at least a week to 10mg PO OD. The dose can be further increased, at weekly intervals, to a maximum of 20mg PO OD.
- Alternatively, a 3.9mg transdermal patch can be applied twice weekly (every 3–4 days). The patch should be applied to dry intact skin on the abdomen, hip, or buttock. A new application site should be used for each new patch and the same site should not be used within 7 days.

.§ Dose adjustments

Elderly

- For the standard-release formulations, manufacturers recommend lower initial doses (e.g. 2.5mg PO BD) as elderly patients are more susceptible to undesirable effects. In particular, the elderly may have an increased risk for cognitive decline and dementia.

Hepatic/renal impairment

- No specific guidance available. Use the lowest effective dose.

Additional information

- Plasma concentration of oxybutynin declines within 1–2 hours after removal of the transdermal patch.
- For Lyrinel® XL, the tablet membrane may pass through the GI tract unchanged.
- Standard-release tablets can be dispersed in water immediately prior to use if necessary (elixir would be preferable).

◈ Pharmacology

Oxybutynin is an anticholinergic drug which competitively antagonizes acetylcholine at post-ganglionic sites including smooth muscle, secretory glands, and CNS sites. It is extensively metabolized by the liver, primarily by CYP3A4; there is an active metabolite that has similar actions to oxybutynin.

Oxycodone

Standard release

OxyNorm® (CD POM)
Capsule: 5mg (*orange/beige*, 56); 10mg (*white/beige*, 56); 20mg (*pink/beige*, 56)
Oral solution (*sugar-free*; *alcohol-free*): 5mg/5mL (250mL); 10mg/mL (120mL)
Injection: 10mg/mL (5); 20mg/2mL (5); 50mg/mL (5)

Modified release

OxyContin® (CD POM)
Tablet: 5mg (*blue*, 28); 10mg (*white*, 56); 20mg (*pink*, 56); 40mg (*yellow*, 56); 80mg (*green*, 56)

Targinact® (CD POM)
Tablet: 5mg/2.5mg oxycodone/naloxone (28); 10mg/5mg oxycodone/naloxone (56); 20mg/10mg oxycodone/naloxone (56); 40mg/20mg oxycodone/naloxone (56)

Oxycodone is a Schedule 2 controlled drug. Refer to 📖 Legal categories for medicines, p.23 further information. Both parenteral and oral products **can** be prescribed by nurse independent prescribers (📖 Independent prescribing: palliative care issues, p.25).

Indications
- Moderate to severe pain in patients with cancer.
- Postoperative pain (**not** Targinact®).
- Severe pain requiring the use of a strong opioid.
- ¥ Dyspnoea
- For end-of-life care issues see 📖 Use of drugs in end-of-life care, p.53.

Contraindications and precautions
- If the dose of an opioid is titrated correctly, it is generally accepted that there are no absolute contraindications to the use of such drugs in palliative care, although there may be circumstances where one opioid is favoured over another (e.g. renal impairment, constipation). Nonetheless, the manufacturer states that oxycodone is contraindicated for use in patients with:
  - acute abdomen
  - chronic bronchial asthma
  - chronic constipation
  - chronic obstructive airways disease
  - concurrent administration of MAOIs or within 2 weeks of discontinuation of their use
  - cor pulmonale
  - delayed gastric emptying
  - head injury
  - hypercarbia

- • moderate to severe hepatic impairment
- • nonopioid induced paralytic ileus
- • respiratory depression
- • severe renal impairment (creatinine clearance <10mL/min)
- • Use with caution in the following instances:
  - • acute alcoholism
  - • Addison's disease (adrenocortical insufficiency)
  - • delirium tremens
  - • diseases of the biliary tract
  - • elderly patients
  - • hepatic impairment (see above)
  - • history of alcohol and drug abuse
  - • hypotension
  - • hypothyroidism
  - • hypovolaemia
  - • inflammatory bowel disorders
  - • pancreatitis
  - • prostatic hypertrophy
  - • raised intracranial pressure
  - • renal impairment
  - • severe pulmonary disease
  - • toxic psychosis.
- • Oxycodone may modify reactions and patients should be advised not to drive (or operate machinery) if affected.

☺ Undesirable effects

- • Strong opioids tend to cause similar undesirable effects, albeit to varying degrees (see also 📖 Morphine, p.340).

Very common
- • Constipation (not Targinact®)
- • Dizziness
- • Drowsiness
- • Fatigue
- • Nausea
- • Pruritus
- • Somnolence
- • Vomiting

Common
- • Abnormal thoughts
- • Anxiety
- • Asthenia
- • Confusion
- • Dry mouth
- • Dyspepsia (give with food if problematic)
- • Headache
- • Postural hypotension
- • Rash
- • Restlessness
- • Sedation

- Sweating
- Tremor
- Yawning

Uncommon
- Biliary spasm
- Dyspnoea
- Hiccups
- Insomnia
- Miosis
- Vasodilatation
- Vertigo

Rare
- Convulsions (particularly in patients with epilepsy)
- Stomatitis
- Long-term use may result in sexual dysfunction (e.g. amenorrhea, decreased libido, erectile dysfunction)

Drug interactions

Pharmacokinetic
- Metabolized mainly by CYP3A4; a minor pathway involves CYP2D6.
- The clinical significance of co-administration with CYP3A4 inhibitors (📖 end cover) is unknown. The prescriber should be aware of the potential for interactions. Clinical reports are lacking; in theory this interaction may lead to an increased risk of toxicity because of possible increases in the plasma concentration of oxycodone and an increase in metabolism by CYP2D6 to the active metabolite, oxymorphone. Dose adjustments may be necessary.
- The clinical significance of co-administration with CYP3A4 inducers, (📖 end cover) is unknown. The prescriber should be aware of the potential for possible reduced analgesic benefit and that dose adjustments may be necessary.
- Avoid excessive amounts of grapefruit juice as it may increase the bioavailability of oxycodone through inhibition of intestinal CYP3A4.

Pharmacodynamic
- *Antihypertensives*—increased risk of hypotension.
- *CNS depressants*—risk of excessive sedation.
- *Haloperidol*—may be an additive hypotensive effect.
- *Ketamine*—there is a potential opioid-sparing effect with ketamine and the dose of oxycodone may need reducing.
- *Levomepromazine*—may be an additive hypotensive effect.
- *MAOIs and linezolid*—avoid concurrent use (📖 Morphine, p.340).
- *SSRIs*—serotonin syndrome has been reported with oxycodone and various SSRIs.

♣ Dose
Pain

The initial dose of oxycodone depends upon the patient's previous opioid requirements. Refer to ⏛ Opioid substitution, p.33 for information regarding opioid dose equivalences see ⏛ Breakthrough cancer pain for guidance relating to BTcP.

Oral

- Standard release
  - For opioid-naive patients, the initial dose is 5mg PO every 4–6 hours and PRN. The dose is then increased as necessary until a stable dose is attained. The patient should then be converted to a modi-fied-release formulation.
- Modified release
  - For opioid-naive patients, the initial dose is 5–10mg PO BD. The dose can then be titrated as necessary.
- Targinact®
  - For opioid-naive patients, the initial dose is 10mg/5mg oxycodone/ naloxone PO BD. This can be increased to 20mg/10mg PO BD if needed.
  - ¥ The dose can be increased further as necessary, although higher doses are presently unlicensed.

Subcutaneous

- Initial dose in opioid-naive patients is 5mg SC 4-hourly PRN. Alternatively, 7.5mg via CSCI over 24 hours and increase as necessary.

¥ *Dyspnoea*
Oral

- Standard release
  - For opioid-naive patients, initial dose is 2.5mg PO PRN. A regular prescription every 4 hours plus PRN may be necessary.
  - In patients established on opioids, a dose that is equivalent to 25% of the current PRN rescue analgesic dose may be effective. This can be increased up to 100% of the rescue dose in a graduated fashion.

Subcutaneous

- For opioid-naive patients, initial dose is 1.25–2.5mg SC PRN. If patients require more than two doses daily, a CSCI should be considered.
- In patients established on opioids, a dose that is equivalent to 25% of the current PRN rescue analgesic dose may be effective. This can be increased up to 100% of the rescue dose in a graduated fashion.

♣ Dose adjustments
Elderly

- No specific guidance available, although lower starting doses in opioid-naive patients may be preferable. Dose requirements should be indi-vidually titrated.

Hepatic/renal impairment
- In patients with mild hepatic impairment, the plasma concentration is expected to be increased. Lower doses may be needed and the starting dose is suggested to be 2.5mg PO every 6 hours and titrate to pain relief. The manufacturer contraindicates the use of oxycodone in patients with moderate to severe hepatic impairment. Nonetheless, oxycodone is used in this group of patients and the dose should be titrated carefully to the patient's need.
- In patients with mild to moderate renal impairment, the plasma concentration of oxycodone is likely to be increased. The initial dose is suggested to be 2.5mg PO every 6 hours and titrate to pain relief. The use of oxycodone in patients with severe renal impairment is contraindicated. Nonetheless, oxycodone is used in this group of patients and the dose should be titrated carefully to the patient's need.

Additional information
- OxyNorm® 10mg/mL oral solution may be mixed with a soft drink to improve taste.
- OxyNorm® 5mg/5mL and 10mg/mL oral solutions do not contain alcohol as an excipient.
- OxyContin® tablets provide an initial immediate release of oxycodone, coupled with the modified release. There is no need to administer a dose of OxyNorm® at the same time.
- Ultra-rapid metabolizers of CYP2D6 may at risk of toxicity because of the potential increase in formation of the active metabolite oxymorphone.
- Oxycodone via CSCI is stated to be compatible with clonazepam, dexamethasone, glycopyrronium, haloperidol, hyoscine butylbromide, hyoscine hydrobromide, ketamine, ketorolac, levomepromazine, metoclopramide, midazolam, octreotide, ondansetron, and ranitidine. There is a concentration-dependent compatibility issue with cyclizine; unlike diamorphine, the exact concentrations have not yet been identified. Refer to Dickman A et al., *The Syringe Driver* (2nd edn), Oxford University Press, 2005, for further information.

♦ Pharmacology
Oxycodone is a strong opioid with similar properties to morphine. It acts primarily via μ-opioid receptors, although it is also stated to have affinity for δ- and κ-opioid receptors. Following oral administration, oxycodone is well absorbed with a bioavailability of up to 87%. It is metabolized principally to the inactive metabolite noroxycodone by CYP3A4. A minor metabolic pathway involves CYP2D6, with the active metabolite oxymorphone being produced. In general, the contribution of oxymorphone to the overall analgesic benefit of oxycodone is minimal since it is usually present in the plasma at low concentrations. However, ultra-rapid CYP2D6 metabolizers or patients receiving CYP3A4 inhibitors can respond to oxycodone at lower than expected doses. Approximately 10% of oxycodone is excreted unchanged, and can accumulate in patients with renal impairment.

Pamidronate disodium

Aredia Dry Powder® (POM)
Injection (*powder for reconstitution*): 15mg; 30mg; 90mg

Generic (POM)
Injection (*concentrate solution*):
- 3mg/mL: 5mL vial (15mg); 10mL vial (30mg); 20mL vial (60mg); 30mL vial (90mg)
- 6mg/mL: 10mL vial (60mg)
- 9mg/mL: 10mL vial (90mg)
- 15mg/mL: 1mL ampoule (15mg); 2mL ampoule (30mg); 4mL ampoule (60mg); 6mL ampoule (90mg)

Indications
- Tumour-induced hypercalcaemia.
- Bone pain and osteolytic lesions due to metastases associated with breast cancer or multiple myeloma.
- Paget's disease of bone (not discussed).

Contraindications and precautions
- Pamidronate must be given as an infusion as described above and not as a bolus injection.
- Assess renal function and electrolytes (e.g. calcium, magnesium) before each dose and ensure adequate hydration (especially hypercalcaemia).
- Use with caution in the following circumstances:
  - cardiac disease (risk of fluid overload)
  - elderly
  - patients who have undergone thyroid surgery (risk of hypocalcaemia if hypoparathyroidism)
  - renal impairment (see 📖 *Dose adjustments,* p.384)
  - severe hepatic impairment (see 📖 *Dose adjustments,* p.384).
- Assess the need for calcium and vitamin D supplements in patients receiving pamidronate other than for hypercalcaemia.
- Consider dental examination before initiating therapy because of the possibility of inducing osteonecrosis of the jaw.

☺ Undesirable effects

Osteonecrosis of the jaw has been discovered to be a potential complication of bisphosphonate therapy. It has been reported in cancer patients, many of whom had a pre-existing local infection or recent extraction. Cancer patients are more likely to be at risk of osteonecrosis as a result of their disease, cancer therapies, and blood dyscrasias. Dental examination is recommended for patients undergoing repeated infusions of pamidronate (and other bisphosphonates) and dental surgery should be avoided during this treatment period as healing may be delayed.

Very common
- Fever (within 48 hours of treatment; sometimes with rigor, fatigue, and flushes)
- Hypophosphataemia

Common
- Abdominal pain
- Anaemia
- Arthralgia
- Conjunctivitis
- Constipation
- Diarrhoea
- Drowsiness
- Headache
- Hypertension
- Hypokalaemia
- Hypomagnesaemia
- Insomnia
- Infusion site reactions
- Nausea
- Rash
- Transient bone pain
- Thrombocytopenia
- Vomiting

Uncommon
- Acute renal failure
- Agitation
- Dizziness
- Dyspepsia
- Hypotension
- Muscle cramps
- Pruritis
- Seizures
- Uveitis

Drug interactions
Pharmacokinetic
- None known

Pharmacodynamic
- *Aminoglycosides*—may have additive hypocalcaemic effect.
- *Diuretics*—increased risk of renal impairment.
- *NSAIDs*—increased risk of renal impairment.
- *Thalidomide*—increased risk of renal impairment (in treatment of multiple myeloma).

Dose
Tumour-induced hypercalcaemia
- Ensure patients are well hydrated prior to and following administration of pamidronate.
- The dose of pamidronate depends on the patient's initial serum calcium levels. It is usually infused as a single dose (Table 3.12).
- Must be given as an IV infusion at a rate not exceeding 1mg/min.
- Maximum response should be seen within 3–7 days. If an insufficient reduction is obtained within this time, the dose can be repeated.

Osteolytic lesions and bone pain
- 90mg by IV infusion at a rate not exceeding 1mg/min every 4 weeks

Table 3.13 Pamidronate dosage

Initial serum calcium (mmol/L)	Recommended dose (mg)
Up to 3.0	15–30
3.0–3.5	30–60
3.5–4.0	60–90
>4.0	90

Dose adjustments

Elderly
- Usual adult doses can be used.

Hepatic/renal impairment
- Dose adjustment is unnecessary in patients with mild to moderate hepatic impairment. The manufacturer advises caution in patients with severe hepatic impairment because of lack of data.
- For the treatment of osteolytic lesions, if renal function deteriorates, treatment should be withheld until renal function returns to within 10% of the baseline value.
- For the treatment of hypercalcaemia, dose adjustment is unnecessary in patients with mild to moderate renal impairment (CrCl >30mL/min). In severe renal impairment the infusion rate should not exceed 90mg/4hr.

Additional information
- To reconstitute Aredia Dry Powder® the powder in the vials should first be dissolved in sterile WFI (15mg in 5mL; 30mg and 90mg in 10mL).
- The concentrated solution should be diluted to a maximum concentration of 60mg/250mL with infusion fluid (NaCl 0.9% or D5W). One manufacturer (Medac) permits a maximum concentration of 90mg/250mL.

Pharmacology

Pamidronate disodium is an inhibitor of osteoclastic bone resorption. It has been shown to exert its activity by binding strongly to hydroxyapatite crystals, inhibiting their formation and dissolution and suppressing the accession of osteoclast precursors onto the bone. Additionally, and to a greater extent, as the drug binds to bone mineral, this reduces the resorption of osteoclastic bone. It is almost exclusively excreted unchanged by the kidney.

Pantoprazole

Protium® (POM)
Tablet: 20mg (28); 40mg (28)
Injection: 40mg

Generic (POM)
Tablet: 20mg (28); 40mg (28)

Indications
- Treatment of gastric and duodenal ulcer.
- Treatment of moderate and severe reflux oesophagitis.
- Treatment of mild reflux disease and associated symptoms.
- Long-term treatment and prevention of relapse in reflux oesophagitis.
- Prophylaxis of NSAID-associated peptic ulcer disease.

Contraindications and precautions
- Do not administer with atazanavir or erlotinib.
- Treatment with omeprazole may lead to a slightly increased risk of developing GI infections (e.g. *Clostridium difficile*). Therefore avoid unnecessary use or high doses.
- The manufacturer recommends monitoring of LFTs in patients on long-term treatment.
- Rebound acid hypersecretion may occur on discontinuation if the patient has received more than 8 weeks treatment.

☺ Undesirable effects
Common
- Diarrhoea
- Flatulence
- Headache
- Upper abdominal pain

Uncommon
- Nausea and vomiting
- Dizziness
- Visual disturbances
- Pruritus

Rare
- Arthralgia
- Depression
- Dry mouth
- Hallucinations

Drug interactions
Pharmacokinetic
- Pantoprazole is metabolized by CYP2C19; a minor pathway involves CYP3A4. It is a moderate inhibitor of CYP2C8/9.

- Drugs with pH-dependent absorption can be affected:
  - *atazanavir*—avoid combination because of substantially reduced absorption
  - *digoxin*—increased plasma concentrations possible
  - *erlotinib*—avoid combination as bioavailability of erlotinib can be significantly reduced
  - *ketoconazole/itraconazole*—risk of sub-therapeutic plasma concentrations
  - *metronidazole suspension*—pantoprazole may reduce/prevent the absorption of metronidazole.
- *Azole antifungals*—proton pump inhibitors may decrease the absorption of itraconazole and ketoconazole.
- *Clopidogrel*—antiplatelet action may be reduced.
- The clinical significance of co-administration with CYP2C19 inducers or inhibitors (☐ end cover) is unknown. The prescriber should be aware of the potential for interactions and that dose adjustments may be necessary.
- Although the clinical significance is unknown, co-administration of pantoprazole may increase the levels/effects of CYP2C8/9 substrates (☐ end cover). The prescriber should be aware of the potential for interactions and that dose adjustments may be necessary.

Pharmacodynamic
- No clinically significant interactions noted.

⚖ Dose
Treatment of duodenal ulcer and gastric ulcer
- 40mg PO OM for 2–4 weeks (duodenal) or 4–8 weeks (gastric).
- Alternatively, 40mg IV OD until oral treatment is possible.

Treatment of moderate and severe reflux oesophagitis
- 40mg PO OM for 4–8 weeks.
- Alternatively, 40mg IV OD until oral treatment is possible.

Treatment of mild reflux disease and associated symptoms
- 20mg PO OM for 2–8 weeks. After this time, patients can be controlled with 20mg PO OD PRN, switching to regular treatment if necessary.

Long-term treatment and prevention of relapse in reflux oesophagitis
- 20–40mg PO OM

Prophylaxis of NSAID-associated peptic ulcer disease
- 20mg PO OM

⚖ Dose adjustments
Elderly
- No dose adjustments are necessary.

Hepatic/renal impairment
- In patients with severe liver impairment, 20mg OM should not be exceeded and regular LFTs should be performed.
- No dose adjustments are necessary in renal impairment.

Additional information

- Tablets should not be chewed or crushed, but should be swallowed whole.

✥ Pharmacology

Pantoprazole is a gastric proton pump inhibitor, reducing the release of H^+ from parietal cells by inhibiting H^+/K^+-ATPase. It is rapidly inactivated by gastric acid; hence oral formulations are enteric coated. It is extensively metabolized, mainly by CYP2C19 although an alternative pathway involves CYP3A4. Note that CYP2C19 poor metabolizers (or patients taking CYP2C19 inhibitors) can have significantly higher plasma concentrations, leading to unexpected results. Metabolites are virtually inactive and are eliminated mainly by renal excretion, with a small percentage eliminated in faeces.

Paracetamol

Perfalgan® (POM)
Intravenous infusion: 500mg/50mL; 1g/100mL

Generic (POM)*
Tablet: 500mg (16; 32; 100)
Caplet: 500mg (16; 32; 100)
Soluble tablet: 500mg (60)
Oral suspension: 250mg/5mL (100mL); 500mg/5mL (300mL)
Note: sugar-free suspensions are available
Suppository: 60mg, 125mg, 250mg, 500mg

Combination products
See codeine (□ Codeine, p.114), dihydrocodeine (□ Dihydrocodeine, p.150) and tramadol (□ Tramadol, p.466).

Paradote® (POM)
Tablet: co-methiamol 100/500 (24; 96)

Note: available to purchase OTC (**P**) in quantities of 24 tablets or less.

*The legal status of paracetamol depends upon pack size: 16 (**GSL**), 32 (**P**), >100 (**POM**).

Indications
- Mild to moderate pain.
- Pyrexia.

Contraindications and precautions
- Paracetamol is contraindicated for use in severe hepatic impairment.
- It should be used with caution in patients with:
  - alcohol dependence
  - concurrent use of enzyme-inducing drugs (see □ *Drug interactions, (below)*)
  - hepatic impairment
  - renal impairment
  - state of malnutrition (low reserves of hepatic glutathione).

☺ Undesirable effects
Rare
- Abnormal LFTs
- Hypotension (on infusion)

Very rare
- Blood dyscrasias

Drug interactions
Pharmacokinetic
- *Carbamazepine*—increased risk of paracetamol toxicity (especially in overdose).

- *Colestyramine*—absorption of paracetamol is reduced (avoid co-administration by 2 hours).
- *Imatinib*—glucuronidation inhibited by imatinib; potential paracetamol toxicity with prolonged use.
- *Metoclopramide*—increased rate of absorption of paracetamol.
- *Warfarin*—monitor with long-term paracetamol therapy as INR may be raised.

Pharmacodynamic
- None known.

🎵 Dose
Pain and fever
- 0.5–1g PO or PR up to every 4–6 hours. Max. dose 4g in 24 hours.
- Alternatively, if necessary, 1g IV infusion every 4–6 hours. Max. dose 4g in 24 hours.

🎵 Dose adjustments
Elderly
- No dose adjustments are necessary.

Hepatic/renal impairment
- Dose reductions may be necessary in liver impairment; avoid if severe impairment
- For patients with severe renal impairment (CrCl <30mL/min), the dose interval of Perfalgan® should be increased to 6 hours.

Additional information
- Liver damage can occur with small increases of the dose above the 4g recommendation and so it is especially important to ensure that patients are not taking proprietary preparations as well as prescribed paracetamol or combination products.

⊕ Pharmacology
The precise analgesic action of paracetamol is unknown but it is generally accepted that it exerts its analgesic effect by inhibition of prostaglandin synthesis within the CNS. Recent studies have suggested that serotonergic pathways are involved. When used regularly it is an effective and useful analgesic and it can be a useful adjunct at any step on the WHO analgesic ladder.

Paracetamol is quickly absorbed after oral administration with a bioavailability of around 60%. After rectal administration, its bioavailability is considerably lower and absorption is often delayed and erratic. It is largely metabolized by conjugation reactions in the liver, but a minor route of paracetamol metabolism involves CYP1A2 and CYP2E1 which forms a reactive intermediate, *N*-acteyl-*p*-benzoquinimine (NAPQI). Usually, NAPQI is inactivated by conjugation with glutathione in the liver. However, following ingestion of a large amount of paracetamol the hepatic stores of glutathione become depleted so more NAPQI is available to cause hepatic damage and cellular death. Toxicity may occur following ingestion of approximately twice the normal daily dose (i.e. 14–16 paracetamol 500mg tablets in an adult). Drugs that induce CYP1A2 and CYP2E1 may increase the risk of paracetamol toxicity.

Paroxetine

Seroxat® (POM)
- **Tablet** (scored): 10mg (28); 20mg (30); 30mg (30)
- **Oral suspension** (sugar free): 10mg/5mL (150mL)

Generic (POM)
- **Tablet**: 20mg (30); 30mg (30)

Indications
- Anxiety
- Depression
- Panic
- * Pruritus

Contraindications and precautions
- Do not use with an irreversible MAOI, or within 14 days of stopping one, or at least 24 hours after discontinuation of a reversible MAOI (e.g. moclobemide, linezolid). Note that in exceptional circumstances linezolid may be given with paroxetine, but the patient must be closely monitored for symptoms of serotonin syndrome (☐ Box 1.10, p.19).
- Depression is associated with an increased risk of suicidal thoughts, self-harm, and suicide which persists until remission. Note that that the risk of suicide may increase during initial treatment.
- Hyponatraemia should be considered in all patients who develop drowsiness, confusion, or convulsions while taking an antidepressant. Hyponatraemia has been associated with all types of antidepressants, although it is reportedly more common with SSRIs.
- Use with caution in:
  - diabetes (alters glycaemic control)
  - elderly (greater risk of hyponatraemia)
  - epilepsy (lowers seizure threshold)
  - hepatic/renal impairment
  - glaucoma (may cause mydriasis).
- May precipitate psychomotor restlessness, which usually appears during early treatment.
- Avoid abrupt withdrawal as symptoms such as agitation, anxiety, confusion, diarrhoea, dizziness, emotional instability, nausea, and sleep disturbances (including intense dreams) can occur. Although generally mild, they can be severe in some patients. Withdrawal symptoms usually occur within the first few days of discontinuing treatment and they usually resolve within 2 weeks, although they can persist in some patients for up to 3 months or longer. See ☐ Discontinuing and/or Switching Antidepressants, p.45 for information about switching or stopping antidepressants.
- Paroxetine may increase the risk of haemorrhage (see ☐ Drug interactions, p.391).
- The oral suspension contains parabens, sunset yellow, and sorbitol which may cause allergic reactions in susceptible patients.

- Paroxetine may increase the risk of haemorrhage (see 📖 *Drug interactions*, p.391).
- It may modify reactions and patients should be advised not to drive (or operate machinery) if affected.

☺ Undesirable effects

Very common
- Nausea
- Sexual dysfunction

Common
- Agitation
- Appetite reduced
- Asthenia
- Diarrhoea
- Dizziness
- Drowsiness
- Dry mouth
- Headache
- Insomnia
- Sweating
- Tremor
- Weight gain
- Yawning

Uncommon
- Abnormal bleeding (e.g. bruising)
- Confusion
- Extrapyramidal symptoms
- Hallucinations
- Mydriasis

Rare
- Anxiety (mainly during initial treatment)
- Hyponatraemia
- Seizures

Very rare
- SIADH

Drug interactions

Pharmacokinetic
- Paroxetine is a potent CYP2D6 inhibitor and a moderate CYB2B6 inhibitor; it is metabolized by CYP2D6 and inhibits its own metabolism.
- *Codeine*—reduced analgesic benefit.
- *Haloperidol*—increased risk of undesirable effects from both drugs due to inhibition of CYP2D6. The clinical significance of co-administration with other inhibitors of CYP2D6 (📖 end cover) is unknown, but plasma concentrations of paroxetine may increase. The prescriber should be aware of the potential for interactions and that dose adjustments may be necessary.

- *Risperidone*—metabolism inhibited by paroxetine; increased risk of undesirable effects.
- *Tramadol*—reduced analgesic benefit.
- *Tricyclic antidepressants*—metabolism may be inhibited by paroxetine.
- The clinical significance of co-administration with other substrates of CYP2D6 (📖 end cover) is unknown. Caution is advised if paroxetine is co-administered with drugs that are predominantly metabolized by CYP2D6. The prescriber should be aware of the potential for interactions and that dose adjustments may be necessary, particularly for drugs with a narrow therapeutic index.
- The clinical significance of co-administration with substrates of CYP2B6 (📖 end cover) is unknown. The prescriber should be aware of the potential for interactions and that dose adjustments may be necessary, particularly for drugs with a narrow therapeutic index.
- Drugs that affect gastric pH (e.g. PPIs, H_2 antagonists, antacids) can reduce the absorption of the oral suspension. Dose increases may be necessary if swapping from the tablet formulation.

Pharmacodynamic

- *Anticoagulants*—potential increased risk of bleeding.
- *Carbamazepine* – increased risk of hyponatraemia.
- *Cyproheptadine*—may inhibit the effects of paroxetine.
- *Diuretics*—increased risk of hyponatraemia.
- *MAOIs*—risk of serotonin syndrome (see *Contraindications and precautions*).
- *NSAIDs*—increased risk of GI bleeding.
- *Serotonergic drugs* (e.g. duloxetine, methadone, mirtazapine, tricyclic antidepressants, tramadol and trazodone)—risk of serotonin syndrome (📖 Box 1.10, p.19).

💊 Dose

It is recommended that doses are taken with or after food.

Anxiety and depression

- Initial dose 20mg PO OM, increased gradually up to a maximum of 50mg PO OM in 10mg increments according to the patient's response.

Panic

- Initial dose 10mg PO OM, increased to a usual maximum of 40mg PO OM in 10mg increments according to the patient's response. Further dose increases up to 60mg PO OM may be required.

¥ Pruritus

- Initial dose 5mg PO OM, increased to a maximum of 20mg PO OM. Any beneficial effect may be short lived.

💊 Dose adjustments

Elderly

- Normal initial doses can be used, but the maximum dose should not exceed 40mg PO daily.

Hepatic/renal impairment
- Increased plasma concentrations of paroxetine occur in patients with hepatic impairment or those with severe renal impairment (CrCl <30mL/min). Wherever possible, doses at the lower end of the range should be used. Patients may be more susceptible to undesirable effects.

Additional information
- Remember that up to 10% of the Caucasian population are classified as poor CYP2D6 metabolizers which will have implications for treatment.
- If withdrawal symptoms emerge during discontinuation, increase the dose to prevent symptoms and then start to withdraw more slowly.
- Withdrawal symptoms may be more likely with paroxetine than with other SSRIs.
- Symptoms of anxiety or panic may worsen on initial therapy. This can be minimized by using lower starting doses.

❖ Pharmacology
Paroxetine is a potent and highly selective inhibitor of neuronal serotonin reuptake, with only very weak effects on noradrenaline and dopamine neuronal reuptake. It has a weak affinity for muscarinic receptors, but little affinity for α_1, α_2, D_2, 5-HT$_1$, 5-HT$_2$, and H$_1$ receptors. Paroxetine is metabolized primarily by CYP2D6 to virtually inactive metabolites which are excreted by the kidneys; it is a potent inhibitor of CYP2D6 and a moderate inhibitor of CYP2B6.

Phenobarbital

Generic (CD No Register POM)
Tablet: 15mg (28); 30mg (28); 60mg (28)
Elixir: 15mg/5mL (some products contain alcohol)
Injection (as phenobarbital sodium): 200mg/mL (10)

> Phenobarbital is a Schedule 3 controlled drug. Refer to 🕮 Legal categories of medicines, p.23 for further information.
>
> Note: Independent prescribers are **NOT** authorized to prescribe phenobarbital (🕮 Independent prescribing: palliative care issues, p.25).

Indications
- Epilepsy (not absence seizures).
- Status epilepticus.
- ⁑ Terminal agitation (in patients who have failed to be controlled by usual interventions).
- For end-of-life care issues see 🕮 Use of drugs in end-of-life care, p.53.

Contraindications and precautions
- Avoid phenobarbital in the following circumstances:
  - acute intermittent porphyria
  - severe respiratory depression
  - severe hepatic/renal impairment.
- Suicidal ideation and behaviour have been reported with anti-epileptics.
- Use with caution in:
  - children
  - elderly
  - hepatic impairment (avoid if severe)
  - hypothyroidism (increased metabolism of levothyroxine)
  - renal impairment (avoid if severe)
  - respiratory depression (avoid if severe).
- Avoid sudden withdrawal (may precipitate seizures).
- Phenobarbital may modify reactions and patients should be advised not to drive (or operate machinery) if affected.
- Phenobarbital sodium injection is strongly alkaline and **must** be diluted with 10 times its own volume of WFI before administration via IV injection or CSCI.

☺ Undesirable effects
The frequency is not defined, but reported undesirable effects include:
- Ataxia
- Cholestasis
- Confusion
- Drowsiness
- Hepatitis
- Hyperkinesia and behavioural disturbances in children
- Lethargy

- Local necrosis following SC injection (avoid)
- Megaloblastic anaemia (due to folate deficiency)
- Memory and cognitive impairment (especially in the elderly)
- Nystagmus
- Osteomalacia (with long-term treatment)
- Paradoxical excitement
- Respiratory depression
- Restlessness

Drug interactions

Pharmacokinetic

- Metabolized by CYP2C19. Induces CYP1A2, CYP2B6, CYP2C8/9 and CYP3A4.
- Affects many drugs through enzyme induction: 📖 end cover for potential list of affected drugs.
- *Clonazepam*—effect of clonazepam may be reduced.
- *Corticosteroids*—effect of corticosteroids reduced; higher doses necessary (possibly double or more).
- *Haloperidol*—effect of haloperidol reduced.
- *Fentanyl*—risk of reduced analgesic benefit.
- *Levothyroxine*—increased metabolism may precipitate hypothyroidism.
- *Mirtazapine*—effect of mirtazapine may be reduced.
- *Modafinil*—effect of modafinil may be reduced; may enhance effect of phenobarbital.
- *Oxycodone*—possible risk of reduced analgesic benefit.
- *Paracetamol*—may increase the risk of hepatoxicity of paracetamol.
- *Tramadol*—reduced analgesic benefit.
- The clinical significance of co-administration with other substrates of CYP1A2, CYP2B6, CYP2C8/9, and CYP3A4 (📖 end cover) is unknown. Caution is advised if phenobarbital is co-administered with drugs that are predominantly metabolized by these isoenzymes. The prescriber should be aware of the potential for interactions and that dose adjustments may be necessary, particularly for drugs with a narrow therapeutic index.
- The clinical significance of co-administration with CYP2C19 inducers or inhibitors (📖 end cover) is unknown. The prescriber should be aware of the potential for interactions and that dose adjustments may be necessary.

Pharmacodynamic

- *Antipsychotics*—seizure threshold lowered
- *Antidepressants*—seizure threshold lowered
- *CNS depressants*—risk of excessive sedation
- *MAOIs*—Avoid concurrent use
- *Tramadol*—seizure threshold lowered

♣ Dose

Epilepsy

- 60–180mg PO ON
- ¥ Alternatively, 200–400mg (11–22mL after dilution with 10 times own volume) via CSCI over 24 hours. If necessary, give stat dose of 100mg by IV injection (ensure dilution with 10 times own volume, i.e. dilute 0.5mL with 5mL WFI)

Status epilepticus

- 10mg/kg by IV injection at a rate of not more than 100mg/min. Ensure dilution with 10 times own volume of WFI.

¥ Terminal agitation

- Initial dose 100–200mg IM (undiluted) or IV (diluted with 10 times own volume) injection. Continue treatment with 200–600mg (11–33mL after dilution with 10 times own volume) via CSCI over 24 hours. Higher doses may be used, but the volume of infusion will necessitate 12-hourly infusions.

♣ Dose adjustments

Elderly

- No specific dose adjustments are suggested. Use the lowest dose possible and monitor the patient closely since the elderly are more susceptible to undesirable effects.

Hepatic/renal impairment

- Phenobarbital is contraindicated for use in severe hepatic or renal impairment. In mild to moderate impairment, no guidance is available; use the lowest effective dose and monitor for undesirable effects.

Additional information

- Phenobarbital sodium injection is incompatible with most drugs via CSCI. Unless compatibility information is available, it should be administered via a separate CSCI.
- The CSCI may be diluted with either WFI or NaCl. Dilution with NaCl may improve site tolerance.
- Therapeutic plasma concentration range: 15–40mg/L or 65–170µmol/L

⊕ Pharmacology

Phenobarbital is sedative anti-epileptic which acts on $GABA_A$ receptors, increasing synaptic inhibition by modulation of chloride currents through receptor channels. It may also affect calcium channels. It is extensively hepatically metabolized, principally by CYP2C19, and it is a potent inducer of CYP1A2, CYP2B6, CYP2C8/9, and CYP3A4. Many drugs are affected (see 📖 *Drug interactions*, p.395).

Pramipexole

Standard release

Mirapexin® (POM)
Tablet: 88mcg (30); 180mcg (scored—30; 100); 350mcg (scored—30; 100); 700mcg (scored—30; 100)

Prolonged release

Mirapexin® (POM)
Tablet: 0.26mg (30); 0.52mg (30); 1.05mg (30); 2.1mg (30); 3.15mg (30)

Indications
- Parkinson's disease (PD).
- Restless legs syndrome (RLS) (up to 540mcg daily).

Contraindications and precautions
- Use with caution in patients with:
  - psychotic disorders (antagonism between drugs)
  - renal impairment
  - severe cardiovascular disease (risk of hypotension—monitor BP during initiation).
- Dopamine receptor agonists can cause excessive daytime sleepiness and sudden onset of sleep.
- Behavioural symptoms of impulse control disorders and compulsions such as binge eating and compulsive shopping can occur. Dose reduction/tapered discontinuation should be considered.
- Pramipexole may modify reactions and patients should be advised not to drive (or operate machinery) if affected.
- Because of the risk of visual disturbances, ophthalmological monitoring is recommended at regular intervals
- Pramipexole must not be suddenly discontinued due to the risk of neuroleptic malignant syndrome. This only applies to PD as the dose for RLS does not exceed 0.54mg daily (although rebound symptoms can develop). The recommended withdrawal schedule is as follows:
  Standard release
  - taper dose at a rate of 0.54mg daily until the dose has been reduced to 0.54mg
  - reduce the dose thereafter by 0.264mg per day
  Modified release
  - taper dose at a rate of 0.52mg daily until the daily dose has been reduced to 0.52mg
  - reduce the dose thereafter by 0.26mg per day

☺ Undesirable effects
Undesirable effects are generally dose related. Therefore they are more likely to be experienced by patients receiving pramipexole for PD than for RLS.

Very common
- Dizziness
- Drowsiness
- Dyskinesia
- Hypotension
- Nausea

- Headache
- Insomnia
- Peripheral oedema
- Restlessness
- Vomiting
- Visual disturbance

Common
- Abnormal dreams
- Amnesia
- Confusion
- Constipation
- Fatigue
- Hallucinations

Uncommon
- Compulsive shopping
- Delusion
- Hypersexuality
- Paranoia
- Pathological gambling

Drug interactions

Pharmacokinetic
- Pramipexole is mainly eliminated unchanged by the kidneys.
- Drugs that are secreted by the cationic transport system (e.g. diltiazem, quinine, ranitidine, verapamil) have the potential to interact with prami- pexole, increasing plasma concentration. The clinical significance is unknown, and until further information is available the following is suggested:
  - if pramipexole is co-administered with these drugs, a slow and cautious titration is advisable
  - if these drugs are prescribed for a patient already using pramipexole, it is advisable to review the pramipexole dose (lower doses may be required).
- Drugs which affect renal function have the potential to interact with pramipexole. If such drugs are co-administered, regular monitoring of renal function is advisable. Such drugs include:
  - ACE-Is
  - NSAIDs.

Pharmacodynamic
- *Alcohol*—additive sedative effect.
- *CNS depressants*—additive sedative effect.
- *Dopamine antagonists (e.g. antipsychotics, metoclopramide)*—may decrease the efficiency of pramipexole because of dopamine antagonism.

⚗ Dose

Parkinson's disease

Standard release
- Initial dose 88mcg PO TDS. The dose can be doubled every 5–7 days if necessary and tolerated to 350mcg PO TDS;
- The dose can be further increased if necessary by 180mcg PO TDS at weekly intervals to a maximum of 3.3mg daily in 3 divided doses (i.e. 3 x 350mcg TDS)

Modified release
- Initial dose 0.26mg PO OD. The dose can be doubled every 5–7 days if necessary and tolerated to 1.05mg PO OD. If a further dose increase is necessary the daily dose should be increased by 0.52mg at weekly intervals up to a maximum dose of 3.15mg PO OD.

Restless legs syndrome
- Initial dose 88mcg PO 2–3 hours before bedtime

- The dose can be doubled every 4–7 days if necessary to 350mcg PO daily
- The dose can be further increased after 4–7 days to a maximum of 540mcg PO daily

⚑ Dose adjustments

Elderly

- No specific guidance available. Dose requirements should be individually titrated.

Hepatic/renal impairment

- Dose adjustment in patients with hepatic impairment is not required.
- The elimination of pramipexole depends on renal function. The manufacturer gives advice on dosing that is dependent on condition being treated:
- Parkinson's disease:
  - Patients with a CrCl > 50mL/min require no reduction in dose.

Standard release

- For a CrCl >50mL/min, initial dose should be 88mcg PO BD. A maximum daily dose of 1.57mg PO OD should not be exceeded.
- If CrCl >20mL/min, the recommended dose is 88mcg PO OD. A maximum dose of 1.1mg PO OD should not be exceeded.
- If renal function deteriorates during treatment, reduce the dose by the same percentage as the decline in creatine clearance.

Prolonged release

- For a CrCl 30–50mL/min, initial dose 0.26mg PO ALT DIE, increasing to 0.26mg PO OD after 7 days. If necessary, the dose may be further increased by 0.26mg at weekly intervals up to a maximum dose of 1.57mg PO OD.
- For a CrCl <30mL/min, treatment with prolonged release tablets is not recommended and the use of the standard release formulation should be considered.
- Restless legs syndrome:
  - Patients with CrCl >20mL/min require no reduction in dose
  - For patients with CrCl <20mL/min, a dose reduction will be necessary, although the initial dose cannot practically be reduced.

Additional information

- Pramipexole is given orally as the dihydrochloride monohydrate (DHCM) salt but doses are described in terms of the base. Dose equivalents are:
  - pramipexole base 88mcg = pramipexole DHCM 125mcg
  - pramipexole base 180mcg = pramipexole DHCM 350mcg
  - pramipexole base 350mcg = pramipexole DHCM 500mcg
  - pramipexole base 700mcg = pramipexole DHCM 1mg.
- Tablets can be crushed and mixed with water immediately prior to administration if necessary

⊙ Pharmacology

Pramipexole is a dopamine agonist which binds with high selectivity and specificity to dopamine receptors; it has a preferential affinity for D_3 receptors. The mechanism of action of pramipexole as treatment for PD or RLS is unknown, although in the former case it is believed to be related to its ability to stimulate dopamine receptors in the striatum. Pramipexole is completely absorbed after oral administration. It is metabolized to a small extent, with the majority of the dose being renally excreted.

Prednisolone

Generic (POM)
Tablet: 1mg (28); 5mg (28); 25mg (56)
Tablet (*enteric-coated*): 2.5mg (30); 5mg (30)
Soluble tablet: 5mg (30)

Indications
- Suppression of inflammatory and allergic disorders.
- Also inflammatory bowel disease, asthma, immunosupression, rheumatic disease, adjunct to chemotherapy.

Contraindications and precautions
- The use of dexamethasone is contraindicated in systemic infection unless specific anti-infective therapy is employed.
- Patients without a definite history of chickenpox should be advised to avoid close personal contact with chickenpox or herpes zoster.
- Caution is advised when considering the use of systemic corticosteroids in patients with the following conditions:
  - concurrent use of NSAIDs (see 📖 *Drug interactions*, p.402)
  - congestive heart failure
  - diabetes mellitus (risk of hyperglycaemia—close monitoring of blood glucose recommended)
  - epilepsy (see 📖 *Drug interactions*, p.402)
  - glaucoma
  - hypertension
  - hypokalaemia (correct before starting dexamethasone)
  - liver or renal impairment (see 📖 *Dose adjustments*, p.403)
  - osteoporosis (see *BNF* for bisphosphonate guidance)
  - peptic ulceration
  - psychotic illness (symptoms can emerge within a few days or weeks of starting the treatment).

☺ Undesirable effects
The frequency is not defined. Undesirable effects are generally predictable and related to dose, timing of administration, and the duration of treatment. They include the following.
- Endocrine:
  - diabetes mellitus
  - hirsutism
  - hyperlipidemia
  - weight gain
- Fluid and electrolyte disturbances:
  - congestive heart failure
  - hypertension
  - hypokalaemia
  - sodium and water retention
- Gastrointestinal:
  - acute pancreatitis
  - dyspepsia peptic ulceration with perforation

Prednisolone withdrawal

In patients who have received more than physiological doses of systemic corticosteroids (i.e. >7.5mg prednisolone) for >3 weeks, withdrawal should be gradual in order to avoid acute adrenal insufficiency. Abrupt withdrawal of doses of up to 40mg daily of prednisolone for 3 weeks is unlikely to lead to clinically relevant HPA suppression in the majority of patients. In the following cases, withdrawal may need to be more gradual:

- Patients who have had repeated courses of systemic corticosteroids, particularly if taken for >3 weeks.
- Patients receiving doses of systemic corticosteroid >40mg daily of prednisolone.
- Patients repeatedly taking doses in the evening.

There is no evidence as to the best way to withdraw corticosteroids and it is often performed with close monitoring of the patient's condition. The dose may initially be reduced rapidly (e.g. by halving the dose daily) to physiological doses (approximately 7.5mg prednisolone) and then more slowly (e.g. 1mg per week for 1–2 weeks). A 'withdrawal syndrome' may also occur including fever, myalgia, arthralgia, rhinitis, conjunctivitis, painful itchy skin nodules, and loss of weight.

In dying patients, once the decision is made to withdraw corticosteroids, they can be discontinued abruptly. Patients with brain tumours may require additional analgesia as raised intracranial pressure can develop and may manifest as worsening headache, or terminal restless-ness.

- haemorrhage
- Musculoskeletal:
  - aseptic necrosis of femoral head
  - avascular necrosis
  - loss of muscle mass
  - osteoporosis
  - proximal myopathy
  - tendon rupture
- Neurological:
  - aggravation of epilepsy
  - anxiety
  - confusion
  - depression
  - insomnia
  - mood elevation
  - psychotic reactions
- Other:
  - glaucoma

- impaired wound healing
- Increased susceptibility and severity of infections (signs can be masked)
- sweating

Drug interactions

Pharmacokinetic

- Prednisolone is metabolized by CYP3A4.
- Note that low activity of CYP3A4 (e.g. through inhibition) can contribute to the development of osteonecrosis of the femoral head.
- *Carbamazepine*—effect of prednisolone likely to be reduced; consider doubling the prednisolone dose and monitor the response.
- *Colestyramine*—may decrease the absorption of prednisolone.
- *Erythromycin*—may increase the effects of prednisolone through inhibition of CYP3A4.
- *Phenytoin*—effect of prednisolone likely to be reduced; consider doubling the prednisolone dose and monitor the response.
- The clinical significance of co-administration with other inducers or inhibitors of CYP3A4 (🕮 end cover) is unknown. The prescriber should be aware of the potential for interactions and that dose adjustments may be necessary.

Corticosteroid-induced osteoporosis

- Patients aged over 65 years and with prior or current exposure to oral corticosteroids are at increased risk of osteoporosis and bone fracture. Treatment with corticosteroids for periods as short as 3 months may result in increased risk. Three or more courses of corticosteroids taken in the previous 12 months are considered to be equivalent to at least 3 months of continuous treatment.
- Prophylactic treatment (e.g. bisphosphonate, calcium and vitamin D supplements, hormone replacement therapy) should be considered for all patients who may take an oral corticosteroid for ≥3 months.

- Avoid excessive amounts of grapefruit juice as it may increase the bioavailability of prednisolone through inhibition of intestinal CYP3A4.

Pharmacodynamic

- *Anticoagulants*—increased risk of bleeding.
- *Anti-hypertensives*—effect antagonized by prednisolone.
- *Ciclosporin*—additive immunosuppressive effect; convulsions reported with combination.
- *Diuretics*—effect antagonized by prednisolone; increased risk of hypokalaemia and hyperglycaemia.
- *Hypoglycaemic drugs*—effect antagonized by prednisolone.
- *NSAIDs*—increased risk of GI toxicity.
- *SSRIs*—increased risk of bleeding.

⚕ Dose

- Initial dose up to 10–20mg PO OD (severe disease up to 60mg PO daily) preferably in the morning

- With acute conditions, the dose can usually be reduced after a few days but may need to be continued for several weeks or months, tapering to the lowest effective dose
- Maintenance dose is usually 2.5–15mg PO OD

Dose adjustments

Elderly
- No specific dose adjustments are necessary. Use the lowest dose for the shortest duration possible since the elderly are more susceptible to undesirable effects.

Hepatic/renal impairment
- No specific guidance available. The lowest effective dose should be used for the shortest duration possible.

Additional information

- Prednisolone is less commonly used in palliative care than dexamethasone as it has a slightly higher mineralocorticoid activity.
- Consider oral hygiene with prednisolone use. The patient may develop oral thrush and need a course of nystatin.
- Oral anti-inflammatory corticosteroid equivalences are:
  - dexamethasone 750mcg = hydrocortisone 20mg = prednisolone 5mg.

Pharmacology

Prednisolone is a synthetic corticosteroid used as a replacement or adjunctive therapy in a wide range of inflammatory or allergic conditions. It is rapidly and almost completely absorbed after oral administration. Prednisolone is metabolized primarily in the liver by CYP3A4 to inactive metabolites which, together with small amounts of unchanged drug, are excreted renally.

Pregabalin

Lyrica® (POM)
Capsule: 25mg (56; 84), 50mg (84), 75mg (56), 100mg (84), 150mg (56), 200mg (84), 225mg (56), 300mg (56)

Indications
- Central and peripheral neuropathic pain
- Generalized anxiety disorder
- Adjunctive therapy for partial seizures
- ¥ Malignant bone pain
- ¥ Sleep improvement

Contraindications and precautions
- Avoid sudden withdrawal. Discontinue gradually over at least a week in order to avoid undesirable effects such as nausea, vomiting, flu syndrome, anxiety, and insomnia. These withdrawal effects have been reported even after short-term use.
- Suicidal ideation and behaviour have been reported with anti-epileptics.
- Caution in renal impairment—dose adjustments may be necessary (see 📖 *Dose adjustments,* p.405).
- Use with caution in patients with congestive heart failure.
- Diabetic patients may need to adjust hypoglycaemic treatment as weight gain occurs.
- If affected by drowsiness and dizziness, patients should be warned about driving.

☺ Undesirable effects
Very common
- Dizziness
- Drowsiness

Common
- Blurred vision
- Confusion
- Constipation
- Dry mouth
- Erectile dysfunction
- Fatigue
- Impaired memory
- Increase in appetite
- Paraesthesia
- Peripheral oedema
- Tremor
- Vomiting
- Weight gain (effect may plateau after 3–4 months)

Uncommon
- Agitation
- Hallucinations

- Myoclonus
- Panic
- Sweating

Unknown
- Congestive heart failure
- Headache
- Loss of vision

Drug interactions

Pharmacokinetic
- No clinically significant pharmacokinetic drug interactions.

Pharmacodynamic
- Opioids—possible opioid-sparing affect, necessitating opioid dose review.
- CNS depressants—increased risk of CNS undesirable effects.

♪ Dose

- Initially 75mg PO BD, increased weekly by 150mg to a maximum dose of 300mg PO BD after 2 weeks.
- May only need to take dose at bedtime if used for sleep improvement.
- The licensed schedule is shown in the Table 3.13. This may be poorly tolerated by elderly patients or those with cancer, and a more cautious titration is suggested for these patients. Whichever strategy is adopted, undesirable effects are more common around the time of dose escalation but usually resolve in a few weeks. The slower titration may be preferred in the elderly or cancer population, although it may take longer to appreciate the therapeutic benefit.

Table 3.13 Dose schedules for pregabalin

	Licensed dose		Suggested dose
Day 1	75mg PO BD	Day 1	25mg PO ON
Days 3–7	150mg PO BD	Day 2	25mg PO BD
Day 10–14	300mg PO BD	Days 6–7	75mg PO BD
Increase dose according to response. Maximum dose 600mg/day. Dose can be given TDS if needed		Increase dose by 25mg BD every 2 days as needed to a maximum of 600mg/day	

♪ Dose adjustments

Elderly
- May require a more cautious titration as described in Table 3.13, or may need a dose reduction due to renal impairment (Table 3.14).

Renal impairment
- Dose adjustments are necessary for patients in renal failure or undergoing haemodialysis (Table 3.14).

Table 3.14 Pregabalin dosage for patients with renal impairment

Creatinine clearance (mL/min)	Maximum dose
≥60	300mg PO BD
≥30 – <60	150mg PO BD
≥15 – <30	75mg PO BD or 150mg PO OD
<15	75mg PO OD

A supplementary dose should be given immediately after every 4 hour haemodialysis treatment.

Additional information

- Neuropathic pain and anxiety can improve within a week.
- Pregabalin can be readily dissolved in water. If necessary, the capsules can be opened and mixed with water prior to use, although the solution may have a bitter taste. There are no problems flushing the solution down an enteral feeding tube.
- Avoid TDS dosing—treatment costs increase without offering significant improvement in outcome.

✦ Pharmacology

Pregabalin is an anti-epileptic which reduces the release of neurotransmitters through an interaction with the $\alpha_2\delta$ subunit of voltage-dependent calcium channels. Its bioavailability is >90% which, unlike gabapentin, is independent of dose. Pregabalin is excreted by the kidneys, with 98% of an administered dose being excreted unchanged in urine, so dose adjustment is required in renal impairment.

Propantheline

Pro-Banthine® (POM)
Tablet: 15mg (112)

Indications
- Smooth muscle spasm (e.g. bladder, bowel).
- Sweating.
- Urinary frequency.

Contraindications and precautions
- Propantheline is contraindicated in patients with:
  - hiatus hernia associated with reflux oesophagitis
  - myasthenia gravis
  - narrow-angle glaucoma
  - obstructive diseases of the GI or urinary tract
  - paralytic ileus
  - prostatic enlargement
  - pyloric stenosis
  - severe ulcerative colitis
  - toxic megacolon.
- It should be used with caution in patients with the following:
  - cardiac arrhythmias
  - congestive heart failure
  - coronary heart disease
  - dementia
  - Down's syndrome
  - elderly (see 📖 Dose adjustments)
  - GI reflux disease
  - hepatic impairment
  - hypertension
  - hyperthyroidism
  - pyrexia (reduces sweating)
  - renal impairment
  - ulcerative colitis.
- Propantheline may modify reactions and patients should be advised not to drive (or operate machinery) if affected.

☺ Undesirable effects
The frequency is not defined, but reported undesirable effects include:
- Confusion
- Difficulty in micturition
- Dizziness
- Drowsiness
- Dry mouth
- Inhibition of sweating
- Palpitations
- Tachycardia
- Visual disturbances

◈ Drug interactions

Pharmacokinetic

- No recognised pharmacokinetic interactions.

Pharmacodynamic

- *Donepezil*—effect may be antagonized.
- *β_2-agonists*—increased risk of tachycardia.
- *Cyclizine*—increased risk of undesirable anticholinergic effects.
- *Domperidone*—may inhibit prokinetic effect.
- *Galantamine*—effect may be antagonized.
- *Metoclopramide*—may inhibit prokinetic effect
- *Nefopam*—increased risk of undesirable anticholinergic effects.
- *Rivastigmine*—effect may be antagonized.
- *TCAs*—increased risk of undesirable anticholinergic effects.

◈ Dose

Tablets should be taken at least 1 hour before food:

- Initial dose 15mg PO BD–TDS, increased if necessary up to maximum of 30mg PO QDS.

◈ Dose adjustments

Elderly

- No specific guidance available. Use the lowest effective dose as the elderly may be more susceptible to undesirable effects. In particular, there is an increased risk for cognitive decline and dementia.

Hepatic/renal impairment

- No specific guidance available. Use the lowest effective dose.

Additional information

- Tablets may be dispersed in water immediately prior to administration if necessary.

◈ Pharmacology

Propantheline is an anticholinergic drug which blocks the action of acetylcholine at post-ganglionic sites including smooth muscle, secretory glands, and CNS sites. It inhibits peristalsis, reduces gastric acid secretion, and decreases pharyngeal, tracheal, and bronchial secretions. Propantheline is extensively metabolized, mostly in the small intestine prior to absorption.

Quinine sulphate

Generic (POM)
Tablet: 200mg (28); 300mg (28)

Indications
- Nocturnal leg cramps.
- Falciparum malaria—not discussed.

Contraindications and precautions
- Quinine is contraindicated for use in patients with:
  - glucose 6-phosphate dehydrogenase (G6PD) deficiency (*use not justified for the treatment of leg cramps*)
  - haemoglobinuria
  - myasthenia gravis
  - optic neuritis
  - tinnitus.
- Quinine should be used with caution in patients with:
  - atrial fibrillation
  - cardiac conduction defects
  - heart block.

☺ Undesirable effects
The frequency is not defined, but reported undesirable effects include:
- Cinchonism (related to dose and duration of therapy)
- Confusion
- Diarrhoea
- Hypersensitivity (e.g. angio-oedema)
- Nausea
- Severe headache
- Tinnitus
- Visual disturbances (e.g. blurred vision, night blindness, diplopia)
- Vomiting

> Quinine is extremely toxic in overdose. Urgent advice must be sought if overdose is suspected.

Drug interactions
Pharmacokinetic
- Quinine is metabolized by CYP3A4. It is an inhibitor of CYP2D6 and CYP2C8/9.
- *Digoxin*—plasma concentration of digoxin can rise by >50% (reduce digoxin dose and monitor levels).
- *Warfarin*—INR may increase due to inhibition of CYP2C8/9.
- The clinical significance of co-administration with substrates of CYP2D6 or CYP2C8/9 (📖 end cover) is unknown. Caution is advised if quinine is co-administered with drugs that are predominantly metabolized by CYP2D6 or CYP2C8/9. The prescriber should be aware of the potential for interactions and that dose adjustments may be necessary, particularly for drugs with a narrow therapeutic index.

- The clinical significance of co-administration with pro-drug substrates of CYP2D6 (e.g. codeine, tramadol) is unknown. The prescriber should be aware of the potential for interactions and that dose adjustments may be necessary.
- Inhibitors of CYP3A4 (📖 end cover) may increase plasma concentrations of quinine; other factors may be necessary before this interaction becomes clinically significant (e.g. co-administration of other interacting drugs).
- Grapefruit juice is not believed to affect quinine significantly. Nonetheless, avoid excessive intake.
- The clinical significance of co-administration of inducers of CYP3A4 (📖 end cover) is unknown. The effect of quinine may be reduced.

Pharmacodynamic
- Quinine can cause dose-related prolongation of the QT interval. There is a potential risk that co-administration with other drugs that also prolong the QT interval (e.g. amiodarone, erythromycin, haloperidol) may result in an increased risk of developing ventricular arrhythmias.

⚕ Dose
Take evening dose with a snack or milk to reduce GI irritation. The tablets must be swallowed whole.

Nocturnal leg cramps
- 200–300mg PO ON.

⚕ Dose adjustments
Elderly
- No specific guidance is available. Use the lowest effective dose.

Hepatic/renal impairment
- No specific guidance is available for either hepatic or renal impairment. Since reduced clearance may occur in hepatic impairment, the patient should be monitored for signs of excessive dose. Renal clearance accounts for <20% of total clearance, but accumulation may occur as renal function deteriorates.

Additional information
- May need a trial of up to 4 weeks before benefit is seen. Discontinue if no benefit.
- Treatment should be interrupted at intervals of approximately 3 months to assess the need for further treatment.
- As quinine has an irritant nature, the tablet should not be crushed.

➔ Pharmacology
Quinine is believed to affect calcium distribution within muscle fibres and also decrease the excitability of the motor endplate region. It is well absorbed orally (80%) and undergoes extensive hepatic metabolism, with the major metabolic pathway thought to involve glucuronidation, although CYP3A4 is also involved.

Rabeprazole

Pariet® (POM)
Tablet: 10mg (28); 20mg (28)

Indications
- Treatment of benign gastric and duodenal ulcer.
- Treatment and maintenance of gastro-oesophageal reflux disease.
- ¥ Treatment and prophylaxis of NSAID-associated peptic ulcer disease.

Contraindications and precautions
- Treatment with rabeprazole may lead to a slightly increased risk of developing GI infections (e.g. *Clostridium difficile*). Therefore avoid unnecessary use or high doses.
- Do not administer with atazanavir or erlotinib.
- Use with caution in patients with severe hepatic dysfunction (see 📖 *Dose adjustments*, p.413).
- Rabeprazole may modify reactions and patients should be advised not to drive (or operate machinery) if affected.
- Rebound acid hypersecretion may occur on discontinuation if the patient has received treatment for more than 8 weeks.

☺ Undesirable effects
Common
- Abdominal pain
- Asthenia
- Cough
- Diarrhoea
- Dizziness
- Flatulence
- Headache
- Influenza-like illness
- Insomnia

Uncommon
- Abnormal LFTs
- Arthralgia
- Drowsiness
- Dry mouth
- Myalgia
- Rash

Rare
- Blood dyscrasias
- Depression
- Hepatitis
- Jaundice
- Pruritus
- Visual disturbance
- Weight gain

Unknown
- Confusion
- Gynaecomastia
- Oedema

Drug interactions

Pharmacokinetic
- Rabeprazole is metabolized by CYP2C19 and CYP3A4; it has a weak-moderate inhibitory effect on CYP2C19.
- Drugs with pH-dependent absorption can be affected:
  - *atazanavir*—avoid combination because of substantially reduced absorption
  - *digoxin*—increased plasma concentrations possible
  - *erlotinib*—avoid combination as bioavailability of erlotinib can be significantly reduced
  - *ketoconazole/itraconazole*—risk of sub-therapeutic plasma concentrations
  - *metronidazole suspension*—rabeprazole may reduce/prevent the absorption of metronidazole
- *Antacids*—should be given at least 1 hour before rabeprazole (reduced bioavailability).
- *Azole antifungals*—proton pump inhibitors may decrease the absorption of itraconazole and ketoconazole.
- *Clopidogrel*—antiplatelet action may be reduced.
- The clinical significance of co-administration with CYP2C19 or CYP3A4 inducers or inhibitors (☐ end cover) is unknown. The prescriber should be aware of the potential for interactions and that dose adjustments may be necessary.
- Although the clinical significance is unknown, co-administration of rabeprazole may increase the levels/effects of CYP2C19 substrates (☐ end cover). The prescriber should be aware of the potential for interactions and that dose adjustments may be necessary.

Pharmacodynamic
- No clinically significant interactions noted.

↯ Dose

Treatment of benign gastric and duodenal ulcer
- 20mg PO OM for 4–8 weeks.

Treatment of gastro-oesophageal reflux disease
- 20mg PO OM for 48 weeks.

Maintenance of gastro-oesphageal reflux disease
- 10–20mg PO OM.

¥ Treatment and prophylaxis of NSAID-associated peptic ulcer disease
- 20mg PO OM.

⚖ Dose adjustments

Elderly
- No dose adjustments are necessary.

Hepatic/renal impairment
- No dose adjustments are necessary for patients with liver or renal impairment.

Additional information
- Tablets should not be chewed or crushed, but should be swallowed whole.

⟿ Pharmacology
Rabeprazole is a gastric proton pump inhibitor which reduces the release of H^+ from parietal cells by inhibiting H^+/K^+-ATPase. It is rapidly inactivated by gastric acid; hence oral formulations are enteric coated. It is extensively metabolized by CYP2C19 and CYP3A4 and the metabolites are excreted principally in the urine. Note that CYP2C19 poor metabolizers (or patients taking CYP2C19 inhibitors) can have significantly higher plasma concentrations, leading to unexpected results.

Ranitidine

Zantac® (POM)
Tablet: 150mg (60); 300mg (30)
Effervescent tablet: 150mg (60); 300mg (30)
Syrup (*sugar-free*): 75mg/5mL (300mL)
Injection: 50mg/2mL (5)

Generic (POM)
Tablet: 150mg (60); 300mg (30)
Effervescent tablet: 150mg (60); 300mg (30)
Oral solution: 75mg/5mL (300mL)

Note: Ranitidine can be sold in pharmacies for the short-term symptomatic relief of heartburn, dyspepsia, and hyperacidity, and for the prevention of these symptoms when associated with consumption of food or drink in those aged over 16 years at a maximum single dose of 75mg and a maximum daily dose of 300mg.

Indications
- Treatment of duodenal and benign gastric ulcers.
- Prevention of NSAID-associated duodenal ulcers.
- * Prevention of NSAID-associated gastric ulcers.
- Oesophageal reflux disease.
- Chronic episodic dyspepsia.
- Symptomatic relief in gastro-oesophageal reflux disease.
- Zollinger–Ellison syndrome.
- For end-of-life care issues see 📖 Use of drugs in end-of-life care, p.53.

Contraindications and precautions
- Use with caution in patients with renal impairment (see 📖 Dose adjustments, p.416).
- Ranitidine should be avoided in patients with a history of acute porphyria.
- The elderly may be at a greater risk of developing community-acquired pneumonia when prescribed ranitidine.
- Zantac® effervescent tablets contain aspartame—avoid in phenylketonuria (check individual generic products).

☺ Undesirable effects
Common
- Diarrhoea
- Dizziness
- Headache

Uncommon
- Hypersensitivity reactions
- Reversible blurred vision
- Skin rash

Rare
- Depression

Unknown
- Acute interstitial nephritis
- Acute pancreatitis
- Alopecia
- Arthralgia
- Bradycardia
- Confusion
- Gynaecomastia
- Galactorrhoea
- Hallucinations
- Hepatitis
- Jaundice
- Leucopenia
- Thrombocytopenia

Drug interactions

Pharmacokinetic
- Elimination of ranitidine is mainly as unchanged drug via the kidneys. Several minor metabolic pathways involve CYP1A2, CYP2C19, and CYP2D6. It is unlikely to be involved in cytochrome-related interactions.
- Drugs with pH-dependent absorption can be affected:
  - *atazanavir*—avoid combination because of substantially reduced absorption.
  - *digoxin*—increased plasma concentrations possible.
  - *erlotinib*—take erlotinib at least 2 hours before or 10 hours after H_2 antagonist.
  - *ketoconazole/itraconazole*—risk of sub-therapeutic plasma concentrations.
  - *metronidazole suspension*—ranitidine may reduce/prevent the absorption of metronidazole.

Pharmacodynamic
- No clinically significant interactions noted.

Dose

Treatment of duodenal ulcer and benign gastric ulcer
- 150mg PO BD or 300mg PO ON for at least 4 weeks.
- A further 4 week course may be necessary; 8 weeks' treatment may be required for ulcers associated with NSAIDs.

Prevention of NSAID-associated duodenal ulcers
- 300mg PO BD.
- ☀ Alternatively, 150–300mg via CSCI over 24 hours.

¥ *Prevention of NSAID-associated gastric ulcers*
- 300mg PO BD
- Alternatively, 150–300mg via CSCI over 24 hours.

Oesophageal reflux disease
- 150mg PO BD or 300mg PO ON for 8–12 weeks.

Dose can be increased to 150mg PO QDS in severe cases
- ¥ Alternatively, 150–300mg via CSCI over 24 hours

Chronic episodic dyspepsia
- 150mg PO BD for up to 6 weeks
- ¥ Alternatively, 150–300mg via CSCI over 24 hours

Gastro-oesophageal reflux disease
- 150mg PO BD for 2 weeks
- ¥ Alternatively, 150–300mg via CSCI over 24 hours

Zollinger–Ellison syndrome
- 150mg PO TDS, increased as necessary up to a maximum of 6g PO daily in divided doses.

♣ Dose adjustments
Elderly
- No dose adjustments are necessary. However, given the risk of developing community-acquired pneumonia, ranitidine should be used at the lowest dose and for the shortest duration possible.

Hepatic/renal impairment
- For liver impairment, no specific guidance is available. However, ranitidine is excreted via the kidneys mainly as the free drug, so dose adjustments are unlikely.
- In patients with CrCl <50mL/min, the daily dose of ranitidine should be 150mg PO ON. This can be increased to 150mg PO BD if necessary and reviewed after 4–8 weeks.

Additional information
- Ranitidine is generally considered a second-line option gastro-protective agent; PPIs remain the first choice. However, in certain circumstances, such as intolerable adverse effects, ranitidine may be preferred.
- By CSCI, ranitidine is compatible with cyclizine, diamorphine, glycopyrronium, haloperidol, hyoscine butylbromide, hyoscine hydrobromide, ketorolac, octreotide, and oxycodone. It is incompatible with levomepromazine, midazolam and phenobarbital.

⊕ Pharmacology
Ranitidine is a non-imidazole histamine H_2 receptor antagonist which blocks the action of histamine on parietal cells in the stomach, thereby decreasing gastric acid secretion.

Reboxetine

Edronax® (POM)

Tablet (*scored*): 4mg (60)

Indications
• Major depression

Contraindications and precautions
• Use with caution in patients with epilepsy because of the risk of seizures.
• Clinical experience with reboxetine in patients affected by comorbidity is limited. Close supervision should be applied in patients with current evidence of:
  • cardiac disease
  • glaucoma
  • prostatic hypertrophy
  • urinary retention.
• Depression is associated with an increased risk of suicidal thoughts, self-harm, and suicide which persists until remission. Note that that the risk of suicide may increase during initial treatment.
• Use with caution in the elderly as experience is limited.
• Avoid abrupt withdrawal, although there does not appear to be a withdrawal syndrome.
• Do not use with an MAOI, or within 14 days of stopping one; avoid concomitant use with linezolid or moclobemide. At least a week should elapse after stopping reboxetine therapy before starting an MAOI.

☺ Undesirable effects

Very common
• Insomnia
• Dry mouth
• Constipation
• Sweating

Common
• Vertigo
• Tachycardia
• Palpitation
• Vasodilation
• Postural hypotension
• Loss of appetite
• Urinary hesitancy (treat with an α_1-antagonist such as tamsulosin)
• Urinary tract infections
• Sexual dysfunction (including ejaculatory and testicular pain, impotence)

Unknown
- Aggression
- Agitation
- Allergic dermatitis/rash
- Anxiety
- Cold extremities
- Hallucination
- Hypertension
- Hypokalaemia
- Irritability
- Nausea
- Paraesthesia
- Suicidal ideation
- Vomiting

Drug interactions

Pharmacokinetic
- Reboxetine is metabolized by CYP3A4. It may have weak inhibitory actions on CYP2D6 and CYP3A4, but at concentrations which exceed those in clinical use.
- The clinical significance of co-administration with CYP3A4 inducers or inhibitors (📖 end cover) is unknown. The prescriber should be aware of the potential for interactions and that dose adjustments may be necessary.
- Avoid excessive amounts of grapefruit juice as it may increase the bio-availability of reboxetine through inhibition of intestinal CYP3A4.

Pharmacodynamic
- *Diuretics*—increased risk of hypokalaemia.
- *MAOIs*—risk of serotonin syndrome (see *Contraindications and precautions*).
- *Tramadol*—increased risk of seizures.

Dose
- 4mg PO BD increased if necessary after 3–4 weeks to 10mg PO daily in divided doses; maximum dose 12mg PO daily.

Dose adjustments

Elderly
- Manufacturer does not recommend use in the elderly because of insufficient data.

Hepatic/renal impairment
- Initial dose in patients with liver or renal impairment should be 2mg PO BD, which can be increased as necessary and as tolerated, but must not exceed 12mg PO daily.

Additional information

- If necessary, the tablets can be crushed and dispersed in water prior to use.
- Onset of therapeutic action is usually not immediate, but is often delayed 2–4 weeks.
- Although some undesirable anticholinergic effects may appear, reboxetine does not directly antagonize cholinergic receptors. These effects are due in some degree to α_1-receptor activation, causing acetylcholine release.
- May have beneficial analgesic effects when combined with an opioid.

⮿ Pharmacology

Reboxetine is a selective noradrenaline reuptake inhibitor (NaRI). It has a weak effect on serotonin reuptake but no effect on dopamine reuptake. Reboxetine has no significant affinity for muscarinic receptors. It is predominantly metabolized by CYP3A4, with approximately 10% of the dose excreted unchanged in urine.

Repaglinide

Prandin® (POM)

Tablet: 500mcg (30, 90); 1mg (30, 90); 2mg (90)

Indications

- Type 2 diabetes mellitus (as monotherapy or in combination with metformin when metformin alone is inadequate).

Contraindications and precautions

- Contraindicated for use in patients with:
  - concurrent use of gemfibrozil (see 📖 *Drug interactions, (below)*)
  - ketoacidosis
  - severe hepatic impairment.
- Repaglinide should be used with caution or be avoided in patients receiving drugs which affect CYP2C8.
- Use with caution in:
  - debilitated or malnourished patients (lower initial doses recommended)
  - renal impairment (increased insulin sensitivity).

☺ Undesirable effects

Common

- Abdominal pain
- Diarrhoea
- Hypoglycaemia

Rare

- Constipation
- Visual disturbances
- Vomiting

Drug interactions

Pharmacokinetic

- Is mainly metabolized by CYP2C8. A minor pathway involves CYP3A4 (which becomes important if CYP2C8 is inhibited). Repaglinide is a substrate for active hepatic uptake via organic anion transporting (OAT) protein. Certain drugs may interfere with this process.
- *Ciclosporin*—increases the effect of repaglinide, possibly through inhibition of OAT.
- *Gemfibrozil*—combination contraindicated (CYP2C8 inhibition).
- The clinical significance of co-administration with other CYP2C8 inhibitors or inducers (📖 end cover) is unknown. The prescriber should be aware of the potential for interactions and that dose adjustments may be necessary.

Pharmacodynamic

- *Metformin*—increased risk of hypoglycaemia.
- Drugs that may precipitate hyperglycaemia may interfere with blood glucose control, e.g.
  - corticosteroids
  - diuretics
  - nifedipine.

♣ Dose

- Initial dose 500mcg PO within 30 minutes of main meals; starting dose of 1mg is recommended if transferring from another oral hypoglycaemic
- Patients who skip a meal (or add an extra meal) should be instructed to skip (or add) a dose for that meal.
- The dose is titrated individually according to response at intervals of 1–2 weeks
- Up to 4mg may be given as a single dose; maximum dose 16mg PO daily

♣ Dose adjustments

Elderly

- No specific guidance is available. Use the lowest effective dose.

Hepatic/renal impairment

- No specific guidance is available for use in mild to moderate hepatic impairment. Use the lowest effective dose. Repaglinide is contraindicated for use in patients with severe hepatic impairment.
- Repaglinide is mainly excreted via hepatic metabolism, so renal impairment is unlikely to cause problems. Nonetheless, the manufacturer advises caution in renal impairment because of an increase in insulin sensitivity.

Additional information

- Tablets can be crushed and mixed with water immediately prior to administration if necessary.

⊹ Pharmacology

Repaglinide closes ATP-dependent potassium channels in the β-cell membrane. This depolarizes the β cell, leading to opening of the calcium channels. The resulting increased calcium influx induces insulin secretion. The net effect is an acute lowering of blood glucose. Note that repaglinide requires functioning β cells if it is to work. It is rapidly absorbed orally and virtually completely metabolized to inactive compounds. The majority of the dose is excreted in bile.

Risperidone

Risperdal® (POM)
Tablet (*scored*): 500mcg (20); 1mg (20, 60); 2mg (60); 3mg (60); 4mg (60); 6mg (28)
Liquid: 1mg/mL (100mL)

Risperdal Quicklet® (POM)
Orodispersible tablet: 500mcg (28); 1mg (28); 2mg (28), 3mg (28); 4mg (28)

Generic (POM)
Tablet: 500mcg (20); 1mg (20, 60); 2mg (60); 3mg (60); 4mg (60); 6mg (28)
Orodispersible tablet: 500mcg (28); 1mg (28); 2mg (28); 3mg (28); 4mg (28)
Liquid: 1mg/mL (100mL)

Indications
Short term (up to 6 weeks) management of aggression in Alzheimer's dementia
- Psychosis.
- ¥ Delirium.
- ¥ Anti-emetic (refractory nausea and vomiting).
- ¥ Major depression.

Warning
Risperidone can be used for the short-term (up to 6 weeks) management of aggression in patients with Alzheimer's dementia where there is a risk of harm to the patient and others. Note that there is a clear risk of CVA and small increased risk of mortalilty when antipsychotics are used in elderly people with dementia.
- Risperidone should not be used to treat behavioural symptoms of dementia. Elderly patients with dementia-related psychosis treated with risperidone are at an increased risk of CVA.
- For acute psychosis, risperidone may be used for short-term treatment only, under specialist advice. The risks associated with CVA (e.g. diabetes, hypertension, smoking) should be assessed before commencing treatment with risperidone.
- Avoid combination of risperidone and furosemide. Treatment with this combination is associated with a higher mortality than with either drug alone.

Contraindications and precautions
- Phenylketonuria—*Risperdal Quicklet*® contains aspartame, a source of phenylalanine.
- Use with caution in:
  - diabetes (risk of hyperglycaemia in elderly)
  - epilepsy (seizure threshold may be lowered)
  - hepatic/renal impairment (see 🕮 *Dose adjustments*, p.424)

• Parkinson's disease (risperidone may interfere with treatment).
• Orthostatic hypotension may occur during initiation.
• Avoid sudden withdraw treatment as this may lead to recurrence of symptoms or, rarely, acute withdrawal symptoms such as nausea, vomiting, and sweating.
• Electrolyte disturbances (e.g. hypokalaemia) must be corrected.
• Risperidone may modify reactions and patients should be advised not to drive (or operate machinery) if affected.

☺ Undesirable effects

Very common
• Agitation
• Anxiety
• Extrapyramidal symptoms (dose-dependent)
• Headache
• Insomnia
• Weight gain (may be >5%)

Common
• Constipation
• Cough
• Dizziness
• Dry mouth
• Fatigue
• Hypotension
• Nausea and vomiting
• Restlessness
• Rhinitis
• Sedation
• Sexual dysfunction
• Tremor

Uncommon
• Hyperglycaemia

Drug interactions

Pharmacokinetic
• Risperidone is metabolized mainly by CYP2D6; a minor pathway involves CYP3A4.
• *Carbamazepine* significantly reduces the plasma concentrations of both risperidone and the active metabolite (CYP3A4 induction). The dose of risperidone may need to be titrated accordingly when carbamazepine is added or discontinued.
• The clinical significance of co-administration with other CYP3A4 inducers or inhibitors (📖 end cover) is unknown. The prescriber should be aware of the potential for interactions and that dose adjustments may be necessary.
• Co-administration with inhibitors of CYP2D6 (📖 end cover) may increase plasma concentrations of risperidone, potentially increasing the benefit, but also the risk of undesirable effects. The prescriber

should be aware of the potential for interactions and that dose adjustments may he necessary.

Pharmacodynamic

- Risperidone can cause dose-related prolongation of the QT interval. There is a potential risk that co-administration with other drugs that also prolong the QT interval (e.g. amiodarone, erythromycin, quinine) may result in ventricular arrhythmias.
- *Antiepileptics*—may need to be increased to take account of the lowered seizure threshold.
- *CNS depressants*—additive sedative effect.
- *Levodopa and dopamine agonists*—effect antagonized by risperidone.
- *Levomepromazine*—increased risk of extrapyramidal symptoms.
- *Metoclopramide*—increased risk of extrapyramidal symptoms.

Unknown

- *Furosemide*—increased risk of death in elderly patients with dementia.

Dose

Psychosis

- Initial dose 1mg PO BD, increasing on the second day to 2mg PO BD. Some patients may benefit from a slower dose increase (see 📖 *Dose adjustments*). Dose can be increased further to a usual maximum of 3mg PO BD. Higher doses are possible, but should be used under expert supervision.

¥ *Delirium*

- Initial dose 500mcg PO BD, increased as necessary by 500mcg PO daily to a usual maximum of 1mg PO BD. Unusual to require higher doses.

¥ *Refractory nausea and vomiting*

- Initial dose 500mcg PO ON. Usual maximum of 1mg PO ON.

¥ *Major depression*

- Initial dose 1mg PO ON, increased to 1mg PO BD or 2mg PO ON if necessary after 1–2 weeks. To be used in conjunction with standard antidepressant monotherapy.

Dose adjustments

Elderly

- For psychosis and delirium, an initial dose of 500mcg PO BD is suggested. Increase by 500mcg PO once or twice daily to a maximum of 2mg PO BD.
- For major depression or refractory nausea and vomiting, an initial dose of 250–500mcg PO ON is suggested. No more than 1mg PO ON should be necessary.

Hepatic/renal impairment

- The manufacturer advises caution in this group of patients because data are lacking. For all indications, starting and consecutive dosing should be halved, and dose titration should be slower for patients with hepatic or renal impairment.

Additional information

- Weight gain generally occurs during the first 6–12 months of treatment.
- The solution can be mixed with water, black coffee, or orange juice prior to administration.
- In the absence of the oral solution, risperidone tablets should be crushed and dispersed in water immediately prior to use. The resulting suspension will easily pass through an NG tube.
- Risk of extrapyramidal effects with risperidone is lower than with haloperidol.
- Risperidone may be a useful anti-emetic for refractory nausea and vomiting (D_2 and 5-HT_2 receptor antagonist).

⊕ Pharmacology

Risperidone is a benzisoxazole antipsychotic which acts as a 5-HT_2 and D_2 receptor antagonist. The serotonin antagonism is believed to improve negative symptoms of psychoses and reduce the incidence of undesirable extrapyramidal effects. Risperidone is also an antagonist at α_1, α_2, and H_1 receptors, with no activity at muscarinic receptors. It is rapidly absorbed well orally and extensively metabolized by CYP2D6 to the active metabolite, 9-hydroxyrisperidone. A minor metabolic pathway involves CYP3A4, but significant induction can reduce the effectiveness of risperidone (see 📖 *Drug interactions*, p.423). Since risperidone metabolism involves CYP2D6, the effect of drug inhibition and polymorphism must be considered if unexpected results are observed.

Ropinirole

Standard release

Adartrel® (POM)
Tablet: 250mcg (12); 500mcg (28; 84); 2mg (28; 84)

Requip® (POM)
Tablet: 1mg (84); 2mg (84); 5mg (84)
Tablet (*starter pack*): 250mcg (42), 500mcg (42), 1mg (21)
Tablet (*follow-on pack*): 500mcg (42), 1mg (42), 2mg (63)

Modified release

Requip® XL (POM)
Tablet: 2mg (28); 4mg (28); 8mg (28)

Indications

- Restless legs syndrome (*Adartrel®*).
- Parkinson's disease (*Requip®* & *Requip® XL*).

Contraindications and precautions

- Manufacturers state that ropinirole should not be used in patients with severe hepatic or renal impairment (CrCl <30mL/min).
- Ropinirole should be used with caution in patients with:
  - cardiovascular disease (risk of arrhythmias and hypotension—monitor BP during initiation)
  - hepatic impairment
  - major psychotic disorders (antagonism between drugs)
  - renal impairment.
- Paradoxical worsening of restless legs syndrome symptoms can occur; dose adjustment or discontinuation should be considered.
- Dopamine receptor agonists can cause excessive daytime sleepiness and sudden onset of sleep
- Behavioural symptoms of impulse control disorders and compulsions such as binge eating and compulsive shopping can occur. Dose reduction/tapered discontinuation should be considered.
- Ropinirole may modify reactions and patients should be advised not to drive (or operate machinery) if affected.

☺ Undesirable effects

Very common
- Dyskinesia
- Drowsiness
- Nausea

Common
- Abdominal pain
- Confusion
- Constipation
- Dizziness
- Dyspepsia
- Fatigue

- Hallucinations
- Hypotension
- Nervousness
- Peripheral oedema
- Vomiting

Uncommon
- Delirium
- Delusion
- Hypersexuality
- Paranoia
- Pathological gambling

Drug interactions

Pharmacokinetic
- Ropinirole is metabolized by CYP1A2; it may inhibit CYP2D6.
- *Ciprofloxacin*—increased plasma concentrations of ropinirole
- Smoking may increase the clearance of ropinirole. If a patient starts or stops smoking, dose adjustments may be necessary.
- The clinical significance of co-administration with CYP1A2 inducers or inhibitors (📖 end cover) is unknown. The prescriber should be aware of the potential for interactions and that dose adjustments may be necessary.

Pharmacodynamic
- *Alcohol*—additive sedative effect.
- *CNS depressants*—additive sedative effect.
- *Dopamine antagonists* (e.g. antipsychotics, metoclopramide)—may decrease the efficiency of ropinirole because of dopamine antagonism.

ꙮ Dose

Parkinson's disease

Standard release
- Initial dose 250mcg PO TDS. The dose can be increased by increments of 750mcg at weekly intervals to 1mg PO TDS. Further dose increases can be made in increments of up to 3mg per week.
- Usual dose range is 9–16mg PO in three divided doses; maximum dose 24mg PO daily.

Modified release
- To be used in patients with stable Parkinson's disease who are transferring from a standard-release formulation
- Initial dose is based on the previous total daily dose of a standard-release formulation. If patients are taking a total daily dose of ropinirole immediate-release tablets that is different to those available as modified release, they should be switched to the nearest available dose.
- If control of symptoms is not achieved or maintained:

- in patients receiving less than 8mg PO OD, increase in steps of 2mg at intervals of at least 1 week to 8mg PO OD according to response
- in patients receiving more than 8mg PO OD, increase in steps of 2mg at intervals of at least 2 weeks according to response to a maximum of 24mg PO OD

Restless legs syndrome
- Initial dose 250mcg PO ON for 2 days, increased if tolerated to 500mcg PO ON for 5 days. The dose can be increased if necessary to 1mg PO ON for 7 days. Further dose increases of 500mcg per week over a 2 week period to a dose of 2mg PO OD can be made if needed. The maximum daily dose of 4mg is achieved by increasing the dose by 500mcg per week over a 2 week period to 3mg PO OD, followed by an additional 1mg PO OD thereafter.

Dose adjustments
Elderly
- No specific guidance available. The manufacturers state that dose increases should be gradual and titrated against the symptomatic response.

Hepatic/renal impairment
- Use with caution in moderate hepatic impairment, but avoid in patients with severe hepatic impairment.
- Doses adjustment is unnecessary in patients with mild-moderate renal impairment (CrCl 30-50mL/min). Ropinirole is contraindicated for use in patients with severe renal impairment (CrCl <30mL/min).

Additional information
- In the management of restless legs syndrome, if treatment is interrupted for more than a few days, ropinirole should be re-initiated by dose titration as described above.
- Down-titration followed by more gradual up-titration has been shown to be beneficial for patients experiencing intolerable undesirable effects.
- Standard-release tablets can be dispersed in water immediately prior to administration if necessary.

Pharmacology
Ropinirole is a dopamine D_2 and D_3 receptor agonist. The mechanism of action of ropinirole as treatment for Parkinson's disease or restless legs syndrome is unknown, although in the former case it is believed to be related to its ability to stimulate dopamine receptors in the striatum. Ropinirole is completely absorbed after oral administration. It is extensively metabolized by CYP1A2 to inactive metabolites that are mainly excreted in the urine.

Rosiglitazone

Avandia® (POM)

Tablet: 4mg (28; 56); 8mg (28)

With metformin

Avandamet® (POM)

Tablet: rosiglitazone 2mg, metformin hydrochloride 500mg (112); rosiglitazone 2mg, metformin hydrochloride 1g (56); rosiglitazone 4mg, metformin hydrochloride 500mg (56).

Indications

- Type 2 diabetes mellitus (alone or combined with metformin or with a sulphonylurea or with both); particularly useful for obese patients.

Contraindications and precautions

- Contraindicated for use in patients with:
  - acute coronary syndrome (unstable angina, NSTEMI and STEMI)
  - cardiac failure
  - diabetic ketoacidosis
  - hepatic impairment.
- Avoid combination with insulin (unless under specialist supervision) since the risks of cardiac failure and/or ischaemia increase.
- Use with caution in patients with renal impairment (see 📖 *Dose adjustments*)
- Rosiglitazone has been associated with hepatic dysfunction. Ensure LFTs are checked prior to treatment and periodically thereafter. If the patient develops symptoms such as unexplained nausea, vomiting, abdominal pain, fatigue, anorexia, and/or dark urine, LFTs should be checked. Withdraw treatment if LFTs significantly altered or jaundice develops.
- There is a risk of cardiac ischaemia with rosiglitazone. Therefore use with caution in patients with ischaemic heart disease.
- Patients are more at risk of hypoglycaemia when rosiglitazone is used in combination with a sulphonylurea or insulin.
- When used in combination with metformin and a sulphonylurea, patients are more at risk of developing fluid retention and heart failure, as well as hypoglycaemia.

☻ Undesirable effects

Common

- Altered blood lipids
- Anaemia
- Bone fracture (female patients)
- Cardiac ischaemia
- Constipation
- Increased appetite
- Oedema
- Weight increase (may be fluid retention)

Rare
- Congestive heart failure
- Macular oedema

Drug interactions

Pharmacokinetic
- Metabolized by CYP2C8. It may act as an inhibitor of CYP2C8.
- The clinical significance of co-administration with CYP2C8 inducers, inhibitors, or substrates (□ end cover) is unknown. The prescriber should be aware of the potential for interactions and that dose adjustments may be necessary.

Pharmacodynamic
- *NSAIDs*—increased risk of oedema.
- Drugs that may precipitate hyperglycaemia may interfere with blood glucose control, e.g.
  - corticosteroids
  - diuretics
  - nifedipine.

Dose
- Initial dose 4mg PO OD.
- May be increased after 8 weeks to 8mg PO daily (in 1–2 divided doses) according to response (undertake cautiously in patients also receiving a sulphonylurea—risk of fluid retention).

Dose adjustments

Elderly
- No dose adjustments are necessary based on age alone.

Hepatic/renal impairment
- Rosiglitazone is contraindicated for use in patients with hepatic impairment.
- No dose adjustment is necessary in patients with mild or moderate renal impairment. Rosiglitazone should be used with caution in patients with severe renal insufficiency (CrCl <30mL/min) due to lack of data.

Additional information
- Tablets can be crushed and mixed with water immediately prior to administration if necessary

⊹ Pharmacology
Rosiglitazone is a selective agonist at the peroxisomal proliferator activated receptor gamma (PPARγ) nuclear receptor. It is a member of the thiazolidinedione class of anti-diabetic agents. PPARγ receptors in adipose tissue, skeletal muscle, and liver regulate the transcription of insulin-responsive genes involved in the control of glucose production, transport, and utilization. Therefore rosiglitazone increases tissue sensitivity to insulin. It is well absorbed after oral administration and is completely metabolized, predominantly by CYP2C8. A minor pathway involves CYP2C9.

Salbutamol

Airomir® (POM)
Aerosol inhalation: 100mcg/metered dose (200 dose unit)
Autohaler®: 100mcg/metered dose (200 dose breath-actuated unit)

Asmasal Clickhaler® (POM)
Dry powder for inhalation: 95mcg/metered dose (200 dose unit)

Salamol Easi-Breathe® (POM)
Aerosol inhalation: 100mcg/metered dose (200 dose breath-actuated unit)

Salbulin Novolizer® (POM)
Dry powder for inhalation: 100 mcg/metered dose (200 refillable dose)

Ventolin® (POM)
Dry powder for inhalation: 200 mcg/blister (60 doses via *Accuhaler®*)
Aerosol inhalation: 100 mcg/metered dose (200 dose unit)
Nebulizer solution: 2.5mg/2.5mL (20 unit dose vials); 5mg/2.5mL (20 unit dose vials)
Respirator solution: 5mg/mL (20mL multi-dose bottle)

Generic (POM)
Aerosol inhalation: 100mcg/metered dose (200 dose unit)
Dry powder for inhalation: 100mcg/metered dose (200 dose unit)
Inhalation powder (Cyclocaps® capsules for use with Cyclohaler®): 200mcg (120); 400mcg (120)
Nebulizer solution: 2.5mg/2.5mL (20 unit dose vials); 5mg/2.5mL (20 unit dose vials)

Indications
- Asthma and other conditions associated with reversible airways obstruction.
- Consider nebulizer treatment for patients with persistent symptoms, despite regular inhaler therapy.

Contraindications and precautions
- Potentially serious hypokalaemia may result from β_2-agonist treatment. Caution is required if salbutamol is used in combination with theophylline and its derivatives, corticosteroids, and diuretics.
- Use with caution in patients with:
  - arrhythmias
  - cardiovascular disease
  - diabetes (may need to monitor blood glucose more frequently)
  - hypertension
  - hyperthyroidism
  - susceptibility to QT-interval prolongation.

☺ Undesirable effects

Common
- Tremor
- Headache
- Tachycardia

Uncommon
- Mouth and throat irritation
- Muscle cramps

Rare
- Hypokalaemia

Drug interactions

Pharmacokinetic
- Metabolized by CYP3A4, but there are no clinically significant pharmacokinetic interactions

Pharmacodynamic
- *Corticosteroids*—increased risk of hypokalaemia.
- *Diuretics*—increased risk of hypokalaemia.
- *Non-selective β-blockers* (e.g. propranolol)—antagonize effect of salbutamol; avoid concurrent use.
- *Theophylline*—risk of hypokalaemia.

♣ Dose

Dry powder inhalation
- 200–400mcg PRN up to QDS

Aerosol inhalation
- 100–200mcg PRN up to QDS.

Nebulized solution
- 2.5–5mg PRN up to QDS.
- Can be given more frequently in severe cases (maximum dose 40mg daily), but monitor for undesirable effects

♣ Dose adjustments

Elderly
- Usual adult doses can be used. However, note that the elderly are more susceptible to undesirable effects.

Hepatic/renal impairment
- No specific dose reductions stated.

Additional information
- If dilution of the unit dose vials is necessary, use only sterile NaCl 0.9%.
- Angina may be precipitated with high doses of nebulized salbutamol in susceptible patients.
- The patient should be reminded to clean the aerosol inhaler at least once a week by to prevent blockages.

✈ Pharmacology

Salbutamol is a selective β_2-adrenoceptor agonist which produces a cascade of intracellular events terminating in smooth muscle relaxation. Following inhalation, up to 20% of the dose is deposited in the lungs, with the majority being swallowed (and undergoes significant first-pass metabolism).

Salmeterol

Serevent® (POM)
Dry powder for inhalation: 50 mcg/blister (60 doses via Accuhaler® or 4x15 dose via Diskhaler®)
Aerosol inhalation: 25mcg/metered dose (120 dose unit)

Compound formulations

Seretide® 100, 250, and 500 Accuhaler® (POM)
Dry powder for inhalation, containing salmeterol 50mcg/blister and increasing doses of fluticasone (100, 250, and 500mcg/blister) (60 blisters per Accuhaler®).

Seretide® 50, 125 and 250 Evohaler® (POM)
Aerosol inhalation, containing salmeterol 25mcg/metered dose and increasing doses of fluticasone (50, 125, and 250mcg/metered dose) (120 dose unit).

Indications
- Add-on treatment of reversible airways obstruction.
- COPD.
- Prevention of exercise-induced asthma.

Contraindications and precautions
- Potentially serious hypokalaemia may result from β_2-agonist treatment. Caution is required if salbutamol is used in combination with theophylline and its derivatives, corticosteroids, and diuretics.
- Use with caution in patients with:
  - arrhythmias
  - cardiovascular disease
  - diabetes (may need to monitor blood glucose more frequently)
  - hypertension
  - hyperthyroidism
  - susceptibility to QT-interval prolongation.
- Use with caution in patients receiving CYP3A4 inhibitors (see 📖 *Drug interactions*, p.435).
- Salmeterol should not be used for relief of acute exacerbations of breathlessness.

☻ Undesirable effects

Common
- Headache
- Muscle cramps
- Palpitations
- Tremor

Uncommon
- Nervousness
- Tachycardia

Rare
- Dizziness
- Hypokalaemia

Drug interactions

Pharmacokinetic

- Metabolized by CYP3A4. Despite very low systemic levels, there is a potential for drug interactions.
- *Erythromycin*—interaction is unlikely to be clinically significant. Caution if additional CYP3A4 inhibitors are prescribed.
- *Ketoconazole*—avoid combination; risk of salmeterol toxicity.
- The clinical significance of co-administration with CYP3A4 inducers or inhibitors (🕮 end cover) is unknown. The prescriber should be aware of the potential for interactions and that dose adjustments may be necessary.

Pharmacodynamic

- *Corticosteroids*—increased risk of hypokalaemia.
- *Diuretics*—increased risk of hypokalaemia.
- *Non-selective β-blockers* (e.g. propranolol)—antagonize effect of salbutamol; avoid concurrent use.
- *Theophylline*—risk of hypokalaemia.

⚕ Dose

Serevent®

- Usual dose 50mcg BD.
- In severe cases, dose can be increased to 100mcg BD.

Seretide®

- Usual dose 50mcg salmeterol/100mcg fluticasone BD (via *Accuhaler®*) *or* 25mcg salmeterol/50mcg fluticasone BD (via *Evohaler®*).
- Dose can be increased as necessary to maximum 50mcg salmeterol/500mcg fluticasone BD (via *Accuhaler®*) *or* 25mcg salmeterol/250mcg fluticasone BD (via *Evohaler®*).

⚕ Dose adjustments

Elderly

- Usual adult doses can be used. However, note that the elderly are more susceptible to undesirable effects.

Hepatic/renal impairment

- No specific dose reductions stated for patients with hepatic impairment.
- Manufacturer states that dose adjustments are unnecessary in patients with renal impairment.

Additional information

• The patient should be reminded to clean the aerosol inhaler at least once a week by to prevent blockages.
• Review need for steroid card with *Seretide*® preparations.

❖ Pharmacology

Salmeterol is a selective long-acting β_2-adrenoceptor agonist with a duration of action of approximately 12 hours.

Senna (sennosides)

Senokot® (P)
Tablet: 7.5mg (60)
Syrup (*sugar-free*): 7.5mg/5mL (500mL)

Generic (P)
Tablet: 7.5mg (60)
Note: Senna is available as a GSL medicine provided that the maximum dose does not exceed 15mg.

Indications
- Management of constipation.

Contraindications and precautions
- Contraindicated in intestinal obstruction.
- Avoid in patients with abdominal pain of unknown origin.

☺ Undesirable effects
- May cause abdominal cramps.

Drug interactions
Pharmacokinetic
- No known pharmacokinetic interactions.

Pharmacodynamic
- *Anticholinergics*—antagonizes the laxative effect.
- *Cyclizine*—antagonizes the laxative effect.
- *Opioids*—antagonizes the laxative effect.
- *5-HT$_3$ antagonists*—antagonizes the laxative effect.
- *Tricyclic antidepressants*—antagonizes the laxative effect.

Dose
- Initial dose 7.5–15mg PO ON, usually in combination with a stool softener.
- Higher doses may be necessary for patients receiving opioids. The licensed maximum dose is 30mg PO ON, but as much as 60mg in divided doses may be required

Dose adjustments
Elderly
- No specific dose adjustments recommended by the manufacturer

Hepatic/renal impairment
- No specific dose adjustments recommended by the manufacturer

Additional information
- Laxative effect is usually evident within 8–12 hours.

⊹ Pharmacology

Sennosides are inactive glycosides that pass through to the large intestine, where they are hydrolysed by bacteria to the active anthraquinone fraction. This stimulates peristalsis via the submucosal and myenteric nerve plexuses. Very little reaches the systemic circulation.

Sertraline

Lustral® (POM)
Tablet (*scored*): 50mg (28); 100mg (28)

Generic (POM)
Tablet: 50mg (28); 100mg (28)

Indications
- Depression (including anxiety).
- Obsessive–compulsive disorder.
- ⌀ Cholestatic pruritus.

Contraindications and precautions
- Do not use with an irreversible MAOI, or within 14 days of stopping one, or at least 24 hours after discontinuation of a reversible MAOI (e.g. moclobemide, linezolid). At least 14 days should elapse after discontinuing sertraline before starting an MAOI or reversible MAOI. Note that in exceptional circumstances linezolid may be given with sertraline, but the patient must be closely monitored for symptoms of serotonin syndrome (📖 Box 1.10, p.19).
- Contraindicated for use in patients with significant hepatic impairment.
- Depression is associated with an increased risk of suicidal thoughts, self-harm, and suicide which persists until remission. Note that that the risk of suicide may increase during initial treatment.
- Hyponatraemia should be considered in all patients who develop drowsiness, confusion, or convulsions while taking an antidepressant. Hyponatraemia has been associated with all types of antidepressants, although it is reportedly more common with SSRIs.
- Use with caution in:
  - diabetes (alters glycaemic control)
  - elderly (greater risk of hyponatraemia)
  - epilepsy (lowers seizure threshold)
  - hepatic/renal impairment (see below).
- Avoid abrupt withdrawal as symptoms such as anxiety, dizziness, headache, nausea, and paraesthesia can occur. Although generally mild, they can be severe in some patients. Withdrawal symptoms usually occur within the first few days of discontinuing treatment and they usually resolve within 2 weeks, although in some patients they can persist for up to 3 months or longer. Refer to 📖 Discontinuing and/or switching antidepressants, p.45 for information about switching or stopping antidepressants.
- Sertraline may increase the risk of haemorrhage (see 📖 *Drug interactions*, p.440).
- It may modify reactions and patients should be advised not to drive (or operate machinery) if affected.

☺ Adverse effects

The frequency is not defined, but reported undesirable effects include:

- Abnormal bleeding
- Anorexia
- Anxiety
- Diarrhoea
- Dizziness
- Drowsiness
- Dry mouth
- Dyspepsia
- Headache
- Insomnia
- Nausea
- Sexual dysfunction
- Sweating
- Tremor

Drug interactions

Pharmacokinetic

- Sertraline is a moderate inhibitor of CYP2B6, CYP2C19, CYP2D6, and CYP3A4. It is metabolized by CYP2C19 and CYP2D6, and a minor pathway involves CYP3A4.
- The clinical significance of co-administration with inducers, inhibitors, or other substrates of CYP2C19 (□ end cover) is unknown. The prescriber should be aware of the potential for interactions and that dose adjustments may be necessary.
- The clinical significance of co-administration with inhibitors or other substrates of CYP2D6 (□ end cover) is unknown. Caution is advised if sertraline is co-administered with drugs that are predominantly metabolized by CYP2D6 (e.g. haloperidol, risperidone, tricyclic antidepressants). The prescriber should be aware of the potential for interactions and that dose adjustments may be necessary, particularly for drugs with a narrow therapeutic index.
- The clinical significance of co-administration with prodrug substrates of CYP2D6 (e.g. codeine, tramadol) is unknown. The prescriber should be aware of the potential for interactions and that dose adjustments may be necessary.
- The clinical significance of co-administration with CYP3A4 inducers or substrates (□ end cover) is unknown. The prescriber should be aware of the potential for interactions and that dose adjustments may be necessary.
- The clinical significance of co-administration with substrates of CYP2B6 (□ end cover) is unknown. The prescriber should be aware of the potential for interactions and that dose adjustments may be necessary.

Pharmacodynamic

- *Anticoagulants*—potential increased risk of bleeding.
- *Carbamazepine*—increased risk of hyponatraemia.
- *Cyproheptadine*—may inhibit the effects of setraline.
- *Diuretics*—increased risk of hyponatraemia.
- *MAOIs*—risk of serotonin syndrome (see *Contraindications and precautions*).
- *NSAIDs*—increased risk of GI bleeding.
- *Serotonergic drugs* (e.g. duloxetine, methadone, mirtazapine, tricyclic antidepressants, tramadol and trazodone)—risk of serotonin syndrome (□ Box 1.10, p.19).

♪ Dose

Anxiety and depression
- Initial dose 50mg PO OD, increased if necessary to 200mg PO OD. Usual maintenance dose is 50mg PO OD.

Obsessive–compulsive disorder
- Initial dose 50mg PO OD, increased if necessary to 200mg PO OD. Usual maintenance dose is 50mg PO OD.

¥ *Cholestatic pruritus*
- Initial dose 50mg PO OD, increased as necessary after 7 days to a usual maintenance of 75–100mg PO OD. Note that the effect may be short-lived.

♪ Dose adjustments

Elderly
- The usual adult dose can be recommended.

Hepatic/renal impairment
- Sertraline is extensively metabolized and is contraindicated for use in patients with significant hepatic impairment.
- The manufacturer states that a lower or less frequent dose of sertraline should be used in patients with hepatic impairment.
- In renal impairment, doses at the lower end of the range should be used wherever possible.

Additional information

- Tablets can be dispersed in water prior to administration if necessary. However, they do not disperse easily.
- Remember that up to 10% of the Caucasian population are classified as poor CYP2D6 metabolizers which may have implications for treatment.
- If withdrawal symptoms emerge during discontinuation, increase the dose to prevent symptoms and then start to withdraw more slowly.
- Symptoms of anxiety or panic may worsen on initial therapy. This can be minimized by using lower starting doses.

♪ Pharmacology

Sertraline is a potent and specific inhibitor of neuronal serotonin uptake but has little affinity for adrenergic, benzodiazepine, dopaminergic, GABA, histaminergic, muscarinic or serotonergic receptors. Sertraline and its major metabolite are extensively metabolized, and the resultant metabolites are excreted in faeces and urine in equal amounts. Only a very small amount of unchanged sertraline is excreted in the urine.

Sevelamer

Renagel (POM)
Tablet: 800mg (180)

Indications
- Hyperphosphataemia in adult patients receiving haemodialysis or peritoneal dialysis.

Contraindications and precautions
- Contraindicated for use in patients with bowel obstruction.

☺ Undesirable effects
Very common
- Nausea
- Vomiting

Common
- Abdominal pain
- Constipation
- Diarrhoea
- Dyspepsia
- Flatulence

Unknown
- Bowel obstruction
- Ileus

Drug interactions
Pharmacokinetic
- Sevelamer should not be given with the following drugs:
  - *ciclosporin*—reduced absorption
  - *ciprofloxacin*—reduced oral absorption by up to 50%
  - *mycophenolate*—reduced absorption
  - *tacrolimus*—reduced absorption.

Pharmacodynamic
- None known.

🥄 Dose
- Initial dose 800mg—1.6g PO TDS with meals, then adjusted according to plasma phosphate concentration.
- Usual range 2.4–12g PO daily in three divided doses.

🥄 Dose adjustments
Elderly
- No specific dose adjustments recommended by the manufacturer.

Hepatic/renal impairment
• No specific dose adjustments recommended by the manufacturer.

⊕ Pharmacology

Sevelamer is a phosphate-binding drug used to prevent hyperphosphataemia in patients with chronic renal failure. It is taken with meals and binds to dietary phosphate, thereby preventing its absorption.

Spironolactone

Aldactone® (POM)
Tablet: 25mg (100); 50mg (100); 100mg (28)

Generic (POM)
Tablet: 25mg (28); 50mg (28); 100mg (28)

Unlicensed special (POM)
Oral suspension (*sugar-free*): 5mg/5mL, 10mg/5mL, 25mg/5mL, 50mg/5mL, 100mg/5mL (see 📖 *Additional information* for supply issues.

Indications
- Congestive cardiac failure (NYHA class III or IV disease)
- Ascites associated with cirrhosis or malignancy.
- Nephrotic syndrome.
- Primary aldosteronism.

Contraindications and precautions
- Contraindicated in patients with:
  - acute renal insufficiency
  - Addison's disease
  - anuria
  - hyperkalaemia, or baseline serum K^+ >5mmol/l
  - severe renal impairment (e.g. SECr >220µmol/l).
- Monitor urea and electrolyte status regularly. May cause hyperkalaemia, hyponatraemia, and a reversible hyperchloraemic metabolic acidosis.
- Spironolactone may modify reactions and patients should be advised not to drive (or operate machinery) if affected.

☺ Undesirable effects
The frequency is not defined, but reported undesirable effects include:
- Confusion
- Dizziness
- Drowsiness
- Gynaecomastia (related to dose and duration of therapy; usually reversible)
- Headache
- Hyperkalaemia
- Hyponatraemia
- Nausea
- Sexual dysfunction

Drug interactions

Pharmacokinetic

- *Digoxin*—half-life of digoxin is increased by spironolactone (plasma concentration increased <30%).

Pharmacodynamic

- *ACE inhibitors*—increased risk of hyperkalaemia and additive hypotensive effect.
- *Angiotensin II antagonists*—increased risk of hyperkalaemia and additive hypotensive effect.
- *Potassium-sparing diuretics*—increased risk of hyperkalaemia and additive hypotensive effect.
- *Potassium supplements*—increased risk of hyperkalaemia.
- *NSAIDs*—may attenuate the natriuretic efficacy of diuretics because of inhibition of intra-renal synthesis of prostaglandins

Dose

It is recommended that doses are taken with or after food. Renal function should be closely monitored during treatment. There is a lag of 3–5 days between initiation of spironolactone and the onset of the natriuretic effect.

Congestive cardiac failure

- Spironolactone should only be used in moderate to severe heart failure on the recommendation of specialist advice. There is no evidence that spironolactone is particularly effective in mild heart failure.
- Initial dose 25mg PO OM, increased if necessary to 50mg PO OM. Higher doses are indicated, but are not recommended.
- If K^+ rises to 5.5mmol/l or creatinine rises to >220µmol/l reduce dose to 25mg PO on alternate days.
- If K^+ ≥6.0mmol/l or creatinine ≥310µmol/l, stop spironolactone immediately and seek specialist advice.
- Check U&Es at 1, 4, 8, and 12 weeks; 6, 9, and 12 months; 6 monthly thereafter.

Ascites

- Initial dose 100mg PO OM. Increase as necessary to a maximum of 400mg PO daily (in divided doses).
- Stop if Na^+ <120mmol/l.
- Consider adding furosemide if not achieving the desired effect.

⚖ Dose adjustments

Elderly
- No specific guidance available. Dose requirements should be individually titrated.

Hepatic/renal impairment
- No specific guidance available. Dose requirements should be individually titrated. Severe hepatic and renal impairment may affect metabolism and excretion.

Additional information

- Spironolactone can interfere with digoxin assays.
- Excessive liquorice intake could reduce the effectiveness of spironolactone.
- An oral suspension is available from Rosemont Pharmaceuticals Ltd as an unlicensed special (Tel: 0113 244 1999).
- Tablets may be dispersed in water immediately prior to use if necessary.
- Advise patients not to self-medicate with NSAIDs.
- As with all diuretics, if vomiting or diarrhoea develops, the patient should stop taking spironolactone and consult a doctor.

⊕ Pharmacology

Spironolactone and two active metabolites are competitive aldosterone antagonists. They increase sodium and water excretion whilst reducing potassium loss at the distal renal tubule. Spironolactone has a gradual onset of action, and it may be up to a week before effects are seen.

Sucralfate

Antepsin® (POM)
Tablet (*scored*): 1g (50)
Suspension: 1g/5mL (250mL)

Indications
- Treatment of duodenal and gastric ulcer.
- Chronic gastritis.
- Prophylaxis of GI haemorrhage from stress ulceration.
- ⌅ Surface bleeding.

Contraindications and precautions
- Use with caution in patients with renal impairment (see 📖 *Dose adjustments*).
- Sucralfate may modify reactions and patients should be advised not to drive (or operate machinery) if affected.
- Bezoars (insoluble masses in the intestine) have been reported, especially in the seriously ill or those receiving enteral feeds.

☻ Undesirable effects
The frequency is not defined, but reported undesirable effects include:
- Back pain
- Bezoar formation (see *Contraindications and precautions*)
- Constipation
- Diarrhoea
- Dizziness
- Drowsiness
- Dry mouth
- Flatulence
- Gastric discomfort
- Headache
- Indigestion
- Nausea and vomiting
- Rash

Drug interactions
Pharmacokinetic
- Sucralfate can affect the absorption of several drugs (see below), and administration should be separated by 2 hours:
  - ciprofloxacin
  - digoxin
  - furosemide
  - ketoconazole
  - levothyroxine
  - phenytoin
  - ranitidine
  - tetracycline
  - theophylline
  - warfarin

- Other drugs may be affected; if there are unexpected outcomes, consider separating administration by ? hours
- Sucralfate and enteral feeds by nasogastric tube should be separated by 1 hour in order to prevent bezoar formation

Pharmacodynamic
- No known pharmacodynamic interactions

♂ Dose
Treatment of duodenal and gastric ulcer and chronic gastritis
- 2g PO BD (on rising and at bedtime) or 1g PO QDS 1 hour before meals and at bedtime
- Should be taken for 4–6 weeks, or up to 12 weeks in resistant cases
- Dose can be increased if necessary to a maximum of 8g daily

Stress ulceration
- Usual dose 1g PO six times a day; can be increased to a maximum of 8g PO daily.

¥ Surface bleeding
- 1–2g PO BD (as suspension) rinsed around mouth for oral bleeding
- 2g (crushed tablets) in suitable agent (e.g. Intrasite® gel) for bleeding wounds (other alternatives may be preferred, e.g. adrenaline, tranexamic acid).

♂ Dose adjustments
Elderly
- No specific adjustments are required, but the lowest effective dose should be used.

Hepatic/renal impairment
- No specific guidance is available for patients with hepatic impairment. Use the lowest effective dose.
- The manufacturer recommends that sucralfate should be used with extreme caution and only for short-term treatment in patients with severe renal impairment. This is unlikely to apply to topical use (surface bleeding).

Additional information
- Tablets can be crushed and dispersed in water if necessary.

⊕ Pharmacology
Sucralfate is a complex of sucrose and aluminium sulphate. In solutions with a low pH (e.g. gastric acid) it forms a thick paste that has a strong negative charge. It then binds to exposed positively charged proteins located within or around ulcers, forming a physical barrier which protects the ulcer from further direct injury. Sucralfate is poorly absorbed from the GI tract. Any amounts that are absorbed are excreted primarily in the urine.

Tamoxifen

Nolvadex D® (POM)
Tablet: 20mg (30)

Generic (POM)
Tablet: 10mg (30); 20mg (30)
Oral solution: 10mg/5mL (150mL)

Indications
- Breast cancer.
- Anovulatory infertility.

Contraindications and precautions
- Tamoxifen is linked to an increased risk of endometrial changes including hyperplasia, polyps, cancer, and uterine sarcoma. Any patient with unexpected or abnormal gynaecological symptoms, especially vaginal bleeding, should be investigated.
- There is a 2–3× increase in risk of venous thromboembolism (VTE) in patients taking tamoxifen. Long-term anticoagulant prophylaxis may be necessary for some patients who have multiple risk factors for VTE.
- Increased bone pain, tumour pain, and local disease flare are sometimes associated with a good tumour response shortly after starting tamoxifen, and generally subside rapidly.
- Avoid combination with CYP2D6 inhibitors (see 📖 *Drug interactions*, p.450).

☺ Undesirable effects
The frequency is not defined, but reported undesirable effects include:
- Alopecia
- Fluid retention
- Headache
- Hot flushes
- Hypercalcaemia (may occur on initiation of therapy)
- Light-headedness
- Liver enzyme changes
- Mood changes (e.g. depression)
- Nausea
- Pruritus vulvae
- Tumour flare (e.g. bone pain)
- Vaginal bleeding
- Vaginal discharge

Drug interactions

Pharmacokinetic

- Tamoxifen is metabolized by CYP2C8/9, CYP2D6, and CYP3A4.
- Co-administration with certain CYP2D6 inhibitors (e.g. paroxetine) has been shown to reduce the plasma levels of the potent anti-oestrogen endoxifen. The clinical significance of this interaction is presently unknown, but patients who are poor CYP2D6 metabolizers may possibly have poorer than expected outcomes with tamoxifen.
- The clinical significance of co-administration with CYP2C8/9 inducers or inhibitors (🛏 end cover) is unknown. The prescriber should be aware of the potential for interactions and that dose adjustments may be necessary.
- The clinical significance of co-administration with CYP3A4 inducers or inhibitors (🛏 end cover) is unknown. The prescriber should be aware of the potential for interactions and that dose adjustments may be necessary.

Pharmacodynamic

- *Warfarin*—increased anticoagulant sensitivity. Mechanism unknown.

⨶ Dose

Breast cancer

- 20mg PO OD. No evidence exists for superiority of higher doses.

⨶ Dose adjustments

Elderly

- Usual adult doses can be used.

Hepatic/renal impairment

- No specific guidance is available for use in liver impairment. In view of the extensive metabolism of tamoxifen, patients with liver impairment may be more susceptible to undesirable effects and/or treatment failure.
- No dose adjustments are necessary for patients with renal impairment.

⧎ Pharmacology

Tamoxifen is a nonsteroidal antiestrogen that has both oestrogen antagonist and agonist activity. It acts as an antagonist on breast tissue and as an agonist on the endometrium, bone and lipids. The precise mechanism of action is unknown, but the effect of tamoxifen is mediated by its metabolites, 4-hydroxytamoxifen and endoxifen. The formation of these active metabolites is catalysed by CYP2D6. It is also metabolised by several other cytochrome P450 isoenzymes (CYP2C8/9 and CYP3A4).

Tamsulosin

Modified release
Flomaxtra® XL (POM)
Tablet: 400mcg (30)

Generic (POM)
Capsule: 400mcg (30)

Indications
- Benign prostatic hyperplasia.

Contraindications and precautions
- Contraindicated for use in patients with:
  - postural hypotension
  - severe hepatic impairment.
- Use with caution in patients with severe renal impairment.

☺ Undesirable effects
Common
- Asthenia
- Dizziness
- Headache
- Sexual dysfunction

Uncommon
- Constipation
- Diarrhoea
- Nausea
- Palpitations
- Rhinitis
- Vomiting

Unknown
- Blurred vision
- Drowsiness
- Dry mouth
- Intraoperative floppy iris syndrome (caution before cataract surgery)
- Oedema

Drug interactions
Pharmacokinetic
- Tamsulosin is metabolized by CYP2D6 and CYP3A4. There have been no documented pharmacokinetic interactions.
- Nonetheless, the clinical significance of co-administration with CYP2D6 inhibitors or CYP3A4 inducers/inhibitors (📖 end cover) is unknown. The prescriber should be aware of the potential for interactions and that dose adjustments may be necessary.
- Avoid excessive amounts of grapefruit juice as it may increase the bio-availability of tamsulosin through inhibition of intestinal CYP3A4.

Pharmacodynamic
- The following drugs can potentially increase the risk of postural hypotension:
  - Antihypertensives
  - Diuretics
  - Levomepromazine
  - Sildenafil
  - Tadalafil.

Dose
- 400mcg PO OD.

Dose adjustments
Elderly
- Dose adjustments are unnecessary.

Hepatic/renal impairment
- No specific guidance is available for patients with hepatic impairment. Given that tamsulosin is extensively metabolized, the patient should be closely monitored.
- The manufacturer recommends that patients with severe renal impairment (CrCl <10mL/min) should be treated with caution.

Pharmacology
Tamsulosin is a selective antagonist of α_{1A}-adrenoceptors, which results in relaxation of the smooth muscle of the prostate and bladder neck. Tamsulosin is extensively metabolized by CYP2D6 and CYP3A4, but the complete pharmacokinetic profile has not been established.

Temazepam

Generic (CD No Register POM)

Tablet: 10mg (28); 20mg (28)
Oral solution: 10mg/5mL (300mL)
Sugar-free formulations are available
Note: Discard 3 months after opening

Note: Temazepam is a Schedule 3 controlled drug. Refer to 📖 Legal categories, p.23 for further information.

Note: Independent prescribers are **NOT** authorized to prescribe temazepam (📖 Independent prescribing—palliative care issues, p.25).

Indications
• Short-term treatment of sleep disturbances.

Contraindications and precautions
• Temazepam is contraindicated for use in patients with the following conditions:
    • acute narrow-angle glaucoma
    • mild anxiety states
    • myasthenia gravis
    • phobic or obsessional state
    • severe hepatic insufficiency
    • severe respiratory insufficiency
    • sleep apnoea syndrome.
• Temazepam should not be used alone in the treatment of depression or anxiety associated with depression because of the risk of precipitation of suicide.
• Use with caution if there is a history of drug or alcohol abuse.
• Dose reductions may be necessary in elderly (see 📖 *Dose adjustments*).
• Avoid abrupt withdrawal, even if short-duration treatment. The risk of dependence increases with dose and duration of treatment. Prolonged use of benzodiazepines may result in the development of dependence with subsequent withdrawal symptoms on cessation of use, e.g. agitation, anxiety, confusion, headaches, restlessness, sleep disturbances (e.g. broken sleep with vivid dreams; may persist for several weeks after withdrawal), sweating, and tremor. Gradual withdrawal is advised.
• The oral solution contains 10% v/v ethanol.
• Temazepam may modify reactions and patients should be advised not to drive (or operate machinery) if affected.

☺ Undesirable effects

The frequency is not defined, but reported undesirable effects include:

- Anterograde amnesia
- Ataxia
- Confusion
- Depression
- Dizziness
- Drowsiness
- Fatigue
- Hallucinations
- Headache
- Muscle weakness
- Nightmares
- Paradoxical events such as agitation, irritability and restlessness
- Respiratory depression
- Sexual dysfunction
- Sleep disturbance
- Visual disturbances

Drug interactions

Pharmacokinetic

- Mainly undergoes conjugation reactions and is unlikely to be affected by inducers/inhibitors.
- Pharmacokinetic interactions are likely to be minimal compared with other benzodiazepines.

Pharmacodynamic

- *Alcohol*—may precipitate seizures.
- *Antidepressants*—reduced seizure threshold.
- *Antipsychotics*—reduced seizure threshold.
- *Baclofen*—increased risk of sedation.
- *CNS depressants*—additive sedative effect.

⚚ Dose

- 10–20mg PO ON. This can be increased to 30–40mg PO ON as necessary.

⚚ Dose adjustments

Elderly

- Half the usual adult dose is suggested.

Hepatic/renal impairment

- No specific guidance is available. The dose of temazepam must be carefully adjusted to individual requirements.

Additional information

- Tablets may be crushed and dispersed in water immediately prior to administration if necessary.

⟐ Pharmacology

Potentiates action of GABA, resulting in increased neuronal inhibition and CNS depression, especially in limbic system and reticular formation. Temazepam is well absorbed and undergoes extensive hepatic metabolism through conjugation. Enterohepatic recirculation is anticipated.

Thalidomide

Thalidomide Pharmion® (POM)
Capsule: 50mg (28)

Indications
- Multiple myeloma
- ¥ Cancer cachexia
- ¥ Paraneoplastic sweating
- ¥ Management of tumour-related gastric bleeding

Contraindications and precautions
- Must not be used in the following circumstances:
  - pregnant women
  - women of childbearing potential unless all the conditions of the Thalidomide Pharmion Pregnancy Prevention Programme are met (see manufacturer's SmPC)
- The conditions of the Thalidomide Pharmion Pregnancy Prevention Programme (see manufacturer's SmPC) must be satisfied for all male and female patients.
- Deep venous thrombosis, pulmonary embolism, and peripheral neuropathy have been reported to occur with thalidomide. Use cautiously with drugs that may increase the risk of thromboembolism or peripheral neuropathy (see 📖 *Drug interactions*, p.456).
- For women of childbearing potential, prescriptions for thalidomide should not exceed 4 weeks. Dispensing should occur within 7 days of the date of issue. For other patients, supply should be limited to 12 weeks.
- Unused capsules should be returned to a pharmacy.
- Thalidomide may modify reactions and patients should be advised not to drive (or operate machinery) if affected.

- Thromboprophylaxis should be administered for at least the first 5 months of treatment, especially in patients with additional thrombotic risk factors (e.g. LMWH, warfarin). Thalidomide must be discontinued if the patient experiences a thromboembolic event. Once the patient is stabilized on appropriate anticoagulant treatment, thalidomide can be restarted. The anticoagulant must be continued throughout the course of thalidomide treatment.
- Peripheral neuropathy can present with the following symptoms:
  - abnormal coordination
  - dysaesthesia
  - paraesthesia
  - weakness.
- Patients presenting with these symptoms should be assessed according to the manufacturer's SmPC. Treatment may be withheld or discontinued.

☺ Undesirable effects

Very common

- Anaemia
- Constipation
- Dizziness
- Drowsiness
- Dysaesthesia
- Leucopenia
- Lymphopenia

- Neutropenia
- Paraesthesia
- Peripheral neuropathy
- Peripheral oedema
- Thrombocytopenia
- Tremor

Common

- Asthenia
- Bradycardia
- Cardiac failure
- Confusion
- Depression
- Dry mouth
- Dyspnoea

- Malaise
- Nausea and vomiting
- Pneumonia
- Pulmonary embolism
- Pyrexia
- Toxic skin eruptions

Drug interactions

Pharmacokinetic

- Thalidomide does not appear to be metabolized by the liver. Clinically significant pharmacokinetic drug interactions have not been reported.

Pharmacodynamic

- *Anti-arrhythmics*—increased risk of bradycardia.
- *Bisphosphonates*—increased risk of renal impairment (in treatment of multiple myeloma).
- *CNS depressants*—risk of excessive sedation.
- *Dexamethasone*—may increase the risk of toxic skin reactions, immunosuppression, and thromboembolic events.
- *Epoetins*—increased risk of thromboembolic events.
- *NSAIDs*—theoretical increased risk of thromboembolic events.

♪ Dose

Multiple myeloma

- 200mg PO ON for 6 week cycle. Patient can receive a maximum of 12 cycles.

¥ *Cancer cachexia*

- 100–200mg PO ON

¥ *Paraneoplastic sweating*

- 100–200mg PO ON

¥ *Management of tumour-related gastric bleeding*

- 100–300mg PO ON
- Used in combination with other agents such as sucralfate and PPIs.

♣ Dose adjustments

Elderly
• No dose adjustments are necessary.

Hepatic/renal impairment
• There are no specific instructions for dose adjustment in liver or renal impairment. The lowest effective dose should be prescribed and the patient should be closely monitored.

Additional information
• The capsule must not be broken or opened; it must be swallowed whole.

♦ Pharmacology
Thalidomide is an immunomodulatory agent that also has anti-inflammatory and anti-angiogenic properties. The mechanism of action of thalidomide is not completely understood, although it has been shown to inhibit the synthesis of tumour necrosis factor α (TNF-α) and modulates the effects of other cytokines. The exact metabolic pathway of thalidomide is unknown, but it is believed not to involve the cytochrome P450 system. Rather, it undergoes non-enzymatic hydrolysis in plasma.

Theophylline

It is not possible to ensure the interchangeability of different makes of modified release. Therefore it is recommended that patients should remain on the same product once treatment has been stabilized. Inclusion of the brand name on the prescription is suggested.

Standard release

Unlicensed Special (P)
Liquid: 60mg/5mL (300mL)

Modified release

Nuelin SA® (P)
Tablet: 175mg (60); 250mg (*scored*, 60)

Slo-Phyllin® (P)
Capsule: 60mg (56); 125mg (56); 250mg (56)

Uniphyllin® (P)
Tablet (*scored*): 200mg (56); 300mg (56); 400mg (56)

Aminophylline

Modified release
Phyllocontin Continus® (P)
Tablet: 225mg (56); 350mg (56)

Indications

• Prophylaxis and treatment of reversible bronchospasm.

Contraindications and precautions

• Contraindicated for use in patients with porphyria.
• Potentially serious hypokalaemia may result from theophylline treatment, particularly if used in combination with β_2-agonists, corticosteroids, and diuretics.
• Use with caution in the following circumstances:
  • acute febrile illness
  • cardiac arrhythmias
  • chronic alcoholism
  • congestive heart failure (increased half-life)
  • elderly (increased half-life)
  • hepatic impairment (increased half-life)
  • hyperthyroidism
  • peptic ulcer
  • severe hypertension.

☹ Undesirable effects

The frequency is not defined, but reported undesirable effects include:

- Abdominal discomfort
- Diarrhoea
- Gastric irritation
- Headache
- Hypotension
- Insomnia
- Nausea/vomiting
- Palpitations

Drug interactions

Pharmacokinetic

- Metabolized by CYP1A2 and CYP2E1; it is also metabolized by CYP3A4 and xanthine oxidase to a lesser extent.
- Theophylline may be affected by many drugs; several interactions are listed below, but refer to 📖 end cover for a list of drugs that may potentially affect theophylline.
- *Allopurinol*—may increase the plasma concentration of theophylline.
- *Amiodarone*—may increase the plasma concentration of theophylline.
- *Carbamazepine*—reduces the plasma concentration of theophylline.
- *Ciprofloxacin*—may increase the plasma concentration of theophylline.
- *Erythromycin*—may increase the plasma concentration of theophylline.
- *Phenobarbital*—reduces the plasma concentration of theophylline.
- *Phenytoin*—reduces the plasma concentration of theophylline.
- *Rifampicin*—reduces the plasma concentration of theophylline.
- Note that smoking and chronic alcohol consumption increase the clearance of theophylline (induce CYP1A2/CYP2E1). If a patient stops smoking, ensure that the dose of theophylline is closely monitored (see 📖 Box 1.9, p.17
- The clinical significance of co-administration with other CYP1A2 or CYP2E1 inducers or inhibitors (📖 end cover) is unknown. The prescriber should be aware of the potential for interactions and that dose adjustments may be necessary.

Pharmacodynamic

- *β_2-agonists*—increased risk of hypokalaemia.
- *Corticosteroids*—increased risk of hypokalaemia.
- *Diuretics*—increased risk of hypokalaemia.

♨ Dose

Standard release

● Usually initiate treatment with m/r formulation and use liquid for patients with difficulty swallowing. Administer TDS. When converting to liquid, monitor plasma concentrations.

Modified release

Nuelin SA®

● Initial dose 175mg PO BD. The dose is adjusted according to plasma concentrations.

Slo-Phyllin®

● Initial dose 250mg PO BD. The dose is adjusted according to plasma concentrations.

Uniphyllin®

● Initial dose 200mg PO BD. The dose is adjusted according to plasma concentrations.

Phyllocontin Continus®

● Initial dose 225mg PO BD. The dose is adjusted according to plasma concentrations.

♨ Dose adjustments

Elderly

● The lowest initial doses should be prescribed, with any dose adjustments based on plasma concentration.

Hepatic/renal impairment

● Theophylline is hepatically metabolized. Although no information exists, it is advisable to initiate treatment with low doses with close monitoring of plasma concentrations.
● No dose adjustments should be necessary in renal impairment.

Additional information

● Plasma theophylline concentration for optimum response is 10–20mg/L (55–110µmol/L). Samples should be taken 4–6 hours after a dose and at least 5 days after starting treatment. There is a narrow margin between therapeutic and toxic dose.
● Unlicensed liquid formulation is available from a variety of manufacturers.

⟐ Pharmacology

Theophylline is a xanthine derivative that is chemically similar to caffeine. It competitively inhibits type III and type IV phosphodiesterase (PDE) and also binds to the adenosine A_2B receptor, blocking adenosine-mediated bronchoconstriction.

Tiotropium

Spiriva® (POM)
Inhalation powder, hard capsule (for use with *HandiHaler*® device): 18mcg (30)

Spiriva Respimat® (POM)
Solution for inhalation: 2.5mcg/metered dose (60 dose unit)

Indications
- Maintenance treatment of COPD

Contraindications and precautions
- Tiotropium should be used with caution in patients with:
  - angle-closure glaucoma
  - bladder outflow obstruction
  - prostatic hyperplasia
  - renal impairment (see 📖 *Dose adjustments*, p.462).
- If eye pain, blurred vision, or visual halos develop, treatment should be discontinued and specialist advice sought immediately

😣 Undesirable effects
Common
- Dry mouth

Uncommon
- Bronchospasm
- Cough
- Dizziness
- Headache
- Oral candidiasis
- Taste disorder

Rare
- Visual disturbances

Unknown
- Dental caries
- Glaucoma
- Sinusitis

Drug interactions
Pharmacokinetic
- Although it is metabolized by CYP2D6 and CYP3A4, no interactions of clinical significance have been noted

Pharmacodynamic
- *Anticholinergics*—concurrent use with ipratropium may increase risk of adverse events

Dose

Dry powder inhalation
- 10mcg OD. This dose should not be exceeded.

Solution for inhalation
- 5mcg OD. This dose should not be exceeded.

Dose adjustments

Elderly
- No dose adjustment is necessary

Hepatic/renal impairment
- No dose reduction is necessary in patients with hepatic impairment.
- Tiotropium may accumulate in patients with renal impairment. In patients with moderate to severe renal impairment (CrCl ≤50mL/min), tiotropium should be used only if the expected benefit outweighs the potential risk. There is no information for severe renal impairment.

Additional information

- The bronchodilatory effect may not occur for up to 2 hours. Tiotropium must not be used for acute episodes of breathlessness.
- If nebulized ipratropium therapy is initiated, ensure that tiotropium is withdrawn

Pharmacology

Tiotropium bromide is a long-acting specific muscarinic receptor antagonist acting mainly on M3 muscarinic receptors located in the airways to produce smooth muscle relaxation. Following inhalation, a small proportion of the dose is deposited in the lungs, but the majority is swallowed. The GI absorption is negligible. Ipratropium is metabolized to inactive compounds, although the majority of the dose is excreted unchanged by the kidneys.

Tolterodine

Standard release
Detrusitol® (POM)
Tablet: 1mg (56); 2mg (56)

Modified release
Detrusitol® XL (POM)
Capsule: 4mg (28)

Indications
- Urinary frequency.
- Urinary incontinence.

Contraindications and precautions
- Tolterodine is contraindicated for use in patients with:
  - myasthenia gravis
  - narrow-angle glaucoma
  - severe ulcerative colitis
  - toxic megacolon
  - urinary retention.
- It should be used with caution in patients with the following:
  - autonomic neuropathy
  - cardiac arrhythmia
  - concomitant use with other drugs known to prolong QT interval and/or inhibit CYP3A4 (see 📖 *Drug interactions*, p.464)
  - congestive heart failure
  - elderly (see 📖 *Dose adjustments*, p.465)
  - GI reflux disease
  - hepatic impairment
  - hiatus hernia
  - history of QT-interval prolongation
  - hyperthyroidism
  - prostatic hypertrophy
  - pyrexia (reduces sweating)
  - renal impairment
- Tolterodine may modify reactions and patients should be advised not to drive (or operate machinery) if affected.

☺ Undesirable effects
Very common
- Dry mouth
- Headache

Common
- Bronchitis
- Constipation
- Diarrhoea (overflow)
- Dizziness
- Drowsiness
- Dyspepsia
- Fatigue
- Palpitations
- Paraesthesia
- Urinary retention
- Visual disturbances
- Vertigo

Uncommon
- Gastro-oesophageal reflux
- Memory impairment
- Tachycardia

Unknown
- Confusion
- Hallucinations

Drug interactions

Pharmacokinetic
- Tolterodine is metabolized by CYP3A4 and CYP2D6.
- Co-administration with CYP3A4 inhibitors (📖 end cover) can cause increased pharmacological effect because of increased serum concentrations of the parent drug and active metabolite. The prescriber should be aware of the need for potential dose reductions.
- The clinical significance of co-administration of CYP3A4 inducers (📖 end cover) is unknown, but the prescriber should be aware that the effect of tolterodine may be reduced and that dose adjustments may be necessary.
- The clinical significance of co-administration of CYP2D6 inhibitors (📖 end cover) is unknown, but the prescriber should be aware that the effect of tolterodine may be reduced and that dose adjustments may be necessary.
- Note that the combination of both CYP3A4 and CYP2D6 inhibitors could increase the risk of toxicity from tolterodine because of excessive serum concentrations.
- The effect of grapefruit juice on the bioavailability of tolterodine is unknown.

Pharmacodynamic
- *Donepezil*—effect may be antagonized.
- *β₂-agonists*—increased risk of tachycardia.
- *Cyclizine*—increased risk of undesirable anticholinergic effects.
- *Domperidone*—may inhibit prokinetic effect.
- *Galantamine*—effect may be antagonized.
- *Metoclopramide*—may inhibit prokinetic effect.
- *Nefopam*—increased risk of undesirable anticholinergic effects.
- *Rivastigmine*—effect may be antagonized.
- *TCAs*—increased risk of undesirable anticholinergic effects.

,§ Dose
Standard release
- Initial dose 2mg PO BD; if undesirable effects troublesome, reduce dose to 1mg PO BD.

Modified release
- Initial dose 4mg PO OD; revert to standard release if undesirable effects become troublesome.

,§ Dose adjustments
Elderly
- No dose adjustments are necessary.

Hepatic/renal impairment
- The manufacturer recommends that a dose of 1mg PO BD is used initially for patients with hepatic impairment or renal impairment (GFR <30mL/min). The modified release formulation is not appropriate for use in these patients.

Additional information
- Standard-release tablet can be crushed and dispersed in water immediately prior to administration if necessary.
- A response to treatment should be seen within 4 weeks.

⊕ Pharmacology
Tolterodine is a competitive muscarinic receptor antagonist with selectivity for the bladder. It is metabolized by both CYP3A4 and CYP2D6; metabolism by CYP2D6 produces a metabolite with activity similar to the parent drug which must be borne in mind if a CYP3A4 inhibitor is administered concurrently (see 📖 *Drug interactions*, p.464).

Tramadol

Standard release (POM)

Zamadol®
Capsule: 50mg (100)
Orodispersible tablet: 50mg (60)
Injection: 50mg/mL (2mL ampoule)

Zydol®
Capsule: 50mg (30; 100)
Soluble capsule: 50mg (20; 100)
Injection: 50mg/mL (2mL ampoule)

Generic
Capsule: 50mg (30; 100)
Injection: 50mg/mL (2mL ampoule)

Modified release (POM)

- **12 hour release** tablet formulation: 100mg (60); 150mg (60); 200mg (60)
  - Brands: Dromadol®; Larapam®; Mabron®; Zydol SR®
- **12 hour release** capsule formulation: 50mg (60); 100mg (60); 150mg (60); 200mg (60)
  - Brands: Maxitram SR®; Zamadol SR®

24 hour release tablet formulations
Tradorec XL®: 100mg (30); 200mg (30); 300mg (30)
Zamadol 24hr®: 150mg (28); 200mg (28); 300mg (28); 400mg (28)
Zydol XL®: 150mg (28); 200mg (28); 300mg (28); 400mg (28)

Combination with paracetamol

Tramacet® (POM)
Tablet: tramadol 37.5mg, paracetamol 325mg (60)

Indications

- Moderate to severe pain

Contraindications and precautions

- Do not use with an MAOI, or within 14 days of stopping one.
- Not be used in epilepsy not adequately controlled by treatment.
- Use with caution in patients with:
  - concurrent use of serotonergic drugs, e.g. SSRIs, TCAs (see ▢ *Drug interactions,* p.467)
  - epilepsy
  - head injury,
  - increased intracranial pressure,
  - porphyria
  - severe impairment of hepatic and renal function (see ▢ *Dose adjustments*).
- A withdrawal syndrome may occur with abrupt discontinuation; symptoms include anxiety, diarrhoea, hallucinations, nausea, pain, sweating, and tremor.

- Phenylketonuria—Zamadol® orodispersible tablets contain aspartame, a source of phenylalanine.
- Ultra-rapid metabolizers of CYP2D6 may produce higher plasma concentrations of the active metabolite. Even at usual doses, ultra-rapid metabolizers may experience symptoms of overdose, such as extreme sleepiness, confusion, or shallow breathing.
- Tramadol may modify reactions and patients should be advised not to drive (or operate machinery) if affected.

- Equianalgesic ratios have been suggested but the conversion from tramadol to morphine, or any other strong opioid, cannot be recommended in practice for the following reasons:
  - opioid analgesia derived from tramadol in the clinical situation is unknown because of the dependence upon CYP2D6 activity (see *Pharmacology*).
  - risk of a withdrawal reaction (depends upon duration of therapy and concurrent treatment).
- The prescriber has two options:
  - stop tramadol and titrate the strong opioid using standard-release formulations (e.g. morphine 5–10mg 4 hourly PRN).
  - gradual cross-tapering, e.g. reduce tramadol dose while introducing standard-release morphine 2.5–5mg 4 hourly PRN.

☺ Undesirable effects

Very common
- Dizziness
- Nausea

Common
- Vomiting
- Constipation
- Diarrhoea
- Dry mouth
- Sweating

Uncommon
- Pruritus
- Rash

Rare
- Withdrawal reactions (anxiety, diarrhoea, hallucinations, nausea, pain, sweating, and tremor)

Drug interactions

Pharmacokinetic
- Tramadol is metabolized to the opioid (+)M1 (see *Pharmacology*) by CYP2D6; additional metabolism of tramadol and the active metabolite occurs via CYP3A4.
- The absorption of tramadol also depends on P-gp (inhibitors may increase tramadol plasma concentrations).

- Co-administration with CYP2D6 inhibitors may alter the analgesic effect of tramadol:
  - paroxetine has been shown to reduce the analgesic benefit of tramadol
    - the efficacy of tramadol may be altered by other CYP2D6 inhibitors, such as duloxetine, fluoxetine, haloperidol, and levomepromazine. The clinical implications of co-administration with these drugs are unknown; the prescriber should be aware of the potential for altered response.
- Carbamazepine reduces the analgesic benefit of tramadol through induction of CYP3A4.
- The clinical significance of co-administration of inhibitors of CYP3A4 (🕮 end cover) is presently unknown. The prescriber should be aware of the potential for interactions (increased opioid effect).
- *Warfarin*—possible risk of increased INR in susceptible patients

Pharmacodynamic
- *Antipsychotics*—increased risk of seizures.
- *CNS depressants*—risk of excessive sedation.
- *MAOIs*, including linezolid, should be avoided.
- *Mirtazapine*—increased risk of seizures and serotonin syndrome; may reduce effect of tramadol by blocking 5-HT$_3$-receptor-mediated analgesia.
- *Ondansetron*—reduces effect of tramadol by blocking 5-HT$_3$-receptor-mediated analgesia.
- *Serotonergic drugs*—caution is advisable if tramadol is co-administered with serotonergic drugs (e.g. methadone, methylphenidate, mirtazapine, oxycodone, SSRIs, tricyclic antidepressants, trazodone) because of the risk of serotonin syndrome (🕮 Box 1.10, p.19).
- *Tricyclic antidepressants*—increased risk of seizures.

⚗ Dose
Oral
Slow titration with modified-release formulations has been shown to improve tolerability. Standard-release formulations are generally not as well tolerated.

Modified release
- Initial dose 100mg daily (50mg m/r PO BD or 100mg m/r PO OD) increasing to 200mg daily (100mg m/r PO BD or 200mg m/r PO OD) several days later, with further dose increases up to a maximum of 400mg PO daily.

Standard release
- Initial dose 50mg PO followed by doses of 50–100mg PO not more frequently than 4 hourly, titrating the dose according to pain severity. Maximum dose 400mg PO daily.

Tramacet®
- Initial dose 2 tablets. Additional doses can be taken as needed, not less than 6 hours apart. Total daily dose must not exceed 8 tablets.

Subcutaneous
- Rarely administered via CSCI in the UK.
- ¥ Initial dose 100mg via CSCI, diluted with NaCl or WFI.

🔊 Dose adjustments
Elderly
- Dose as for adults; slow titration advised.
- Patients over the age of 75 years may need a dose reduction.

Hepatic/renal impairment
- In severe hepatic impairment, avoid the modified-release formulation; the dose interval (of the standard-release formulation) should be increased to 12 hourly.
- If CrCl is <30 mL/min, avoid the modified-release formulation; the dose interval (of the standard-release formulation) should be increased to 12 hourly.
- Avoid in patients with CrCl <10mL/min.
- Patients undergoing haemofiltration or haemodialysis will not require post-dialysis because tramadol is removed very slowly.

Additional information
- Zamadol SR® capsules can be opened and the pellets added to jam or yoghurt. Alternatively, they can be deposited on to a spoon. The spoon and pellets should be taken into the mouth, followed by a drink of water to rinse the mouth of all pellets. The pellets must not be chewed or crushed.
- Tramacet® may be useful for patients taking concurrent antidepressants in order to reduce the incidence of undesirable effects.
- Tramadol via CSCI is compatible with dexamethasone, glycopyrronium, haloperidol, hyoscine butylbromide, levomepromazine, metoclopramide, and midazolam.
- Poor CYP2D6 metabolizers cannot produce (+)M1, while ultra-metabolizers may produce excessive amounts. Drug interactions can affect the metabolism of (±)tramadol via enzyme inhibition (CYP2D6) or induction (CYP3A4 only). The clinical consequences of genotype and drug interaction depend upon the type of pain being treated as the monoaminergic and opioid effects both independently produce analgesia. Genetic variations lead to the possibility of a modified undesirable effect profile and varied analgesic response with tramadol.

⟳ Pharmacology
Tramadol is a centrally acting analgesic with a unique and complex pharmacology. Analgesia is produced by a synergistic interaction between two distinct pharmacological effects. Tramadol has a μ-opioid effect and it also activates descending antinociceptive pathways in the spinal cord via inhibition of reuptake of serotonin and noradrenaline and via presynaptic release of serotonin.

Tramadol is available commercially as a racemate consisting of enantiomers, (+)tramadol and (−)tramadol, which have different pharmacological actions. Opioid and serotonergic actions are associated with (+)tramadol, whereas noradrenaline reuptake inhibition is associated with (−)tramadol. The only pharmacologically active metabolite (+)O-desmethyltramadol (or (+)M1) is produced by the polymorphic cytochrome CYP2D6. The opioid effect of (±)tramadol is mostly due to (+)M1. Additional metabolism of (±)tramadol and (+)M1 is catalysed by CYP3A4 and CYP2B6.

Tranexamic acid

Cyklokapron® (POM)
Tablet (*scored*): 500mg (60)
Injection: 500mg/5mL

Generic (POM)
Tablet (*scored*): 500mg (60)

Indications
- ¥ Prophylaxis and control of haemorrhages from small blood vessels.
- ¥ Bleeding from wounds (topical application).

Contraindications and precautions
- Contraindications and precautions should be individually assessed for topical use.
- Tranexamic acid is contraindicated for use in patients with:
  - active thromboembolic disease
  - severe renal failure (risk of accumulation).
- Use with caution in the following:
  - disseminated intravascular coagulation
  - massive haematuria (risk of ureteric obstruction)
  - past history of thromboembolic disease
  - renal impairment.
- If appropriate, patients on long-term treatment should have regular eye examinations and LFTs.

☺ Undesirable effects
The frequency is not defined, but reported undesirable effects include:
- GI disorders (e.g. nausea, vomiting, diarrhoea)
- Thromboembolic events (withdraw treatment)

Drug interactions
Pharmacokinetic
- None recognized.

Pharmacodynamic
- Will counteract the effect of fibrinolytic drugs.

⚕ Dose
¥ *Haemorrhage*
- Initial dose 1g PO TDS. Can be increased as necessary to 1.5g PO QDS. Consider reducing the dose after 7 days once bleeding has stopped.

¥ *Topical*
- 0.5–1g (using injection, or crushed tablets if warranted) directly into wound via suitable dressing and apply pressure. Review after 10–20 minutes.

¿Ó Dose adjustments

Elderly
● Usual adult doses recommended.

Hepatic/renal impairment
● No specific guidance is available for patients with hepatic impairment. Use the lowest effective dose.
● For patients with SeCr 120–249 µmol/L, oral dose should not exceed 15mg/kg BD. For patients with SeCr 250–500 µmol/L, oral dose should not exceed 15mg/kg OD. The drug is contraindicated in patients with severe renal impairment.

Additional information

● Tablets can be dispersed in water immediately prior to use if necessary.

⟳ Pharmacology

Tranexamic acid is an antifibrinolytic drug that competitively inhibits the activation of plasminogen to plasmin.

Trazodone

Molipaxin® (POM)
Capsule: 50mg (84), 100mg (56)
Tablet: 150mg (28)
Liquid: 50mg/5mL (120mL bottle)

Generic (POM)
Capsule: 50mg (84), 100mg (56)
Tablet: 150mg (28)

Indications
- Depression.
- Anxiety.
- ¥ Insomnia.
- ¥ Agitation/delirium.

Contraindications and precautions
- Avoid use with MAOIs, or within 14 days of stopping one; avoid concomitant use with linezolid or moclobemide.
- Avoid sudden discontinuation, although no specific withdrawal syndrome has been reported.
- Use with caution in patients with a history of epilepsy or hepatic disease.
- Closely monitor the patient if drugs known to affect CYP3A4 are co-administered (see 📖 *Drug interactions*, p.474).
- Hyponatraemia should be considered in all patients who develop drowsiness, confusion, or convulsions while taking an antidepressant. Hyponatraemia has been associated with all types of antidepressants, although it is reportedly more common with SSRIs.
- Depression is associated with an increased risk of suicidal thoughts, self-harm, and suicide which persists until remission. Note that that the risk of suicide may increase during initial treatment.
- Trazodone may modify reactions and patients should be advised not to drive (or operate machinery) if affected.
- See 📖 Discontinuing and/or switching antidepressants, p.45 for information about switching or stopping antidepressants.

☺ Undesirable effects
Very common
- Blurred vision
- Dizziness
- Dry mouth
- Headache
- Nausea
- Sedation

Common
- Confusion
- Constipation
- Diarrhoea

- Fatigue
- Oedema
- Postural hypotension
- Tremor

Uncommon
- Agitation
- Rash
- Restlessness

Rare
- Hyponatraemia
- Priapism

Drug interactions
Pharmacokinetic
- Trazodone is significantly metabolized by CYP3A4; additional metabolism occurs via CYP2D6. It is a weak CYP2D6 inhibitor.
- *Carbamazepine*—may reduce effect of trazodone due to CYP3A4 induction. The clinical significance of co-administration with other inducers of CYP3A4 (🕮 end cover) is unknown. Increased doses of trazodone may be required.
- Inhibitors of CYP3A4 and CYP2D6 (🕮 end cover) may increase plasma concentrations of trazodone. The prescriber should be aware of the potential for interactions and that dose adjustments may be necessary.
- Avoid grapefruit juice as it may increase the bioavailability of trazodone through inhibition of intestinal CYP3A4.
- The clinical significance of co-administration with substrates of CYP2D6 (🕮 end cover) is unknown. Caution is advised if duloxetine is co-administered with drugs that are predominantly metabolized by CYP2D6 (e.g. haloperidol, risperidone, tricyclic antidepressants). The prescriber should be aware of the potential for interactions and that dose adjustments may be necessary, particularly for drugs with a narrow therapeutic index.
- The clinical significance of co-administration with prodrug substrates of CYP2D6 (e.g. codeine, tramadol) is unknown. The prescriber should be aware of the potential for interactions and that dose adjustments may be necessary.

Pharmacodynamic
- *CNS depressants*—risk of excessive sedation
- *MAOIs*, including linezolid, should be avoided
- *Serotonergic drugs*—caution is advisable if trazodone is co-administered with serotonergic drugs (e.g. methadone, methylphenidate, mirtazapine, oxycodone, SSRIs, tricyclic antidepressants, tramadol) because of the risk of serotonin syndrome (🕮 Box 1.10, p.19)

⚕ Dose
Depression
- Initial dose 150mg PO ON, increasing as necessary to a usual maximum of 300mg PO ON (or 150mg PO BD).

Anxiety
- Initial dose 75mg PO ON, increasing as necessary to 300mg PO ON (or 150mg PO BD).

Insomnia
- Initial dose 25–50mg PO ON, increasing as necessary to a usual maximum of 100mg PO ON. Some patients may require higher doses.

Agitation/delirium
- Initial dose 25–50mg PO ON, increasing to a maximum of 300mg PO ON.

₰ Dose adjustments

Elderly

Age-related changes in hepatic metabolism can produce significantly higher plasma concentrations of trazodone. Dose reductions are necessary.
- Depression: 100mg PO ON or 50mg PO BD initially and increase as necessary to a maximum of 300mg PO daily.
- Anxiety: 25–50mg PO ON and increase as necessary to a maximum of 300mg PO daily.
- Insomnia: as for anxiety.
- Agitation/delirium: as for anxiety.

Hepatic/renal impairment
- Dose adjustments as detailed above for elderly patients should be considered for patients with liver disease.
- No dose adjustments are necessary in renal impairment.

Additional information
- Onset of action for insomnia can be within 1–3 hours of the initial dose. Onset of action for depression usually occurs within 2–4 weeks.
- The sedative effect of trazodone may persist the following morning, particularly if the dose is too high.
- Although there is a paucity of evidence, trazodone is occasionally used as the drug of choice to treat behavioural symptoms of dementia.

᧨ Pharmacology

Trazodone blocks post-synaptic 5-HT$_{2A}$ and 5-HT$_{2C}$ receptors. At high doses, it selectively inhibits presynaptic serotonin reuptake. Trazodone also antagonizes H$_1$- and α_1-adrenergic receptors. It has no effect on muscarinic receptors. It is well absorbed by mouth, and food delays, but enhances, the amount absorbed. Trazodone is metabolized by CYP3A4 to an active metabolite, which is further metabolized by CYP2D6 to an inactive compound. Elimination is almost exclusively by urinary excretion of metabolites.

Trimethoprim

Generic (POM)

Tablet: 100mg (28); 200mg (28)
Oral Suspension: 50mg/5mL (100mL)

Indications

- Refer to local guidelines.
- Treatment of infections caused by trimethoprim-sensitive organisms, including urinary and respiratory tract infections.
- Long-term prophylaxis of urinary tract infections.

Contraindications and precautions

- Trimethoprim is contraindicated for use in:
  - blood dyscrasias
  - severe renal impairment if blood levels cannot be measured (see 🕮 *Dose adjustments*, p.327).
- Use with caution in the following:
  - elderly patients (see 🕮 *Dose adjustments*, p.477)
  - folate deficiency
  - renal impairment (see 🕮 *Dose adjustments*, p.477).
- With long-term treatment, patients and carers should be told how to recognize signs of blood disorders (e.g. fever, sore throat, rash, mouth ulcers, purpura, bruising, or bleeding) and to seek immediate medical attention if they develop.

☺ Undesirable effects

The frequency is not defined, but reported undesirable effects include:
- Blood dyscrasias (depression of haematopoiesis)
- Hyperkalaemia
- Nausea
- Photosensitivity
- Pruritus
- Skin rashes
- Severe skin sensitivity reactions (e.g. erythema multiforme, toxic epidermal necrolysis)
- Vomiting

Drug interactions

Pharmacokinetic

- Trimethoprim is metabolized by CYP2C8; it is an inhibitor of CYP2C8 and may affect CYP2C9.
- *Rifampicin*—may reduce the effect of trimethoprim.
- *Warfarin*—possible increase in INR.
- The clinical significance of co-administration with substrates of CYP2C8 (🕮 end cover) is unknown. Caution is advised if trimethoprim is co-administered with drugs that are predominantly metabolized by CYP2C8. The prescriber should be aware of the potential for interactions and that dose adjustments may be necessary, particularly for drugs with a narrow therapeutic index.

Pharmacodynamic
- Co-administration with bone marrow depressants (e.g. methotrexate) may increase the risk of bone marrow aplasia

♣ Dose
Standard doses are described here. Refer to local guidelines for specific advice.
- Treatment: 200mg PO BD
- Prophylaxis: 100mg PO ON

♣ Dose adjustments
Elderly
- No specific guidance, but the manufacturer states that the elderly may be more susceptible to the haematopoietic effects and a lower dose may be advisable.

Hepatic/renal impairment
- No specific guidance is available for hepatic impairment.
- Up to 60% of a dose is excreted unchanged. If CrCl is 15–30mL/min, use half the normal dose after 3 days.
- If CrCl <15mL/min, use half the normal dose (monitor plasma trimethoprim concentration if CrCl <10mL/min).

Additional information
- If necessary, tablets can be dispersed in water immediately prior to administration.

♦ Pharmacology
Trimethoprim is a broad-spectrum antibiotic effective *in vitro* against a wide range of Gram-positive and aerobic Gram-negative organisms. Trimethoprim is a dihydrofolate reductase inhibitor which affects folic acid metabolism and interferes with an essential component of bacterial development. It is rapidly and almost completely absorbed after oral administration. Hepatic metabolism occurs via CYP2C8, although 40–60% of a dose is excreted unchanged in the urine within 24 hours.

Venlafaxine

Normal release
Generic (POM)
Tablet: 37.5mg (28; 56); 75mg (28; 56)

Modified release
Efexor XL (POM)
Capsule: 75mg (14; 28); 150mg (14; 28)
Brands include: Foraven XL, Tifaxin XL, and Venaxx XL

Venlalic XL® (POM)
Tablet: 75mg (28); 150mg (28); 225mg (28)

Generic (POM)
Capsule: 75mg (30); 150mg (30)

Venlalic XL (POM)
Tablet: 75mg (28); 150mg (28); 225mg (28)

Indications
- Major depressive episodes.
- Generalized anxiety disorder.
- Generalized social anxiety disorder.

Contraindications and precautions
- Venlafaxine is contraindicated for use in patients with:
  - conditions associated with high risk of cardiac arrhythmia
  - uncontrolled hypertension.
- Do not use with an irreversible MAOI, or within 14 days of stopping one. At least 7 days should be allowed after stopping venlafaxine before starting an irreversible MAOI. Note that in exceptional circumstances linezolid may be given with venlafaxine, but the patient must be closely monitored for symptoms of serotonin syndrome for several weeks (⬚ Box 1.10, p.19).
- Use with caution in the following:
  - concomitant use of drugs that increase risk of bleeding (see ⬚ *Drug interactions*, p.480)
  - elderly (greater risk of hyponatraemia)
  - epilepsy (lowers seizure threshold)
  - glaucoma (may cause mydriasis)
  - heart disease (monitor blood pressure);
  - hepatic and renal impairment (see ⬚ *Dose adjustments*, p.481)
  - history of bleeding disorders.
- Depression is associated with an increased risk of suicidal thoughts, self-harm, and suicide which persists until remission. Note that that the risk of suicide may increase during initial treatment.
- May precipitate psychomotor restlessness, which usually appears during early treatment. The use of venlafaxine should be reviewed.
- Hyponatraemia should be considered in all patients who develop drowsiness, confusion, or convulsions while taking an antidepressant. Hyponatraemia has been associated with all types of antidepressants, although it is reportedly more common with SSRIs.

- Abrupt discontinuation should be avoided because of the risk of withdrawal reactions, e.g. agitation, anxiety, diarrhoea, dizziness, fatigue, headache, hyperhidrosis, nausea and/or vomiting, sensory disturbances (including paraesthesia), sleep disturbances and tremor. When stopping treatment, the dose should be reduced gradually over at least 1–2 weeks. See 📖 Discontinuing and/or switching antidepressants, p.45 for information about switching or stopping anti-depressants.
- Venlafaxine may modify reactions and patients should be advised not to drive (or operate machinery) if affected.

😕 Undesirable effects

Very common
- Asthenia
- Constipation
- Dizziness
- Drowsiness
- Headache
- Hyperhidrosis (including night sweats)
- Insomnia
- Nausea (common at initiation; less likely with m/r products)
- Nervousness
- Sexual dysfunction
- Xerostomia

Common
- Abdominal pain
- Abnormal dreams
- Agitation
- Anorexia
- Anxiety
- Appetite decreased
- Arthralgia
- Confusion
- Diarrhoea
- Dyspepsia
- Dyspnoea
- Hypertension
- Hypertonia
- Myalgia
- Palpitation
- Paraesthesia
- Pruritus
- Pyrexia
- Serum cholesterol increased
- Tremor
- Vasodilatation
- Visual disturbances
- Vomiting
- Yawning

Uncommon
- Arrhythmias
- Hallucinations
- Myoclonus
- Photosensitivity
- Postural hypotension
- SIADH/hyponatraemia

Rare
- Serotonin syndrome (see 📖 *Drug interactions*, p.480)

Drug interactions

Pharmacokinetic

- Venlafaxine is metabolized mainly by CYP2D6. It is also metabolized by CYP3A4 which is important in poor CYP2D6 metabolizers. It is a weak inhibitor of CYP2D6.
- *Haloperidol*—increased risk of haloperidol undesirable effects through inhibition of CYP2D6.
- The clinical significance of co-administration with inhibitors of CYP2D6 (📖 end cover) is unknown, but plasma concentrations of venlafaxine may increase. The prescriber should be aware of the potential for interactions and that dose adjustments may be necessary.
- The clinical significance of co-administration with other CYP3A4 inducers or inhibitors (📖 end cover) is unknown. The prescriber should be aware of the potential for interactions and that dose adjustments may be necessary.
- The clinical significance of co-administration with prodrug substrates of CYP2D6 (e.g. codeine, tramadol) is unknown. The prescriber should be aware of the potential for interactions and that dose adjustments may be necessary.
- Avoid grapefruit juice as it may increase the bioavailability of venla-faxine through inhibition of intestinal CYP3A4.

Pharmacodynamic

- *Anticoagulants*—potential increased risk of bleeding.
- *CNS depressants*—additive sedative effect.
- *Cyproheptadine*—may inhibit the effects of venlafaxine.
- *Diuretics*—increased risk of hyponatraemia.
- *MAOIs*—risk of serotonin syndrome (see *Contraindications and precautions*).
- *NSAIDs*—increased risk of GI bleeding.
- *Serotonergic drugs*—caution is advisable if venlafaxine is co-administered with serotonergic drugs (e.g. methadone, mirtazapine, SSRIs, tricyclic antidepressants, tramadol, trazodone) because of the risk of serotonin syndrome (📖 Box 1.10, p.19).
- *SSRIs*—increased risk of seizures and serotonin syndrome.
- *Tramadol*—increased risk of seizures and serotonin syndrome.

💊 Dose

Depression

- Initial dose 37.5mg PO BD increased if necessary after at least 3–4 weeks to 75mg PO BD. Dose may be increased further on specialist advice if necessary in steps of up to 75mg every 2–3 days to a maximum of 375mg PO daily.
- Alternatively, 75mg m/r PO OD, increased if necessary after at least 2 weeks to 150mg m/r PO OD. Dose can be increased to a maximum of 225mg PO OD.

Generalized anxiety disorder

- 75mg m/r PO OD. Discontinue if no response after 8 weeks.

VENLAFAXINE **481**

Generalized social anxiety disorder
- 75mg m/r PO OD. Discontinue if no response after 12 weeks.

Dose adjustments
Elderly
- No dose adjustment is necessary but, wherever possible, lower doses should be used. The elderly are more susceptible to undesirable effects.

Hepatic/renal impairment
- In patients with moderate hepatic impairment, the dose should be reduced by 50%. Avoid in severe hepatic impairment since no information is available.
- In patients with moderate renal impairment (GFR 10–30mL/min), the dose should be reduced by 50%. Avoid in severe renal impairment (GFR <10mL/min) since no information is available.

Additional information
- Antidepressant therapeutic response is usually seen after 2–4 weeks of treatment.

Pharmacology
Venlafaxine is a serotonin noradrenaline reuptake inhibitor (SNRI). Like duloxetine, it inhibits the reuptake of both serotonin and noradrenaline, with a weaker action on the reuptake of dopamine. It has no action at muscarinic, H_1, or α_1-adrenergic receptors. It is metabolized to its active metabolite O-desmethylvenlafaxine (ODV) by CYP2D6. The clinical significance of inhibition of CYP2D6, or use in poor metabolizers, is unknown. An additional pathway involves CYP3A4.

Warfarin

Generic (POM)

Tablet: 0.5mg (*white*, 28); 1mg (*brown*, 28); 3mg (*blue*, 28); 5mg (*pink*, 28)

Indications

- Prophylaxis of systemic embolism in patients with rheumatic heart disease and atrial fibrillation.
- Prophylaxis after insertion of prosthetic heart valves.
- Prophylaxis and treatment of venous thrombosis and pulmonary embolism.
- Transient attacks of cerebral ischaemia.

Contraindications and precautions

- Warfarin is contraindicated for use in the following circumstances:
  - bacterial endocarditis
  - haemophilia
  - peptic ulcer
  - recent surgery (within 24 hours)
  - severe hepatic impairment (use LMWH)
  - severe renal impairment
  - uncontrolled hypertension.
- INR (international normalized ratio) must be measured daily or on alternate days initially and then at longer intervals depending on response, but usually every 12 weeks.
- For instructions on the management of bleeding – see the current edition of the *BNF*.
- Use with caution in:
  - elderly patients
  - renal impairment
  - hepatic impairment (LMWH may be preferred).

☺ Undesirable effects

The frequency is not defined, but reported undesirable effects include:

- Alopecia
- Diarrhoea
- Hepatic dysfunction
- Hypersensitivity
- Jaundice
- Skin necrosis
- Skin rashes
- Purple toes syndrome
- Unexplained drop in haematocrit

If the following occur, the manufacturer advises that warfarin must be discontinued:

- Epistaxis
- Fever
- Haemothorax
- Nausea
- Pancreatitis
- Purpura
- Vomiting

Drug interactions

There are many potential drug interactions with warfarin, but as the INR is regularly monitored, it is more important to take account of the introduction or discontinuation of concurrent medication. The list below contains only those interactions most likely to be relevant in palliative care. Changes in medical conditions, especially liver involvement, and marked changes in diet are also a potential source of changes in warfarin levels.

Pharmacokinetic
- Warfarin is a substrate of CYP1A2, CYP2C9, and CYP2C19. Several interactions are listed below, but refer to □ end cover for a list of drugs that may potentially affect warfarin.
- The following can enhance the effect of warfarin:
  - alcohol (acute use)
  - amiodarone (may take up to 2 weeks to develop)
  - cephalosporins
  - ciprofloxacin
  - cranberry juice
  - erythromycin
  - fluconazole
  - metronidazole
  - miconazole
  - mirtazapine
  - omeprazole
  - penicillins
  - trimethoprim.
- The following can reduce the effect of warfarin:
  - alcohol (chronic use)
  - carbamazepine
  - menadiol (vitamin k)
  - phenobarbital
  - St John's wort
  - sucralfate.

Pharmacodynamic
- The following drugs increase the risk of bleeding:
  - aspirin
  - corticosteroids
  - NSAIDs
  - SSRIs.

♣ Dose

Refer to local guidelines

Rapid anticoagulation

• 10mg PO on day 1, then subsequent doses based on INR.

Less urgent cases

• Lower loading doses can be introduced over a period of 3–4 weeks.
• The daily dose is usually 3–9mg.

♣ Dose adjustments

Elderly

• No dose reductions necessary. Titrate the dose individually.

Hepatic/renal impairment

• Avoid in severe liver disease, especially if INR is already raised. LMWH may be preferred. In moderate hepatic impairment, more frequent monitoring will be required.
• Avoid in severe renal impairment; LMWH may be preferred.

Additional information

• The use of warfarin in palliative care needs to be balanced with the burden of monitoring and drug interactions. The use of LMWH is often preferred.
• As other pre-existing conditions in may have an effect on INR, monitoring may be needed more frequently than in otherwise healthy patients who are at risk of or requiring treatment for thrombosis
• Recommended ranges of therapeutic anticoagulation are as follows.
   • INR 2–2.5: prophylaxis of DVT including surgery in high risk patients
   • INR 2–3: prophylaxis in hip surgery and fractured femur operations, treatment of DVT, PE, prevention of venous thromoembolism in myocardial infarction, transient ischaemic attacks, mitral stenosis with embolism, tissue prosthetic heart valves
   • INR 3–4.5: recurrent DVT and PE, mechanical prosthetic heart valves, arterial disease including myocardial infarction.

⊘ Pharmacology

Warfarin is one of the coumarin anticoagulants which act by antagonizing the effects of vitamin K. The anticoagulant effects do not develop fully until 48–72 hours after dose initiation, so heparins should also be given during that period. Warfarin is metabolized by CYP2C9 and to a lesser extent by CYP1A2 and CYP2C19. As with other drugs with a narrow therapeutic margin, particular care must be taken when drug regimes are altered. An additional complication is the effect of genetic polymorphism on warfarin metabolism, although monitoring can normalize for this.

Zoledronic acid

Zometa® (POM)

Concentrate for IV infusion: 4mg/5mL

Indications

- Treatment of tumour-induced hypercalcaemia (corrected calcium >3.0mmol/L).
- Prevention of skeletal-related events in patients with advanced malignancies involving bone.
- ¥ Bone pain.

Contraindications and precautions

- Avoid in patients with:
  - severe hepatic impairment (limited data available)
  - renal impairment (see 📖 Dose adjustments, p.487)
  - cardiac disease (avoid fluid overload).
- Assess renal function and electrolytes (e.g. calcium, magnesium) before each dose and ensure adequate hydration (especially hypercalcaemia).
- Consider dental treatment prior to treatment because of the risk of osteonecrosis of the jaw.

☺ Undesirable effects

Osteonecrosis of the jaw has been found to be a potential complication of bisphosphonate therapy. It has been reported in cancer patients, many who had a pre-existing local infection or recent extraction. Cancer patients are more likely to be at risk of osteonecrosis as a result of their disease, cancer therapies, and blood dyscrasias. Dental examination is recommended for patients undergoing repeated infusions of zoledronic acid (and other bisphosphonates) and dental surgery should be avoided during this treatment period as healing may be delayed.

Very common
- Hypophosphataemia

Common
- Anaemia
- Anorexia
- Arthralgia
- Bone pain
- Conjunctivitis
- Fever
- Flu-like syndrome (including fatigue, rigors, malaise, and flushing)
- Headache
- Hypocalcaemia
- Myalgia
- Nausea and vomiting
- Renal impairment

Uncommon
- Abdominal pain
- Acute renal failure
- Constipation
- Diarrhoea
- Dry mouth
- Dyspepsia
- Hypokalaemia
- Hypomagnesaemia
- Leucopenia
- Muscle cramps
- Stomatitis
- Thrombocytopenia

Rare
- Osteonecrosis of the jaw

Drug interactions

Pharmacokinetic
- None known

Pharmacodynamic
- *Aminoglycosides*—may have additive hypocalcaemic effect.
- *Diuretics*—increased risk of renal impairment.
- *NSAIDs*—increased risk of renal impairment.
- *Thalidomide*—increased risk of renal impairment (in treatment of multiple myeloma).

🎝 Dose

The concentrate must be diluted with 100mL NaCl 0.9% or D5W and given in no less than a 15-minute IV infusion.

Treatment of tumour-induced hypercalcaemia
- Ensure patients are well hydrated prior to and following administration of zoledronic acid.
- 4mg by IV infusion as a single dose.

Prevention of skeletal related events
- 4mg by IV infusion every 3–4 weeks.
- Note that calcium 500mg and vitamin D 400 units should also be taken daily.

¥ Bone pain
- 4mg by IV infusion every 3–4 weeks.
- Note that calcium 500mg and vitamin D 400 units should also be taken daily.

♣ Dose adjustments

Elderly
- No dose adjustments are necessary.

Hepatic/renal impairment
- The manufacturer advises caution in severe hepatic impairment because of the lack of data in this population.
- Zoledronic acid is not metabolized and is excreted unchanged via the kidney. For this reason, dose adjustments are necessary:
- Hypercalcaemia:
  - avoid if SeCr >400µmol/L unless benefits outweigh the risks
  - no dose adjustment is necessary if SeCr <400µmol/L.
- Prevention of skeletal-related events and bone pain (Table 3.15).

Table 3.15 Zoledronic acid dosage for prevention of skeletal-related events and bone pain

Baseline creatinine clearance (mL/min)	Recommended dose* (mg)	Volume of concentrate (mL)
>60	4.0	5
50–60	3.5	4.4
40–49	3.3	4.1
30–39	3.0	3.8
<30	Not recommended in severe renal impairment	

*In 100mL NaCl 0.9% or D5W over 15 minutes via IV infusion.

Additional information
- The onset of treatment effect for skeletal-related events is 2–3 months.
- Normocalcaemia is achieved by a median of 4 days and relief from bone pain may take up to 14 days.

♦ Pharmacology
Zoledronic acid is a bisphosphonate that inhibits osteoclast activity, which in turn reduces bone resorption and turnover. It is excreted unchanged by the kidneys.

Zolpidem

Stilnoct® (CD Benz POM)

Tablet: 5mg (28); 10mg (28)

Generic (CD Benz POM)

Tablet: 5mg (28); 10mg (28)

Note: Independent prescribers are **NOT** authorized to prescribe zolpidem (📖 Independent prescribing—palliative care issues, p.25).

Indications

• Short-term treatment of insomnia.

Contraindications and precautions

• Zolpidem is contraindicated for use in patients with:
  • myasthenia gravis
  • obstructive sleep apnoea
  • respiratory failure
  • severe hepatic insufficiency.
• Use with caution in patients with hepatic impairment (see 📖 *Dose adjustments*).
• Lower initial doses should be used in the elderly (see 📖 *Dose adjustments*).
• Sleep-walking and other associated behaviours have been reported with zolpidem and are usually related to concomitant use of alcohol and other CNS depressants, or doses above the recommended.
• Zolpidem treatment can lead to the development of physical and psychological dependence. The risk of dependence increases with dose and duration. Patients with a history of alcohol and or drug abuse also have an increased risk. Withdrawal symptoms that can occur after prolonged treatment include anxiety, hallucinations, insomnia, mood changes, restlessness, sweating, and tremor.
• Zolpidem may modify reactions and patients should be advised not to drive (or operate machinery) if affected.

☺ Undesirable effects

Common
• Agitation
• Anterograde amnesia
• Diarrhoea
• Dizziness
• Drowsiness
• Exacerbated insomnia
• Fatigue
• Hallucination
• Headache
• Nightmare

Uncommon
• Confusional state
• Diplopia
• Irritability

Unknown

- Aggression
- Anger
- Delusion
- Muscular weakness
- Psychosis
- Raised LFTs
- Rash
- Restlessness
- Sleep-walking

Drug interactions

Pharmacokinetic

- Metabolized mainly by CYP3A4 with a minor pathway involving CYP1A2. Drug interactions via cytochrome inhibition may be additive.
- The clinical significance of co-administration with inducers or inhibitors of CYP3A4 or CYP1A2 (📖 end cover) is unknown. The prescriber should be aware of the potential for interactions and the need for dose adjustments.
- The effect of grapefruit juice on the bioavailability of zolpidem is unknown.

Pharmacodynamic

- *CNS depressants*—additive sedative effect.
- *Sertraline*—appears to be an interaction that causes excessive drowsiness and hallucinations.

🥄 Dose

- 10mg PO ON.

🥄 Dose adjustments

Elderly

- Initial dose 5mg PO ON. The dose may be increased to 10mg PO ON if necessary.

Hepatic/renal impairment

- Initial dose in hepatic impairment is 5mg PO ON. The dose can be cautiously increased to 10mg PO ON if necessary. Note that zolpidem is contraindicated for patients with severe hepatic impairment.
- No specific guidance is available for patients with renal impairment.

Additional information

- The tablets can be crushed and dispersed in water immediately before use.

⊙ Pharmacology

Zolpidem is a short-acting non-benzodiazepine hypnotic drug that initiates and sustains sleep without affecting total REM sleep. It interacts preferentially with the GABA receptor via the ω_1-receptor subtype which leads to the sedative effects seen but also the lack of muscle relaxant effects. It is extensively metabolized by CYP3A4, with additional metabolism involving CYP1A2. All metabolites are inactive and are eliminated in urine and faeces.

Zopiclone

Zimovane LS™ (POM)
Tablet: 3.75mg (28)

Zimovane® (POM)
Tablet (scored): 7.5mg (28)

Generic (POM)
Tablet: 3.75mg (28); 7.5mg (28)

Indications
- Short-term treatment of insomnia.

Contraindications and precautions
- Zopiclone is contraindicated for use in patients with:
  - myasthenia gravis
  - respiratory failure
  - severe sleep apnoea syndrome
  - severe hepatic insufficiency.
- Use with caution in patients with hepatic and/or renal impairment (see 📖 *Dose adjustments*).
- Lower initial doses should be used in the elderly (see 📖 *Dose adjustments*).
- Zopiclone treatment can lead to the development of physical and psychological dependence. The risk of dependence increases with dose and duration. Patients with a history of alcohol and or drug abuse also have an increased risk.
- If treatment is limited to 4 weeks or less, discontinuation of therapy should not cause a withdrawal reaction. However, some patients may benefit from a tapered reduction. Withdrawal symptoms that can occur after prolonged treatment include anxiety, hallucinations, insomnia, mood changes, restlessness, sweating, and tremor.
- Sleep-walking and other associated behaviours have been reported with zopiclone and are usually related to concomitant use of alcohol and other CNS depressants, or doses above the recommended.
- Zopiclone may modify reactions and patients should be advised not to drive (or operate machinery) if affected.

☺ Undesirable effects
The frequency is not defined, but reported undesirable effects include:

- Aggressiveness
- Anterograde amnesia
- Bitter or metallic after-taste
- Confusion
- Depressed mood
- Dizziness
- Drowsiness
- Dry mouth
- Hallucinations
- Headache
- Irritability
- Nausea and vomiting
- Sleep walking

Drug interactions
Pharmacokinetic
- Zopiclone is metabolized by CYP3A4 (both metabolites formed) and CYP2C8/9 (to the inactive metabolite). Drug interactions via cytochrome inhibition may be additive.
- *Erythromycin*—increases plasma concentration and effects of zopiclone
- The clinical significance of co-administration with inducers or inhibitors of CYP3A4 or CYP2C8/9 (📖 end cover) is unknown. The prescriber should be aware of the potential for interactions and the need for dose adjustments.
- The effect of grapefruit juice on the bioavailability of zopiclone is unknown.

Pharmacodynamic
- *CNS depressants*—additive sedative effect

♣ Dose
- 7.5mg PO ON.

♣ Dose adjustments
Elderly
- Initial dose 3.75mg PO ON. The dose may be increased to 7.5mg PO ON if necessary.

Hepatic/renal impairment
- Initial dose in hepatic impairment is 3.75mg PO ON. The dose can be cautiously increased to 7.5mg PO ON if necessary. Note that zopiclone is contraindicated for patients with severe hepatic impairment.
- Initial dose in renal impairment is 3.75mg PO ON. The dose can be increased to 7.5mg PO ON if necessary.

Additional information
- The tablets can be crushed and dispersed in water immediately before use.

♦ Pharmacology
Zopiclone is a non-benzodiazepine hypnotic agent that initiates and sustains sleep without affecting total REM sleep. It is unlikely to produce a hangover effect. Its pharmacological properties include hypnotic, sedative, anxiolytic, anticonvulsant, and muscle-relaxant actions (at higher doses). Zopiclone binds with high affinity to the benzodiazepine receptor, although it is believed to act at a different site to the benzodiazepines. Zopiclone is extensively metabolized to two major metabolites, one active (*N*-oxide zopiclone) and one inactive (*N*-desmethyl zopiclone). It is a substrate of CYP3A4 and CYP2C8/9. Both metabolites are excreted via the kidneys.

Index

Index